# Marriage, Family, and Intimate Relationships

# Marriage, Family, and

# Intimate Relationships

Gary S. Belkin
Long Island University

Norman Goodman
State University of New York
at Stony Brook

Rand McNally College Publishing Company
Chicago

Sponsoring Editor: Geoffrey Huck
Project Editors: Gayle Fankhauser and Reeah Parker
Designer: Herbert Jackson

80 81 82 10 9 8 7 6 5 4 3 2 1

To our parents, our wives, and our children

# Table of Contents

# Part TWO

## Intimate Relationships

# Part THREE

## Contemporary Patterns of Bonding

# Part FOUR

## Parenthood: From Marriage to Family Life

# Part FIVE

## Family Troubles and Social Problems

# Photographs

Photo Editor: Shirley Fout Miller

# Preface

This book is designed for use in courses which require an eclectic, functional book on marriage and family life. Its purpose is to introduce the student to a wide range of topics and to generate an interest in the field.

We have attempted throughout the book to integrate sociological and psychological concepts of marriage, family, and intimate relationships, and to apply these concepts to students' lives so that they can better understand and cope with the problems they may be experiencing in their family and interpersonal relationships. Since one author is a sociologist and the other a family counselor, both the psychological and sociological perspectives are given due attention. Although coverage of the subject matter is extensive and thorough, we have tried to present it in an engaging style and to avoid overwhelming the student with encyclopedic detail. Because of the many divergent viewpoints in this field, we have worked toward achieving a balanced presentation, including, and where possible integrating, the major theoretical perspectives. The text is divided into five parts, comprising fourteen chapters. An epilogue ties together much of the material, focusing on the future of marriage and family life in the United States. Some of the features of the book should be noted.

## Writing Style

The book has been written with the student in mind. Special care has been taken, for example, to define terms as they are introduced, to avoid unnecessary jargon, and to develop complex concepts through examples. We have also tried to be sensitive not only in avoiding sexism and racism, but also in avoiding the more subtle prejudice of ageism—the stereotyping of individuals according to their age. This last point is especially important now, when an increasing percentage of the college population is made up of older individuals. Students of both sexes, at all age levels, and of many different ethnic groups should appreciate and find helpful the examples and vignettes that are directed toward them.

## Special Features

Much attention has been paid to the development of useful pedagogical features, through which material becomes meaningful to the student. Some of the helpful features are:
- *Chapter Aims*   Each chapter opens with an explicit aim that identifies for the student the main topics to be covered and the relationship between them.
- *Overview*   Each chapter begins with an interesting series of thought-provoking questions or statements which the student will be reading about in the chapter.
- *Key Terms*   Important new terms are enumerated and defined at the beginning of each chapter, and also included in the glossary at the end of the book.
- *Chapter Summaries*   Each chapter concludes with a summary. The purpose of the summary is to help students review and rethink what they have learned after completing the chapter.
- *Discussion Questions*   At the end of each chapter are included several thought-provoking questions which can be used as a catalyst for class discussion. These questions are specifically designed not only to evaluate the student's understanding of the material, but also to help the student apply the material to his or her life.
- *Illustrations*   Approximately 60 photos, 25 figures, and 30 tables appear throughout the text. These are not included for ornamentation, but to clarify many of the important concepts discussed in the book and to attract students' attention and interest.
- *Suggested Readings*   To enable students to pursue in more depth topics of special interest to them, an annotated list of pertinent supplementary readings is included at the end of each chapter.
- *Glossary*   The glossary at the back of the book contains all

the key terms used throughout, arranged in alphabetical order.

In addition to these pedagogical features, the following characteristics make this a text that helps students as it teaches them:

- *It's up-to-date:* it's contemporary and incorporates the latest research.
- *It's practical:* students can apply the concepts to their own lives.
- *It takes the position that conflicts can be resolved:* it points out causes of conflicts and shows various ways that conflicts can be solved.

## Coverage of Topics

Some of the important content areas of special interest to students which are covered include:

- sex roles in marriage and in dating
- successful adjustment in marriage
- conflict in marriage
- communication—in dating, in the family, and in marriage
- love—its social meaning and why we fall in love
- mate selection and conjugal courtship
- parenthood—social psychological viewpoints
- divorce
- premarital sexual practices and attitudes
- remarriage and the reconstituted family
- aging and the family
- nonnormative sexual practices and the family
- development of gender identity
- reproductive behavior and childbirth

## Acknowledgements

We would like to thank our wives and children who encouraged us in this book and taught us about family life through experience, our students who offered their suggestions as to the kind of book they would enjoy reading, and the reviewers whose comments and insights proved invaluable in the development of the manuscript. We would also like to thank Ms. Carole Roland for her typing and proofreading, etc. and the editorial staff at Rand McNally, especially our editor, Geoffrey Huck, who guided this project from beginning to end, and our production editors, Gayle Fankhauser and Reeah Parker.

# Introduction

Danny Chong has a decision to make, an important one. He loves his father, loves him very dearly in fact. But his father just can't understand how Danny, his ''pride,'' could leave the family home and move out to live with a woman. And a Caucasian woman, at that! To Danny's father, who was born and raised in Shanghai, who came to this country penniless but rich with six thousand years of heritage, and who now finally owns his own hand laundry for which he struggled 20 years, such ''flighty'' and irresponsible behavior is unthinkable and disloyal and goes violently against his family's generations of tradition and continuity. But to Danny, who was born here, who was graduated from the San Francisco public schools and State University, who was raised on American movies and TV—to Danny, what he is doing is natural and normal, although it is causing family conflict.

Marion and Jack Gibbs are having a different problem. Their daughter, Lynda, will be graduating from high school next year, and she can't decide if she wants to go to college or not. Should she attend the local community college or go to State? Or, should she work in her parents' business, starting at the bottom, of course. The Gibbs are not sure how to advise their daughter. In their day it wasn't important for a young woman to go to college, but now, with women's roles changing so much and with such different expectations for women. . . . What should they do? What do they tell her when she comes to them for advice?

"I tell you it's just not right; it's *criminal*," Bob barks at his wife Claire, but unconvincingly, as they both recognize the unalterable fact that his widowed mother, who is becoming more and more helpless, will have to be placed in a home. Bob and Claire have been arguing about this for months now and not effectively communicating their feelings. Yet they will ultimately have to make a decision. It's just difficult for Bob to think of his mother as the helpless invalid she has become and even more difficult for him to discuss his feelings with his wife. Something has happened between them over the years, something that has pulled them apart.

Victor Avinella and Susan Kardonsky have set their wedding date for next September, almost a year away, and the banquet hall is reserved. Both their families are delighted with this match, and the engagement party this summer was a big success. The boxes of gifts they received are in storage in the Kardonsky basement, where they will be safe until Vic and Sue are married and have their own apartment, probably in fashionable downtown. Vic will be finished with law school by next June, and by September he should have a decent job. Sue will be working too, until they have children if they want them. Vic and Sue hope to enjoy the middle-class pleasures of the traditional lifestyle in which they both were raised.

Each of these situations is representative of the kinds of decisions, problems, and circumstances that characterize our study of the individual, marriage, and the family in the contemporary world. They are all distinctly human problems, affected by feelings, social factors, and intellectual beliefs.

We live now in a society where a range of individual choices, options, and possibilities never before seen in history afford us a variety of family organizations and interpersonal arrangements that can be, to a large extent, of our own making. True, we are still beholden to the nuclear family, an institution that has its origins in our ancestral past. But at the same time we should recognize that nothing can be taken for granted anymore: there are too many options and variations. The family in the modern world "has separated from the surrounding community . . . cast off its connections with distant kin and has changed fundamentally even its relationship to close relatives. . . . Whereas once people had been able to answer questions such as who am I by pointing to those who had gone before and come after, in the twentieth century they would have other replies" (Shorter 1975, pp. 3–4). It is the diversity of these replies that will help us understand the organization and purpose of the contemporary family.

## Why This Course?

You probably imagined when you enrolled in this course that you would be learning about individuals within a social order, about the institution of the family in history and in different societies, and about marriage and alternative lifestyles. As you thought about these things, you probably visualized your own family situation, the types of social relationships with which you are familiar, your parents' marriage relationship, and the way you and your siblings were raised. In fact, we all have a tendency to think about dating, marriage, and family life in terms of what we personally have experienced. We know, of course, that other styles and arrangements exist, but because our family life is so ingrained in our thinking, it is very difficult to get away from our preconceptions and our biases and to approach the subject through some kind of objective perspective.

Sociologist Mirra Komarovsky (1974, p. 1) makes the key point at the beginning of a book on life in families. She says,

> Of all social institutions, the family is the one with which every reader of this book has had the most intimate acquaintance. He was born into a family and his deepest emotions are linked to it. Why then, might we ask, should it be necessary to study the family? Does not every person acquire such knowledge naturally through daily participation and observation? Even the young reader who has not yet reached the stage of playing out the adult family roles has normally had opportunities to observe them in his own family and in the families of relatives and friends. . . . *What can the sociologist possibly tell us about the family life of our own society that is not* perfectly obvious on the basis of common sense? (italics ours)

The answer to this question, as we shall see throughout this course, is that there is such a wide variety of family organizations and marriage forms today, comprising so many different cultural components, that the sociology of family life is rarely obvious on the basis of common sense alone. Moreover, because we live in a changing world, filled with options and decisions, and because many of these, although they have historical roots, are different from those of any other time in history, we have to be aware of the variations within our own society. Social commentator Jane Howard (1978), describing the contemporary scene in the United States, points out, "What families are doing, in flamboyant and dumbfounding ways, is changing their size and their shape and their purpose. Only 16.3 percent of this country's 56 million families are conventionally nuclear, with breadwinning fathers, homemaking mothers, and resident children. That leaves 83.7 percent to find other arrangements. . . ." It is to those "other arrangements," as well as to the traditional, that attention must be directed. And to this end, this course should be especially helpful.

## About This Book

This book will attempt to do two things. First, it will show the range of possible arrangements in contemporary society and what we have learned about each of them. Second, it will show historically and psychologically the universality and uniformity of some of these arrangements. We will see that the Dannys, Marions, Jacks, Lyndas, Bobs, Claires, Victors, and Susans are not exceptions in our society, but part of a flexible pattern of rules, institutions, and regulations.

The key point to keep in mind throughout the book is that for the individual living in the United States today there are available not only options but a wider range of observable models of marriage arrangements, family life, and parenting styles than ever before. And, we know from research that much of what we learn comes from closely observing the models around us, and learning new behaviors. Therefore, the preeminence of these varied models will probably lead to even greater changes in the coming years.

We said before that this course is designed to help us see objectively, from a broader perspective, the many systems and functions of family life in our society and throughout history. But there is a second, equally compelling reason for the course and for the book.

Throughout these chapters we will attempt to provide enough information to assist you in your decisionmaking processes. Because we recognize that you, the student, will throughout your life be faced with important choices—choices that require intelligently evaluating the options available to you—we hope to show you, both through the objective information and some brief vignettes, different ways of looking at some of the situations you will face in life.

## Establishing Contexts

As we attempt to understand and describe the contexts in which the individual, the family, and the society interact, we must be careful to acknowledge that there are many ways to go about the task. A number of observers can interpret the exact same thing in different ways, depending on how they view it. Likewise, there are several ways to approach the study of marriage and family life.

The set of assumptions with which we approach our study is called a *conceptual framework*. A conceptual framework is a set of assumptions about how to examine the data we come across. What do we look for? Where do we concentrate our efforts? A conceptual framework also provides a general guideline for interpreting what we find.

There is no one conceptual framework that is universally accepted today. There are a number of competing ones, each offering some clear advantages and some disadvantages. Nye and Berardo (1966) have explicitly detailed the major conceptual frameworks used in family studies, and we will look briefly at some of the ones that will play a part in this book. We will consider how each affects our perception of the family members in interaction with each other and with society.

### The Anthropological Framework

Let us say we are interested in finding out how kinship is recognized by a society. Why is it in some societies that what we call "second cousins" are considered related and in some societies they are not? Are you considered a relative of the man who marries your sister? Of the woman who marries your brother? Is your sister's husband's sister related to you? Could your brother marry her if he wanted to? What about your parents and in-laws; are they related? The anthropologist might try to answer these questions by looking at historical cultures to determine how they dealt with these issues and what purpose their kinship systems served in maintaining their society. In other words, anthropologists look at the human past as well as the present to help us better understand how societies developed into what they have become.

Although we will not emphasize this framework, it should help us to understand the relationship between some of our social "givens" and their historical antecedents.

### The Structure-Functional Framework

In the structure-functional framework, which was developed by sociologist Talcott Parsons, we would still be interested in anthropological evidence, insofar as the past sheds light on the present. But we might also try to find out what purpose is served by our contemporary kinship regulations. How do they affect the interactions between the family and the larger society? What do kinship regulations say about roles and statuses? To find answers to these questions, we might use research on economic realities, on the ratio of men to women in our society, on social class, and so on. In any case, our inquiry would focus on the interplay within the family as a unit, its individual members, and other social institutions. We would examine the complex relationships between the individual family and broader social units, as well as study the relationship between family and personality. It is a comprehensive framework, taking into account the breadth of relevant social forces.

## The Interactional Framework

As a conceptual framework for the study of the family, social interaction provides us with a way of understanding how individual family members' perceptions of themselves and others is related to their functioning inside the family organization. This framework, Manis and Meltzer (1967, p. 137) point out, focuses "attention upon interpersonal relationships, rather than upon whole societies or groups." It is primarily concerned with the social symbolism and personal meaning of the individual's interactions with others.

For example, let's say we wanted to investigate how people develop intimate relationships that lead to marriage. Using this framework, we would consider each act of the courtship as some kind of sign or symbol within a recognized social context. The roles the couple plays with respect to each other could be explored within the context of clearly defined social situations, such as dating formally, dropping by unexpectedly, being alone in private, having sex, and using pet names for each other.

The way that the behavior of one individual affects the behavior of others is also of prime importance in this framework. According to this point of view, family members are always in the process of developing acts to cope with the various situations in which they find themselves (Schvaneveldt 1966). This is not to suggest that family members are not spontaneous and genuine in their interactions. Rather, it implies that a set of expectations and roles is set down for each person and the person learns to enact and respond to these roles.

## The Psychoanalytic Framework

The psychoanalytic framework is based on the writings of Sigmund Freud. The basic assumption is that the family functions according to dynamic— that is, unconscious—forces. In most social situations, according to this framework, there are hidden, underlying reasons behind what we choose to do, behind how we act.

Psychoanalysts believe that what happens during the first five years of life determines one's personality. The child is born a creature of uninhibited impulse (id) and learns through the socialization that takes place in the family how to delay gratification and redirect impulses into constructive and socially acceptable activities. During the process of learning this, the child's ego is developed.

From the psychoanalytic framework, such phenomena as the incest taboo, family roles and statuses, dating behavior, rules of residence, authority, love, and intimacy are all viewed in terms of what meaning they presumably have in the unconscious minds of the participants involved. For instance, they believe in a universal Oedipus complex, in which the young boy falls in love with the mother and views the father as a rival, an enemy. This complex is then used to explain a range of social phenomena.

## The Role-Structure
## Framework

The role-structure framework was not included in Nye and Berardo's collection but appeared separately in several papers and finally was brought together in a book edited by Nye—*Role Structure and Analysis of the Family* (1976). It is an extremely useful position for integrating key insights from several of the above frameworks for the purpose of understanding the family as a unit.

As a conceptual framework for studying the family, it begins by delineating eight family roles: (1) provider, (2) housekeeper, (3) child care, (4) child socialization, (5) sexual, (6) recreational, (7) therapeutic, and (8) kinship. Each of these will be discussed in detail in chapter 7, where we will use this framework.

These are not the only frameworks available, but they are the ones from which we will be drawing at different points in this book. No single one is universally accepted and useful in analyzing all types of situations. We will try to use the framework that is most appropriate to our goal; namely, to provide a practical and accurate discussion of marriage and family life.

# Part ONE

## Marriage and the Family in Perspective

In the opening part of the book we are going to focus directly on the sociological dimensions and implications of the joint institutions of marriage and family. This will provide us with the foundation material, including specialized terminology and key concepts, necessary to understand with increased clarity and relevance the chapters in the following sections.

Two helpful ideas should be kept in mind as you read these chapters. Although you may find many new terms introduced quite rapidly (especially if an introduction to sociology course is not fresh in your mind), they are each clearly defined in the glossary, as well as where they are first discussed in the text. So, if you are in the middle of a chapter and come across the word such as *kinship, unilineal,* or *patrilocal* and forget on what page it was defined, just turn to the glossary at the end of the book and the definition will be there.

The second point is subtler, but even more likely to be of help to you. So much of what we tend to believe about marriage and family life is the result of our own very limited, very distinct experiences. It is difficult for us to relate to some of the family organizations, expectations, and customs different from our own. Yet, if we keep an open mind, we will see that many aspects of totally different institutions are hidden in our own institutions of marriage and family. Here are a few of the things you will find in these three chapters:

- The practice of capturing a bride by force has parallels in our current courtship practices.

# Marriage and the Family in Perspective

**1. Marriage in Perspective**
**2. The Organization and Structure of the Family**
**3. Socialization and the Family**

In the opening part of the book we are going to focus directly on the sociological dimensions and implications of the joint institutions of marriage and family. This will provide us with the foundation material, including specialized terminology and key concepts, necessary to understand with increased clarity and relevance the chapters in the following sections.

Two helpful ideas should be kept in mind as you read these chapters. Although you may find many new terms introduced quite rapidly (especially if an introduction to sociology course is not fresh in your mind), they are each clearly defined in the glossary, as well as where they are first discussed in the text. So, if you are in the middle of a chapter and come across the word such as *kinship, unilineal,* or *patrilocal* and forget on what page it was defined, just turn to the glossary at the end of the book and the definition will be there.

The second point is subtler, but even more likely to be of help to you. So much of what we tend to believe about marriage and family life is the result of our own very limited, very distinct experiences. It is difficult for us to relate to some of the family organizations, expectations, and customs different from our own. Yet, if we keep an open mind, we will see that many aspects of totally different institutions are hidden in our own institutions of marriage and family. Here are a few of the things you will find in these three chapters:

- The practice of capturing a bride by force has parallels in our current courtship practices.

stance, they believe in a universal Oedipus complex, in which the young boy falls in love with the mother and views the father as a rival, an enemy. This complex is then used to explain a range of social phenomena.

## The Role-Structure Framework

The role-structure framework was not included in Nye and Berardo's collection but appeared separately in several papers and finally was brought together in a book edited by Nye—*Role Structure and Analysis of the Family* (1976). It is an extremely useful position for integrating key insights from several of the above frameworks for the purpose of understanding the family as a unit.

As a conceptual framework for studying the family, it begins by delineating eight family roles: (1) provider, (2) housekeeper, (3) child care, (4) child socialization, (5) sexual, (6) recreational, (7) therapeutic, and (8) kinship. Each of these will be discussed in detail in chapter 7, where we will use this framework.

These are not the only frameworks available, but they are the ones from which we will be drawing at different points in this book. No single one is universally accepted and useful in analyzing all types of situations. We will try to use the framework that is most appropriate to our goal; namely, to provide a practical and accurate discussion of marriage and family life.

- Children help socialize their parents, teaching them new behaviors and ideas, at the same time that their parents are socializing them.
- The idea of choosing a marital partner that you love, one whom you *want* to marry, is relatively rare throughout the world.
- In some cultures, only the mother's family is perceived as part of a person's lineage: the father's side is not even considered.
- In societies where polygamy is practiced, it is not usually practiced just for pleasure, but for survival.

In chapter 1, "Marriage in Perspective," we will look at the wide variety of cultural variation that has been identified in the choice of a marriage partner and consider the many marital forms that exist and that have existed throughout the world. We will see, where applicable, how these practices and forms, sometimes remote to our thinking, relate to our own institutions today. Also, we will discuss the possibility of individually written marriage contracts, articulating the couple's philosophy of marriage within its social context, as a contemporary option.

Then, in chapter 2, "The Organization and Structure Of the Family," we will consider the importance of the sociological concept of nuclear family and evaluate its universality and its purpose, historically and in the present. We will also outline the vast range of kinship arrangements and consider their practical implications, in terms of where the newly married live and who is in charge of the family. Finally, we will examine in some detail the taboo against incest.

Finally, in chapter 3, "Socialization and the Family," we will explore many of the ways that we are socialized through our families. We will come to understand the concept of socialization and how it influences virtually every aspect of our behavior and interpersonal functioning.

## Chapter 1

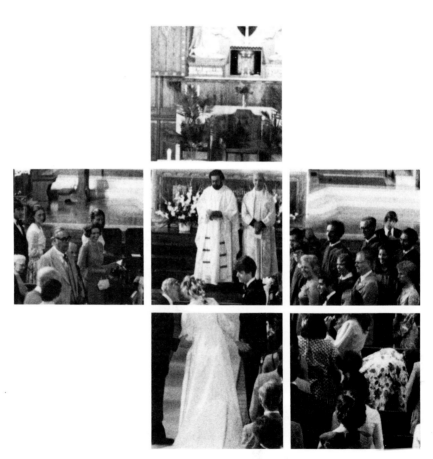

# Marriage in Perspective

## Chapter Aims

1. To show the wide variety of cultural practices that have been identified in the choice of a marriage partner and the many marital forms that exist and have existed throughout the world.

2. To show, where applicable, how these practices and forms relate to our own institutions today.

3. To discuss, as a contemporary option, the possibility of individually written marriage contracts, articulating the couple's philosophy of marriage.

## Overview

Various images come to mind when one thinks of marriage. It is important to remember that these images are colored by your culture and experiences. The range of methods for obtaining a marital partner include capturing a mate, purchasing a mate, having one chosen for you, and, the method common in our society, that of choosing your own mate.

There are also different forms of marriage. You are probably more familiar with marriage between one man and one woman, but in many cultures a marriage may consist of one man and many women, or, less commonly, one woman and many men.

Some couples today prepare their own agreements specifying what they expect of each other in the marriage. These agreements can then be formally written as premarital contracts, which the couples sign.

## Views of Marriage

When you think of the institution of marriage or the process of getting married, you are probably influenced by a series of images that reflect your personal experiences, our culture, or a combination of both. For example, you may conjure up specific fantasies of courtship, the period in which the man and woman get to know each other before making a marriage commitment. You may have an image of marriage as a one-man, one-woman institution, always one husband and one wife together, because this form is what we are used to seeing. You also probably assume

Marriage as a
voluntary decision

that for a marriage to work there should be some kind of chemistry, some physical and emotional attraction between the partners. And, if you have been reared in the culture of the United States, surely you think of the decision to marry as a voluntary decision, one that is within the province of the prospective bride and groom, even though parental permission may be required.

Yet all of these images, although true of our culture, are exceptions rather than the rule in the larger social, cultural, and historical picture. In truth, the institution of marriage assumes many different forms and the selection of a marriage partner has many variations, as do the ceremonies that mark the beginning of marriage.

## Choosing a Marital Partner

Ask people you know how they chose the persons they married or how they plan to choose when they decide to marry. First they will tell you the personal qualities that attracted them: ''I wanted someone intelligent and sensitive.'' Then they will probably tell you some practical reasons. ''. . . and my family liked him.'' It is taken for granted in our culture that people who are getting married choose their marital partners. But how prevalent is this practice throughout the world?

There are actually four major practices of mate selection that have been identified in different cultures. Some of these are mainly of histori-cal interest (capturing a bride by force, for example), some are widely practiced today (marriage by arrangement or by purchase), and one of the practices is clearly recognizable as the predominant way we choose a marital partner in our contemporary American society (marriage by con-sent). The four practices are:

1. marriage by *capture*
2. marriage by *purchase*
3. marriage by *arrangement*
4. marriage by *consent* of two principals, also known as conjugal courtship

Marriage by capture is primarily of historical interest.

## Marriage by Capture

Marriage as a way of balancing sex ratios

*Marriage by capture* is rather rare, apparently occurring most often in hunting societies in which there are many more men than women. Mar-riage by capture is one way of redressing this imbalance of the sex ratio and thus providing better marriage opportunities for the extra men who would otherwise not be able to find mates. Murdock (1949) reports that this form of acquiring a mate is exceedingly rare. He did not find a single case of it among the 250 societies he sampled from the Human Relations Area File. This repository that he helped to set up includes ethnographic reports of societies around the world that are then itemized and cate-gorized along a variety of dimensions of anthropological and sociological interest. However, Stephens (1963, pp. 172–78) provides an interesting description of an unsuccessful attempt at marriage by capture by a young Cheyenne.

As remote as this practice seems, our own contemporary marital prac-tices may reveal some subtle parallels to the historical practice of acquir-ing a mate through capture. We even find such phrases as ''catching'' or ''hooking'' the right man or the right woman as a part of our colloquial language. Many of the parallel practices are viewed in a romantic light. For example, there is the popular practice of the groom carrying the new bride over the threshold. Is it not possible to interpret this action as a sym-bolic re-creation of the man dragging his captured bride off to the marital chamber? Then, there is the wedding ring. Although we tend to interpret the wedding ring in romantic terms, as a ''circle of unbroken love,'' is it not just as plausible to interpret it as a symbol of a miniature shackle—the sign of the capturer?

## Marriage by Purchase

Marriage as an economic contract

In most societies, marriage is not only a social contract but an economic one as well. Therefore, it is not surprising that in some societies *marriage by purchase* occurs. This involves some form of economic exchange between the two individuals, their families, or their tribes. This economic exchange is sometimes regulated by the government to serve some social purpose. For example, a recent Reuters news release reported that in central Java bridegrooms have been ordered to pay a bride price of 25 dead rats for their brides before officially being allowed to marry. Carrying out this order not only shows the man's enthusiasm for his future bride but helps solve the dangerous rat problem in that area. Gypsy families living in urban American centers sometimes earn large amounts through the bride price paid for their daughters. In fact, in some societies the economic factor is so crucial that it may truly be said that what has occurred has been a marriage by purchase.

Stephens (1963) points out that the form of these economic considerations is often quite varied and complicated. He believes, however, that they can essentially be divided into the following five different major categories (pp. 210–11), which comprise all the examples that have been found in different societies:

1. *Bride price:* Payments to the bride's family or other kin by the groom or the groom's family and kin. This is the most common form of marriage payment.
2. *Bride service:* The groom works for his bride's family as a substitute for bride price.
3. *Dowry:* Payments to the groom and his family and kin by the bride's family or kin.
4. *Gift exchange:* Both the groom's kin and the bride's kin make payments or exchange gifts with each other, the groom's kin making bride-price payments and the bride's kin making dowry payments.
5. *Woman exchange:* Two groups or individuals may merely trade women, no other payment being involved. For example, *A* gives his sister to *B,* who takes her as his wife; in return, *B* gives his sister to *A,* who takes *B's* sister as his wife.

In addition to these five types of marriage payments, Stephens continues, marriage finance may take at least two other forms. One is the trousseau, which may consist of payments to the bride by her kin, the groom's kin, or both. The other is the marriage ceremonial or wedding feast, which may be very expensive. The groom and his kin or the bride's kin or both sets of kin may help pay for the event.

**Table 1.1**

**Frequency and Percent of Occurrence
of Marriage by Purchase**

| Form of marriage payment | Murdock (565 societies) | | Stephens (51 societies) | |
|---|---|---|---|---|
| | *f* | % | *f* | % |
| Bride price (substantial or token) | 260 | 48 | 24 | 47 |
| Bride service | 75 | 14 | 10 | 20 |
| Dowry | 24 | 4 | 2 | 4 |
| Gift exchange | 15 | 3 | 13 | 25 |
| Woman exchange | 16 | 3 | 1 | 2 |
| No marriage payment or exchange | 152 | 28 | 1* | 2 |

*Stephens reports one borderline case, the Copper Eskimo, in which a bride price is paid only if the bride is taken from her home territory.

Source: Based on data presented in W. N. Stephens's *The Family in Cross-Cultural Perspective* (New York: Holt, Rinehart, & Winston, 1963), pp. 211–12.

Murdock (1949) and Stephens (1963) have both reported the frequent occurrence of each of these five main types of economic considerations. See table 1.1 for data from their ethnographic surveys. While there are considerable differences between the Murdock and Stephens data in the areas of gift exchange and no marriage payment or exchange, these differences are probably caused by the divergent natures and sizes of the samples involved. However, it is interesting to note the close agreement between the two samples on the relative importance of providing some form of compensation to the bride's family rather than to the groom's. Both Murdock's and Stephens's data, for example, show that almost half the societies require the groom to pay the bride's family. This agreement accords well with the general anthropological literature on this issue.

Other anthropologists have described an array of specific exchanges, some unilateral and others reciprocal. Bronislaw Malinowski (1964, pp. 93–104), for example, depicts the exchanging of gifts among the Trobrianders of New Guinea. This illustrates how clearly defined and ritualistic the practice usually is:

This simple declaration of marriage is followed by that exchange of gifts which is so typical of any social transaction in the Trobriands. . . .

The girl's family have [sic!] to make the first offering to signify their consent to the marriage. Since their agreement is absolutely essential, this gift, in conjunction with the public declaration of the union of the partners, constitutes marriage. It is a small gift, a little cooked food brought in baskets and offered by the girl's father to the boy's parents. . . .

Soon afterwards, usually on the same day, the girl's relatives bring a bigger present. Her father, her maternal uncle, and her brothers . . . each bring a basket of uncooked yam food, and offer it to the boy's parents. This gift is called *pepe'i*. But even this is not enough. A third offering of food is brought to the boy's parents, cooked this time and carried on large platters. This gift is called *kaykaboma.*

The boy's family must not delay long before they reciprocate. The last gift, cooked on trays, is returned almost immediately and in exactly the same form as it was received. A more important gift follows. The boy's father has already prepared certain valuables of the *vaygu'a* type, that is to say, large polished axe-blades of green stone, necklaces of polished spondylus shell discs, and armlets made of the *conus* shell; also, when the second gift of the uncooked food was brought to him by the girl's family, he made a small distribution of it among his own relatives, and they in turn now bring him other valuables to add to his own. All these he presents to the girl's family.

Although the initial sources of these economic considerations are not completely clear, many believe that bride price and bride service, the two most common forms of economic considerations, arose to serve two purposes: compensation to the wife's family for the loss of her services and a reward for guarding her virtue (called the "price of a virgin"). Whatever their reason for being, the economic considerations have certain consequences for marriage and family life. Payment by a family to the bride, the groom, or their families gives the paying family some stake and legitimate claim in the marriage and, particularly, in the offspring. In many respects, this situation is similar to the common practice in a capitalist society of buying some shares of a stock in a particular venture or company.

Payment for the bride has also been viewed as a way of reducing the frequency of divorce. In most cases, the bride price is not refundable; neither is the bride service returnable nor transferrable to a new bride. Hence, husbands, who generally control the divorce mechanisms in most societies, must think a long time before instituting a suit for divorce. The

dowry, on the other hand, besides being relatively rare, was generally refundable upon divorce and thus probably also played the same function
in the ongoing marriage.

There are many remnants, although sometimes subtle, of marriage
by payment in our contemporary American society. The young man who
marries the boss's daughter to get ahead is, in a sense, receiving remu-
neration for doing so by being given a part in the business. Also, when
one of the conditions of a marriage is that the bride's or groom's elderly
mother or father come to live with the couple, this is a price paid to the elderly parent for giving his or her child to the marriage.

*Remnants of the marital
customs of primitive cul-
tures are common in
modern practice. A
bride's father escorting
her to the altar may be a
reference to marriage by
purchase.*

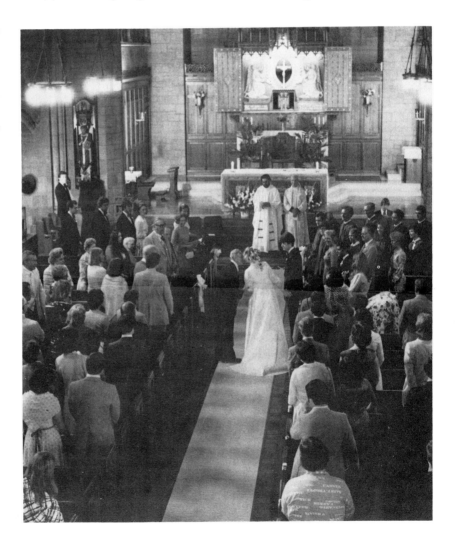

## Marriage by Arrangement

Most societies view marriage as an extremely important social act in which the society has a profound stake. Hence, few societies allow such matches to occur by chance or at the whim of the two, usually young and inexperienced, persons involved. Many societies provide for the choice of a marital partner through the mechanism of *marriage by arrangement.* Usually the arrangements are made by parties other than the two involved and often their consent is not even required. Although both men and women are subject to arranged marriages, it is considerably more likely, as Stephens (1963, p. 190) puts it, for women to be "helpless pawns in the marriage plans of the parents and kin."

In most cases, parents decide and plan the arranged marriages. When others are involved, either on their own or in conjunction with the parents, they are almost always the adult men of the kin group. Thus, we see an example of the second-class status of women in most societies. They are generally considered to be property of the kin group, like land or crops or cattle. And they usually have as much say in the transactions about their marriages as do the land or crops or the cattle in economic transactions involving them!

Marriage as an alliance of families

Most frequently, marriages are arranged because they are viewed as alliances not just between two individuals but between two families. Thus, the family is seen as having a legitimate stake in the choice of mates by one of its members. Also, in many societies, marriage takes place at a relatively young age. In these circumstances, marriage is seen as too important a decision to be left to the young who are considered still too immature socially and too inexperienced to understand the long-run social, economic, and political as well as personal consequences of mate choice. Goodsell (1915, p. 189) quotes a German peasant as saying, "It's not a man that marries a maid, but field marries field, vineyard marries vineyard, cattle marry cattle."

The bases upon which marriages are arranged vary from society to society. However, there is some similarity across societies in the kinds of criteria that are likely to be taken into account. Clearly, the prestige and wealth of the groom's family is an important consideration since it is more often the bride for whom the arrangements are being made. Also, there are occasions in which social obligations require a particular match. Recall Stephens's (1963) fifth category of economic arrangements in mate selection by purchase (women exchange) in which some reciprocal bargains are struck.

Sororate

Two particularly interesting examples of this, the sororate and the levirate, deserve some discussion. These practices involve replacing a deceased marriage partner with a living relative. The *sororate* involves the replacement of a deceased wife with her sister or female kin. In some societies, this replacement is required by law, while in others it is custom. When the sister or female kin is added to an existing marriage, rather than supplied as a replacement for a deceased wife, it is called *sororal polygyny.*

Levirate

The *levirate* involves the man; through this practice he inherits the wife and family of his deceased brother or other male kin. When a male is an addition rather than a replacement of the husband or father, this occurrence is called *fraternal polyandry.*

Finally, in some societies and in some families, the importance of political and economic union becomes a critical factor in the arrangement of marriages. Note, for example, the role these considerations have played in the arrangements of royal families in Western history. Even in the history of American capitalism, there are many instances where the daughter of a steel or oil tycoon was encouraged to marry the son of someone of equal and compatible fortune for the benefit of the business.

Social, economic, and political factors often take precedence over personal wishes in arranged marriages, although the personal is not necessarily excluded entirely. Thus, the importance attributed to personal wishes in the choice of a marital partner in some Western countries, notably the United States, is quite unique, almost deviant, in the broad sweep of the recorded history of marriage.

## Marriage by Consent: Conjugal Courtship

*Marriage by consent,* also called *conjugal courtship,* is the voluntary selection of a marriage partner.

Conjugal courtship

In Stephens's (1963) sample of 53 cases, only 5, other than our own society, permitted free choice of mates by the 2 potential marriage partners without requiring approval of the parents. In addition, 6 others (including Colonial America) permitted free mate choice subject to the approval of the parents or other family elders. To the extent that this sample is reasonably representative, and there is no reason to doubt that it is, it demonstrates quite clearly the unusual amount of freedom accorded North Americans in the choice of their mates. Our system is quite clearly the exception and not the norm.

However, emphasis on the formal freedom to choose a mate tends to underplay the substantial degree of influence that occurs through the parents' role in the socialization process and the more subtle and informal pressures exerted by them on their semidependent and semimature children. We will explore these issues in considerable detail in chapter 6,

*In North America an unusual amount of freedom is accorded in the choice of mates. Our system is the exception, not the norm.*

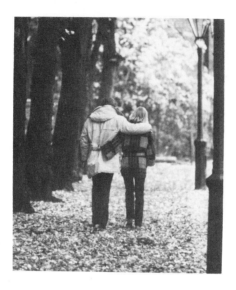

which discusses mate selection. Factors that influence conjugal courtship, factors such as romantic love, will be discussed in chapter 4, which treats intimacy, sexual attraction, and love. Two important points about conjugal courtship should be mentioned here, however.

Larger kin groups

First, there seems to be an association between the importance of the larger kin group and the amount of freedom accorded an individual in the choice of a mate. The more important the larger kin group is, the less freedom the individual is likely to have in the choice of a marital partner. Relatively free choice, requiring the acquiescence if not the approval of parents, seems to be a halfway measure. This transitional tendency can be seen in the change in both the larger kin group and freedom in marital choice from our own colonial past to the present day as indicated in Stephens's data on both periods. Even today, when a prospective bride or groom comes from a very large, closely knit extended family, it is probably necessary to get approval, or at least the acquiescence, from many family members in order to get married.

## Brenda and Eddie

Brenda and Eddie have been dating for about a year and have decided they want to get engaged—and married when she finishes college. Brenda lives in a large brownstone with her parents, paternal grandparents, maternal grandmother, paternal aunt and uncle, a married cousin, and her cousin's two children. There are other relatives, including a brother and two sisters, on the block. Eddie lives alone with his parents, who have little to do with any other family members.

When Brenda and Eddie tell their families their engagement plans, the reactions are mixed. Eddie tells his parents casually, not exactly asking permission, which he doesn't feel he needs, and although they don't object, he can see that they are not too pleased. They've been telling him for some time now that Brenda's family is "low-life," that they are not of the same quality as Eddie's family, who own a successful business. They wish he would marry someone from a better family. But that's about all they have to say.

When Brenda approaches her family; however, it is not to tell them but to ask permission. For she knows that without her family's support she could never go ahead with her plans, no matter how much she loves Eddie. She approaches her parents first, then the grandparents. They are tentative in their responses, cautious, conferring with each other over the next few days. Is Eddie the kind of fellow they want to welcome into the family? Does he look down on them because they are all working people, while he comes from a business family? Will he want children, or will he want Brenda to work since she'll have a college education? Meanwhile, Brenda anxiously awaits their approval.

Brenda is an important part of a large kinship network; Eddie is not. There is a noticeable difference in the effect of the family on their free choices.

Personal fulfillment

Another factor associated with conjugal courtship is the degree to which marriage is seen more as a personal than as a social act, a mode of personal fulfillment rather than a social obligation. In the continually difficult balance between the needs of the individual and the needs of the social group, conjugal courtship is more likely to occur where greater emphasis is placed on the individual. In such circumstances, the needs of the participating individuals are taken into account. As we have mentioned before, such individual freedom is relatively rare in societies throughout the world.

Love, Courtship, and Marriage   No understanding of conjugal courtship is possible without some mention of the concept of love. Since we devote chapter 4 to it, we will mention here only briefly its connection with conjugal courtship.

*Our society, unlike many others, does not enforce strict controls (e.g., a chaperonage system) to regulate the amount of contact between potential marriage partners.*

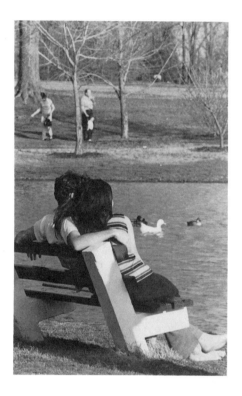

In tracing the history of love to at least the time of Plato, it is clear that its role in relation to marriage has changed considerably over time (see, for example, Reiss 1971). Particularly interesting is the fact that what we have come to call romantic love was believed to be outside of the province of marriage. In contrast to this view is the modern Western, mainly North American, view of love as an absolutely essential ingredient of mate selection and marital life. But, as Reiss points out, this is a recent and not universally accepted view of the role of love in marriage.

Goode (1959) has pointed out another facet of the relationship between love and marriage. Most societies have recognized the power of romantic love as a potentially disruptive force in the control of social structure, particularly in maintaining class distinctions and in regulating kinship lines. Because "love is frequently a basis for and prelude to marriage," Goode argues (p. 41), "it must be controlled or channeled in some way. More specifically, the stratification and lineage patterns would be weakened greatly if love's potentially disruptive effects were not kept in check." Where marriage is primarily an arrangement between families, the introduction of a personal and idiosyncratic element such as love is not only unnecessary, it may well threaten the negotiations (we are reminded of Romeo and Juliet). Though the specific techniques they use may differ, these societies have evolved social mechanisms to keep the phenomenon of love from intruding and hence disrupting the selection of marital partners.

**Child marriages**

Some societies use *child marriages,* where the arrangements for marriage are made while the two potential partners are still children and romantic love is not present as a complicating factor. Under these conditions, social relationships between the two potential marriage partners can begin early and thus serve to exclude other considerations. In some cases, marriages are arranged even before the children are born with due allowance, of course, for alternative arrangements based on the sex of the yet-to-be-born betrotheds. Other societies use a strict *chaperonage system* in which parents, housekeepers, or others supervise the amount and type of contact between potential marriage partners. Still others use ridicule of romantic love as a coercive form of social control over its intrusion into

**Chaperonage system**

mate selection. In short, though the form differs, many societies attempt to control romantic love and to keep it from intruding into the essential social process of mate choice. Once more, our society, where romantic love is glamorized, is a deviant case: the exception, not the rule.

## Marital Forms

The various mate selection practices may result in quite different *marital forms,* that is, the arrangements between the adult members in marriage. Two principal forms of marriage exist: monogamy and polygamy.

## Monogamy

*Monogamous marriage,* that is, marriage between only one man and one woman at a time, is familiar to all of us. It is the only marital form that most of us are likely to know from firsthand experience and close acquaintanceship, although given the increasing divorce and remarriage rate, perhaps our system ought to be labeled *serial monogamy,* which re-

**Serial monogamy**

fers to the process of having a number of spouses, one after another. As far as we can tell from historical and anthropological records, monogamy has been and still is the most widely practiced marital form around the world. Moreover, it is probably the only marital form that is permitted in all societies. However, monogamy is *not* the preferred form of marriage around the world. In a sample of 250 societies, Murdock (1949) found that only 43 of these societies (17 percent) actually considered monogamy the preferred marital arrangement.

When there is about an equal number of men and women of marrying age, monogamy provides the maximum marriage opportunities for the members of society. Theoretically at least, under these conditions there is a man for each woman and a woman for each man. However, considerations of personal taste and social acceptability complicate this somewhat simplistic view of marriage opportunities.

Monogamy also has the consequence of centering all emotional gratification and marital responsibilities on only two people. Whether this situation is viewed as an advantage or a disadvantage depends at least in part on the role of the marital relationship in the broader social structure. To the extent that the partners in the marital relationship are expected to carry a large share of societal responsibilities with little outside help, limiting the number of persons available to carry these responsibilities out may be disadvantageous. On the other hand, the more social responsibilities are assumed by other social institutions the less disadvantageous monogamy may become. Monogamy is advantageous in that it is compatible with the general balance of males and females in a society. In any event, for most of us it is the marital form that seems most natural, most acceptable, and for many the most moral.

## Polygamy

Exotic places, natives running around naked, perpetual ecstasy, frequent orgies—these are the visions often conjured up by the word polygamy for those practicing monogamy.

The reality is actually a lot duller than this fantasy for most of the people who live in polygamous societies. Even though in its common usage *polygamy* refers to a man having many wives, technically, polygamy is a generic term referring to a situation of multiple spouses for *either* or *both* of the sexes.

Multiple spouses

There are in fact three distinct subtypes of polygamy—polyandry, polygyny, and group marriage—each of which we shall discuss separately. However, the important general point that should not be lost in the specific discussions to follow is that marriage not only takes quite diverse forms but that these forms are related to other facets of a society's culture and cannot be separated from it.

Polyandry    *Polyandry* is the marriage of one woman to two or more men at the same time. It is a relatively rare practice, occurring in only 2 cases in Murdock's (1949) sample of 250 societies and in 4 cases in his later (1957) and larger sample of 565 societies. When polyandry does occur, it tends to be associated with a population in which there are more men than women and in which there are the severe economic conditions

One wife, two or more husbands

of a subsistence economy. These conditions suggest that polyandry may be a society's way of adapting to sexual and social conditions that make things difficult for individuals to function any other way. It serves the function of putting a relatively large number of men in the role of wresting a subsistence from a harsh environment for a family that is not much larger than a monogamous one. Three men hunting food for one wife in a sparsely populated area is an economical way of surviving.

Female infanticide

Female infanticide is a frequent concomitant of a polyandrous society. We are thus led to suspect that the imbalanced sex ratio is an artificial product of polyandry and not the other way around. Apparently, it is the nature of a harsh subsistence economy that led to polyandry as an adaptation, with female infanticide used to maintain a favorable sex ratio for its practice while at the same time keeping the birth rate in check and holding down the number of mouths to feed. How clearly this illustrates the relationship between a predominant marital form and economic-environmental factors!

There are two forms of polyandry: *fraternal,* in which the husbands are brothers biologically or by accepted classification, and *nonfraternal,* in

*Monogamy centers all emotional gratification and marital responsibilities on only two people.*

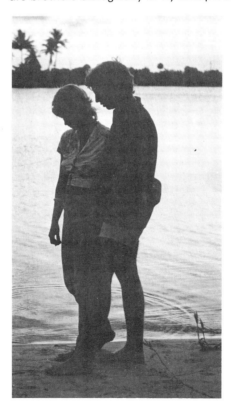

Fraternal polyandry

which the husbands are not related. In the few cases of polyandry that have been found, the fraternal form seems to be more prevalent. Stephens (1963) believes that the fraternal arrangement reduces the amount of jealousy that may arise among men who share a single wife. At least it may temper the way it is handled since the brothers have a history of relationships and attachments with each other and with kinsmen that predates the marriages. We see parallels of this feeling in our society where men who are in the same gang or fraternity may lay claim to certain women and resent anyone outside their circle of ''brotherly'' friendship sharing these women.

It is interesting that polyandry is so rare. One reason that has been suggested is that it is very difficult for men to grant other men sexual access to their wives, which is precisely what is required by polyandry. While there are no clear and unequivocal data to support this suggestion, the rarity of polyandry does seem to lend some credence to this viewpoint.

Polygyny   The marriage of one man to two or more women at the same time is called *polygyny.* It is the most common of the polygamous forms of marriage. In fact in its everyday but technically incorrect usage, it is called polygamy.

One husband, two or more wives

In his earlier sample, Murdock (1949) found that 193 of his 250 societies (81 percent), and in his later sample (1957) 415 of his 565 societies (75 percent), permitted polygyny. The difference in frequency of societal preference between polygyny and polyandry is striking.

While polygyny appears to be the most preferred form of marriage, we have noted earlier that monogamy is the most frequently practiced. The reasons for the difference in preference and actuality have roots in the economics, status systems, and sex ratios of societies. As people in most societies find out, in practice two, and especially four, cannot live as cheaply as one. Extra spouses require extra resources, especially when there is a bride price involved. Thus, even where polygyny is permitted and preferred, it is only a small number of men—usually the older, wealthier, and more prestigious men—who actually take an additional wife or two. Polygynous marriages are associated with wealth and high social status.

Wealth and high social status

Actually the relationship is a mutually supporting one: only those with some degree of wealth and status can afford to marry more than once, and marrying more than once often enhances a man's social status. And sometimes enhanced social status can lead to more control of the scarce resources.

The realities of polygyny are very different from the sexual fantasies

Sexual fantasies vs.
economic realities

of many men in Western society. A polygynous union is based more often on an economic and social decision rather than on a sexual one. In fact, the sexual aspects of polygynous marriages seem to be decidedly secondary to its economic (in the broad sense of acquiring and distributing the goods and services required in the family) and its social-status facets. Additional wives are more often valued for the prestige they bring to the husband and for their role in providing extra labor for family responsibilities than for their inherent sexuality.

## Muran and Bhagtar

Muran was a big and ugly woman, having many scars and no teeth. She never smiled. Bhagtar took her as his third wife because she was strong, could work in the field, and could carry a great deal of wood. His second wife was now pregnant, and he needed someone to help in her place.

Often polygynous societies require a strict rotational system whereby the husband spends an equal time in the dwellings of each of his wives; and, this system holds true whether the wife is young or old, attractive or ugly, pleasant or unpleasant. With the possible exception of the first wife, to whom polygynous societies generally accord somewhat higher status, privileges, and authority, this distribution of attention generally extends to nonsexual matters as well, and thus reduces potential jealousy that may and, according to the anthropological reports, does arise in the polygynous family.

A separate dwelling for each of the wives is another fairly common feature of polygynous societies. This separate habitation also serves to reduce possible friction. It keeps the plural wives out of each other's way on a day-to-day basis and gives each of them an independent sphere of authority and responsibility. Separate houses are less likely under conditions of *sororal polygyny,* where a husband takes sisters as his wives (Murdock and Whiting 1951). Stephens (1963) interprets this finding as signifying that ''siblings can better tolerate, suppress, and live with a situation of sexual rivalry than can nonsiblings'' (p. 67).

An imbalanced ratio with more men than women in a society will severely restrict the possibility of polygyny. For polygyny to be widespread there must be considerably more women than men. Since in most societies the sex ratio hovers between about 95 and 100, that is, with approximately equal numbers of men and women, pervasive polygyny is quite unlikely. Since polygyny does occur in some societies with sex ratios that are unfavorable to its development, some social mechanisms are needed to provide for its occurrence. One such mechanism is the tendency of polygynous societies to have girls marry early and men marry late. Since men die at earlier ages than women, there are fewer men at the upper age levels. Also, the requirements of wealth and social standing reduce the number of men who can expect to take more than one wife. However, as far as we can tell, there are no mechanisms that adequately compensate for the sex ratio. So in most polygynous societies many, if not most, young men will have to content themselves with one wife, and some with none.

**Group Marriage**  One of the theoretically possible but extremely rare forms of polygamy is *group marriage,* where two or more men are collectively married to two or more women at the same time. Murdock (1949) doesn't believe that group marriage exists anywhere as the cultural norm; that is, he knows of no society where group marriage is the preferred form. However, among certain religious cults and fringe groups, it is practiced in contemporary societies. The followers of Charles Manson, for example, are reported to have practiced group marriage, which reinforced their concept of belonging to a family. And reports from Jonestown, Guyana, suggest that bizarre group marriage ceremonies took place there in the weeks and months preceding the mass suicide-murder of over 900 followers of the Reverend Jim Jones.

Stephens (1963) argues that group marriage often goes hand-in-hand with polyandry, especially fraternal polyandry. In fact, he believes that group marriage is essentially an extension of fraternal polyandry with the brothers taking additional wives and bringing them into a common family. However, both Murdock and Stephens, as well as other informed opinion, agree that group marriage is a rare form that occasionally occurs as a variant form within a society generally practicing one or another of the marital forms that we have discussed.

In group marriage, each of the men generally has equal sexual access to each of the women. However, Linton (1936) has pointed out that there is often a primary couple whose marital rights with one another have the highest priority within the group. But as with the other forms of marriage, there are factors other than the sexual. In effect, group marriage is a collective experience that fulfills the sexual, economic, and social needs of the participants.

There is still some discussion among anthropologists as to whether group marriage ever existed as an independent viable marriage form, outside of special circumstances that made it temporarily desirable. It is fascinating, therefore, to observe the current discussions over some semblance of group marriage in the contemporary United States, where such

Two or more men, two or more women

An extension of fraternal polyandry

phenomena as communal living, cohabitation in dormitories, and so forth have gained press attention (see chapter 8). Also, we can note the similarity to group marriage of the arrangements often worked out between specific fraternities and sororities on some college campuses during the period of the 1930s through the 1960s and which is now being revived.

There is still a small contingent of group marriages and communal structures within the United States today (Pomeroy 1973). However, given the overall American value system it is unlikely that this pattern will ever be practiced by more than a select few (Ellis 1973). Despite this, there is increasing attention being paid to those interested in alternative lifestyles (see Constantine and Constantine 1973).

In concluding this section, it should be pointed out that neither monogamy nor polygamy in any of its forms can rightfully be considered the normal, natural, or most moral arrangement of marriage. As Crosby (1976, p. 88) points out,

> Neither belief [that monogamy or polygamy is the natural condition of society] has ever been established. . . . Whether or not monogamy or polygamy is the ''natural'' thing cannot be resolved by looking at the animal world, for the wolf and the tiny gerbil are monogamous, while many other species are not. The appeal to morality depends entirely on the mores of the society in which the appeal is made.
>
> In some instances, a man would be considered lax in his duty if he had only one wife. The appeal to religious authority depends on the religious tradition to which one appeals. The appeal to libidinous [sexual] drives and desires for justification for multiple mates may reveal more about man's psyche than his libido. *The traditions, customs, and mores of a given society together with one's own sense of value and meaning would appear to be the more accurate predictors of ''man's essential nature''* (italics ours).

Now that we have had an opportunity to look at some ways people have traditionally entered marriages and at some of the major marital forms, let us look briefly at a new and important way of entering marriage: by an individual marriage contract.

## Marriage By Contract

At the very opposite pole of marriage by capture is the increasingly popular option of marriage by individual *premarital contract*. This is based on a simple idea. Wherever marriage exists, it is governed by a specific set of laws, either explicit or implicit. These laws serve a variety of purposes that are either significant historically or relevant at a specific moment in time. Customs and laws pertaining to marriage, like all other kinds of laws and customs, are usually created to deal with a specific social problem. As a society changes, often so do its laws and customs.

The relationship between custom and law is so intricate that we often don't realize the difference. For example, consider the common practice of a woman taking her husband's surname. The law does not *require* a woman to do this; rather, it *assumes* the practice so thoroughly that most people think there is no choice in the matter. And the reason the law assumes that a woman will take her husband's name is that until recently the practice was totally pervasive.

These laws may be enforced or generally ignored. In either case, the couple getting married is bound by them. Whenever two people agree to a legally recognized marriage, they agree to abide by these laws, even though often they don't know what the laws are. "Entering marriage without a premarital contract," Brooklyn matrimonial lawyer Saul Edelstein argues, "is like going into a business venture under someone else's rules."

What are some of the rules and laws that we agree to when we marry? Weitzman (1975) has discussed in detail some of the conditions imposed on men and women who enter into legal marriage. She points out that "the marriage contract is unlike most contracts: its provisions are unwritten, its penalties are unspecified, and the terms of the contract are typically unknown to the 'contracting' parties" (p. 531). She goes on to define the terms of this unwritten contract in our contemporary American society.

Unwritten provisions, unspecified penalties

1. *The husband is the head of the family.* Today, when a woman marries, she still loses her independent identity: she assumes her husband's name, his residence, and his status—socially and economically. [p. 532]
2. *The husband is responsible for support.* The traditional marriage contract assumes a strict division of labor within the family. The financial aspects of family life are delegated to the husband. . . . All states, even those with community property systems, place the primary obligation of family support upon the husband. [p. 533]
3. *The wife is responsible for domestic services.* In legal marriage, the man exchanges financial support for his wife's service as a companion, housewife, and mother. [p. 534]
4. *The wife is responsible for child care.* The woman's role as mother remains at the very core of our legal conceptions of her

place in society; it is a basic source of stereotype, the most stubborn and intractable bastion of discrimination. [p. 539]

Recently, some important changes in state law and in case law have affected these four categories by at least giving the parties in matrimonial cases some leeway. For example, in many states the financial and role equality of husbands and wives is spelled out in terms of joint property laws and nonsexist alimony decisions. Also, child custody is no longer automatically awarded to the mother as it had been for years. Still, despite the legal changes, more and more young couples are drawing up their own antenuptial agreements, actually, premarital contracts, to define the rules of their marriage and, often, to declare their philosophy of marriage. For many years, these types of contracts were only used by wealthy older people who were remarrying and wanted to make sure that their estate would be shared with their children of a former marriage or that it would not be shared by the present spouse. In these cases, the agreement was a preventive measure, that is, against exploitation, rather than a positive statement about marriage.

**Contracts to prevent exploitation**

But now, as more and more couples are having contracts drawn up, contracts are beginning to serve a more constructive purpose. A premarriage agreement, suggests David J. Rolfe, who has developed and published a premarriage contract for teenage couples who are living with one of the sets of parents, may be constructively used "to establish an explicit *quid pro quo* [tit for tat]; to itemize and delineate expectations; to protect the rights of privacy of all parties and to spell out the financial commitments of all concerned. . . . The contract serves as an aide in focusing on the realistic and practical aspects of preparing for marriage" (Rolfe 1977, p. 282).

**Constructive use of contracts**

The premarriage contract opens up new opportunities for couples to set the rules by which they will live. There are still pitfalls, however. Wells (1976) has pointed out some of the problems that are raised with the positive qualities; namely, (1) their questionable legality; (2) the fact that people change after marriage and actual areas of conflict are not usually anticipated before the marriage; (3) the fact that they reflect a pessimistic outlook and a lack of flexibility. Still he concludes that premarriage contracts are a step in the right direction toward clarifying expectations and aspirations in marriage.

**Pitfalls of premarriage contracts**

Rather than consider abstractions, let us look at an actual premarriage contract, figure 1.1. This contract was written by the couple in nonlegal language, expressing their feelings and beliefs, and then turned over to their individual lawyers who put it in legal terms. It was signed on their wedding day. Comments in the side column tell how the contract was developed, what conventions it maintains, which customs and laws it attempts to get around and why, and how things actually worked out.

Figure 1.1

## Ante-nuptial Agreement between George Brooke and Marnie Castellano

Preamble:

Whereas, a marriage between the parties is contemplated and each of the parties has fully informed the other of his or her financial situation, including the amount of his or her assets, liabilities, and net income; and

This preamble section is designed to tell the basic purpose of why George and Marnie decided to write the contract.

Whereas, both parties acknowledge their mutual affection to each other contemplating and assuming the relationship of husband and wife and by the instant agreement are seeking to define a marriage relationship that affirms their individuality and equality in the marriage; and

In legalese "instant agreement" simply means this agreement!

Whereas, both parties desire to make fair and reasonable provisions that preserve and promote their individual identities both during the marriage and in the event the marriage is terminated; and

Whereas, the parties hold the following concepts of marriage to be inaccurate, untrue, and not applicable to their intended relationship:

　The husband as head of household and the wife as housewife;

　The husband as supporter and the wife as dependent;

　The husband as authority and the wife as faithful helper and companion;

　The husband gets the rights to the wife's services in return for supporting her; and

Remarkably, court decisions and law have placed women in something of an inferior position in this state (New York). George and Marnie wanted specifically to reject each of these concepts, and the four listed are the one's that Marnie would legally have been required to submit to, a submission the couple found abhorrent.

Whereas, the parties are contemplating their marriage based upon the assumption that each will have contributed equally to the marriage and that the marriage is a partnership contract between two consenting adults and in case of any termination of said contract, both parties intend by this agreement to return to each other a status quo relationship as existed before the marriage; and

Here, George and Marnie begin to state their positive assumptions about marriage.

Whereas, at the time of the contemplated marriage of the parties, both parties are professionals. George is a high school principal and Marnie teaches at a day nursery. It is the intention of Marnie to further her education by completing her masters degree in education and beginning a career in special education counseling.

Now, therefore, in consideration of the aforementioned premises and for other good and valuable consideration, the parties agree as follows:

1. Both parties agree that during the period of their marriage each of them will continue to work and to contribute to their joint assets to the best of their abilities. Neither one of the parties expects to become the sole support of the other. Both parties value the importance and integrity of their respective careers and acknowledge the demands that their careers place upon them, both as individuals and on their parts as partners in the marriage relationship. Both parties recognize themselves as equals in the relationship to the accumulation of income and the responsibility of housework. It is agreed by and between the parties that both will be equal financial contributors to the best of their abilities and both parties agree to assume equal responsibility for the domestic chores such as housework, cooking, shopping, and the like. The parties do not subscribe to the concept that a woman's work is primarily in the home and that a man's work is primarily in the marketplace.

2. George agrees that Marnie may have the right to use her maiden name if she chooses during the marriage and rejects the concept that the wife must adopt the husband's surname.

3. Both parties agree to maintain respect for one another.

4. George hereby waives whatever right he may have to solely determine the legal domicile of the parties.

Here, they outline their future professional plans, so there is no misunderstanding. Marnie, by the way, did complete her degree—and with honors!

This is a key paragraph, in which they again assert their belief that both partners should contribute financially to the marriage.

They are not only going to pursue their respective professions, but as true equals, they are going to share the drudgeries of marriage too, namely, housework.

More and more women are retaining their maiden names after marriage or using a hyphenated name.

Legally, in their state the woman is required to follow the man wherever he chooses to live!

5. Both parties are cognizant of the differences in their cultural upbringings because of the differences in their religions. Marnie has been brought up in the Catholic faith and George has been brought up as a Protestant. Each party agrees to respect the other's individual preference with respect to religion and to make no demands upon the other to change.

6. Both parties represent and warrant to each other that their state of happiness in the impending marriage is not necessarily dependent upon raising a family and having children. Both parties represent to each other and acknowledge that they have not yet made any decision about having children and that their choice to have or not to have children will be a mutual decision, one by choice and not by chance. In the event that the parties decide to have children, whichever partner assumes responsibility for the daily care of said children until the children reach school age will be for all practical purposes assuming a position equal and equivalent to employment that results in pecuniary gain. The parties agree that if they have children, the children will be exposed to the teachings of both parents' religions including their customs and traditions.

7. Both parties recognize that marriage is a road with many difficulties and they are aware that by living together and sharing the deepest of feelings with each other they will inevitably encounter difficulties and conflicts. Recognizing this, the parties agree that, in the case of unresolved conflicts and difficulties between them, they will seek the help of a trained marriage counselor. At the request of either, each shall attend at least seven marriage counseling sessions.

8. If their relationship should terminate either by a separation (de facto or de jure), annulment, or a divorce instituted by either party, regardless of fault, both George and Marnie agree as follows in regard to their respective

George and Marnie discussed at length before marriage their religious beliefs and felt (rightly so) that there would be no conflict between them.

George and Marnie decided, after two years of marriage, that they did want children, very much in fact, and on November 25, 1977, George Edward Brooke, Jr. was born! In retrospect, they were amazed at how their feelings about wanting and then not wanting children fluctuated until they finally made a decision. Now they want at least two more!

George and Marnie know that in the midst of anger it is often difficult to make a sound decision. They decided that they would give marriage counseling an honest try should their relationship get very rocky. Of course, they didn't expect that one of them would take out the contract and wave it at the other, but they did expect that it would remind them of their more "rational" intentions.

property rights arising out of their marriage contract:

A. All assets hereinafter acquired, individually or jointly owned, will be considered as joint property, except such items and material necessary for the conducting of business (e.g., books, typewriter, etc.). All liabilities not connected with the conducting of business shall be considered as joint liabilities except those that are assumed and incurred during three months prior to the actual separation of the parties. Any liability assumed individually without the consent of the other within three months prior to the actual separation of the parties or the dissolution of the partnership as previously defined will be presumed to be the liability of the parties so incurring said liability. If the same were made in good faith not in contemplation of a termination of the marriage, then the same should be a joint liability.

B. All joint property will be divided equally between the partners. All joint liabilities will be divided equally between the partners.

C. In the event that legal action is deemed necessary and the same is undertaken by either of the parties against the other, each partner agrees to assume full responsibility for his or her own legal costs and expenses.

D. Assuming that both parties can upon a termination of their marriage resume their financial status quo, which existed prior to their entry into the marriage relationship, each party waives whatever right he or she may have to alimony and support from the other.

E. If at such time as there may be a child born of this partnership or adopted by the parties, both parties agree to make reasonable provision for the support and education of said child out of their joint income and assets and will determine custody according to the best interests of the child without the traditional bias in favor of the mother.

F. The parties agree that upon any dissolu-

These are some technical restrictions suggested by the lawyer. The couple's primary concern was, in the event that the marriage failed, there would be a fair distribution of property, with neither of them dependent upon the other for support.

Again, these passages emphasize the theme of equal responsibility in the partnership. George and Marnie found this reiteration necessary because of what they viewed as "traditional" roles, which they rejected.

tion of their relationship, either de jure or de facto, the joint division of assets and liabilities equally shall constitute a complete settlement of all their obligations to each other without either party having any claim upon the other for additional alimony, support, monies, settlement, or the like. This particular provision is an extension of their underlying philosophy of marriage: an equal partnership, with equal rights and equal obligations. The parties agree that it is only with this understanding in mind that they are entering the marriage.

9. In the event of a termination of the marriage, the provisions of this agreement shall serve as the final property marital settlement agreement and that the terms and provisions of this agreement shall not be invalidated or otherwise affected by any decree or judgment of annulment, separation, or divorce made by any court in any action that may hereafter be instituted by either party against the other for such marital dissolution, and the obligations and covenants of this agreement shall survive any decree or judgment and shall not merge therein and this agreement shall be enforced independently of such decree. Both parties agree, stipulate, and consent that no judgment, order, or decree in any action for annulment, divorce, or separation, whether brought in the state of New York or any state having jurisdiction of the parties hereto, shall make any provision for financial support nor those that affect property rights inconsistent with the provisions of this agreement. The provisions of this agreement shall take precedence and shall be the primary obligation of both of the parties hereto to each other.

10. The parties represent to each other that both the legal and practical effect of this agreement in each and every respect and the financial status of the parties have been fully explained to both parties by their respective counsel and attorneys. They both acknowledge that it is a fair agreement and is not the result

More legalese, but then after all the lawyers were being paid a total of $300 for their services.

of any duress or undue influence exercised by either party upon the other and both fully intend it to be legally binding upon themselves in consideration of their affection and esteem for each other as equal individuals seeking to define a marriage relationship while they preserve and promote their individual identities as man and woman contracting to live together for mutual benefit and growth. The parties represent to each other that Marnie has been represented by _____ and that George has been represented by _____. Simultaneously with the execution hereof, both parties have individually paid their respective legal fees to their attorneys for their aid in the preparation of the within instrument.

11. Both George and Marnie have been advised of the possibility of some of these provisions being declared at a subsequent date to be invalid or illegal pending the particular state that has jurisdiction of the matter if a controversy exists. Both parties ascribe to the concept that states' interventions in people's marriages may be in violation of Article 1, Section 10, of the United States Constitution that states in part that states are forbidden to pass laws "impairing the obligations of contracts." Both parties are aware of, but do not rely upon, the fact that future legislation may strengthen the legal effect of some of the provisions of the within instrument, through passage of an Equal Rights Amendment or uniform marriage and divorce act. Both parties agree, therefore, that the terms and provisions of the within instrument shall be interpreted and governed, if necessary, by the laws of any state or country in which all or any part that is at issue of the terms and provisions of the within agreement shall be deemed "legal" and agree to be bound prospectively in case of any future litigation that may support the validity of the provisions of the within instrument.

12. In case any provision of this agreement

There is a subtle double standard in the way a judge looks at a premarital agreement. Has the woman, who is presumed to be more eager to get married than the man, given up her legal rights under subtle duress? Has the man said, "Sign this or I..."?

Both lawyers explained that in many parts of the country contracts such as these are unenforceable or are not recognized. This situation is rapidly changing, however, with new court decisions.

shall be held contrary to or invalid under the laws of any country, state, or other jurisdiction, such legality or invalidity shall not affect in any way any other provisions hereof, all of which shall continue nevertheless in full force and effect and any provision that is held to be illegal or invalid in any country, state, or other jurisdiction shall nonetheless remain in full force and effect in any country, state, or jurisdiction in which such provision could be found legal and valid.

13. All matter affecting interpretation and legal effect of this agreement and the rights of the parties hereto shall be governed by the laws of any state that recognizes the validity and enforceability of the provisions herein contained.

14. Any controversy or claim arising out of or relating to this contract or the breach thereof, including the validity of any of the provisions contained therein, shall be settled by arbitration in accordance with the rules of the American Arbitration Association and the judgment upon the award rendered by the arbitrators may be entered in any court having jurisdiction thereof and binding upon the parties.

To avoid expensive litigation, George and Marnie included an arbitration clause, which was recommended by both of their lawyers.

15. The consideration for this agreement is the love and affection of the parties, one to another, as represented by the marriage about to be solemnized.

In witness whereof, the parties have hereunto set their hands this 16th day of July 1975.

_____
Marnie Castellano

_____
Witness

_____
George Brooke

_____
Witness

## Summary

1. In our culture the choice of a marital partner is relatively free and requires the voluntary consent only of the principals. However, this situation does not prevail in all cultures nor did it in all periods of history. There are four major practices used in selecting a mate: marriage by capture, marriage by purchase, marriage by arrangement, and marriage by consent of the principals, also called conjugal courtship. The last is characteristic of our own culture, although it is one of the less common practices throughout the world. While marriage by capture is rare, there are many examples of marriage by purchase and marriage by arrangement. The type of practice found in a particular society may depend upon economic factors or, as in the case of marriage by capture, the ratio of men to women. The involvement of the family versus the importance of the individual also may determine the method of mate selection.

2. There are two major forms of marriage: monogamy, in which one man and one woman are married to each other, and polygamy, in which either a man or a woman or both has more than one mate.

3. In a popular contemporary option, marriage by contract, two people intending to marry write their own agreement regarding their expectations for the marriage. There are certain assumptions made about men and women in marriages, and individual contracts allow couples the opportunity to state which of these they find applicable to their marriages.

**Key Terms**

The following terms were introduced and defined in this Chapter. Definitions also appear in the glossary.

chaperonage system
child marriage
conjugal courtship
fraternal polyandry
group marriage
levirate
marital form
marriage by arrangement
marriage by capture
marriage by consent
marriage by contract

marriage by purchase
monogamy
nonfraternal polyandry
polyandry
polygamy
polygyny
premarital contract
serial monogamy
sororal polygyny
sororate

**Discussion Questions**

1. What kinds of social and economic factors in our culture make conjugal courtship the preferred form of marital choice? Can you envision in the next half a century any changes that may bring in other forms to supplement or supplant conjugal courtship?

2. Aside from conjugal courtship and monogamy, with which you are familiar, what other cultural practice of selecting a marital partner and what other marital form would you personally find most satisfying? What are some of the disadvantages of monogamy and conjugal courtship that would not be inherent in the method and form you selected?

3. What psychological ramifications are there for individuals living in societies where marriage by arrangement and marriage by purchase are the norms. How would you feel in such a society?

4. If you were to draw up a premarital agreement, what specific clauses would you want to be certain were included? What would be your explicit philosophy of marriage at the beginning of the contract?

5. Define the terms monogamy, polygamy, polygyny, and polyandry. What are their relative frequencies throughout the world?

**Suggested Readings**

1. William J. Goode. *World Revolution and Family Patterns*. New York: Free Press, 1963.

An excellent analysis of the diversity of family patterns in a changing world by a renowned sociologist that has become must reading for all students of the family.

2. George P. Murdock. *Social Structure.* New York: Macmillan, 1949.

This classic book on comparative kinship by the premier anthropologist studying the family contains a wealth of descriptive and quantitative data which are used in the course of examining relationships among various aspects of the family structure and practices.

3. William N. Stephens. *The Family in Cross-Cultural Perspective.* New York: Holt, 1963.

An extremely useful, conceptually oriented review of ethnographic reports on family customs of societies around the world.

## Chapter 2

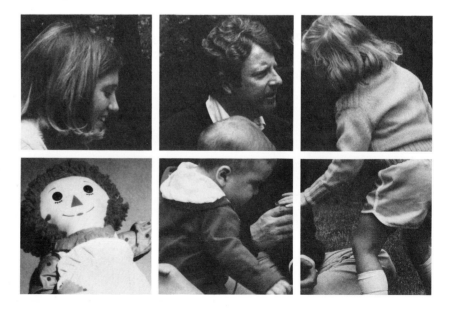

# The Organization and Structure
# of the Family

## Chapter Aims

1. To consider the importance of the sociological concept of nuclear family and to evaluate its universality and its purpose historically and in the present.

2. To delineate the vast range of kinship arrangements and their practical implications, in terms of residence and family authority.

3. To examine in some detail the taboo against incest, in the hope of finding the origins and purpose of the taboo.

## Overview

During our life, most of us are members of two smaller family forms: in one we are the children and in the other we are the parents. Larger family groups are composites of these various parent-child-sibling relationships.

A kinship system is extremely important in every society. Through these systems people's rights, privileges, and positions are defined. Societies have rules of how descent will be determined, through one line or through more than one; where a married couple will live; and who will have the authority in the family.

There has been a great deal of debate about whether or not the family structure of parents and children is universal. This structure does provide a format in which basic intimate, economic, reproductive, and socializing needs can be fulfilled. There is also strong evidence in societies to support a belief in its universality.

Almost all societies prohibit sexual activity between two members of the same family group. There are many interesting theories as to why such a ban has persisted throughout history.

## What Is a Family?

A conjugal union and its kinship ties

Often, when we think of the concept of family, we use our own family life as the model, perhaps the very home in which we were raised, or the family organizations that we saw in the geographical area where we grew up. Our view, in other words, is limited by our experiences. But in fact there is great variation in the different kinds of family forms found throughout the world in different societies.

In this chapter, we will focus on the variation in form taken by the family. We can define the general concept of *family* as the conjugal (marriage) union *and* its kinship ties. The family usually involves consanguineal (blood) ties as well as conjugal relationships, although a family may also consist of two married adults and their adopted children, which would not be consanguineal. Or, as Murdock (1949, p. 1) puts it, the family is a social group consisting of ''adults of both sexes, at least two of whom maintain a socially approved sexual relationship, and one or more children, own or adopted, of the sexually cohabiting adults.'' There are several forms and variations that this organization may take. The key to understanding all of them is the central concept of the nuclear family.

## The Nuclear Family

The primary component of all types of families is the *nuclear family,* which "consists typically of a married man and woman with their off-spring" (Murdock 1949, p. 1). This central unit is the building block for the other two major forms of the family that we will discuss.

There are actually two types of nuclear families, depending on whose perspective is adopted: the child's or the parents'. The *nuclear family of orientation* is the nuclear family as seen through the eyes of the children. It is the social context in which the child receives his or her first and most continuous orientation to life. It consists of the child, the parents, and all siblings. It is the primary agent of socialization through infancy and childhood as well as an extremely important one throughout the person's life.

The *nuclear family of procreation* is the same nuclear family, but viewed from the parents' perspective. Since the roles of the individuals differ, they do not perceive the family in the same social context. The nuclear family of procreation is created through marriage rather than by birth. Parents will typically describe their families in a different light than their children do, even though all of them may believe they are being objective.

Most of us are members of both types of nuclear families throughout a large portion of our lives. Each of us becomes the focal point that unites these two important social groups, each of us the bond between two nuclear families. In fact, some of the problems of married life are caused by the incompatible demands made of us by members of these two important sets of relationships. Some of these problems such as in-law conflicts are discussed in chapter 11.

The nuclear family is central to our understanding of kinship and family organization, and we will consider it in greater depth later in this chapter. First, we will view two major forms of the family: the extended family and the polygamous family.

*The child's viewpoint*

*The parents' viewpoint*

## The Extended Family

The *extended family* is a number of nuclear families, monogamous or polygamous, bound by the parent-child relationship. In its historical form, the members of the extended family all lived under one roof or at least on the same general tract of commonly owned land. Often, it was run by the oldest man, usually the grandfather and consisted of at least three generations of married sons and their families as well as all unmarried dependent children. Married daughters generally joined the extended families of their husband.

Usefulness of the
extended family

For some time now there has been considerable debate in American sociology. There are those who believe that there is an extended family system in contemporary America and that such a system is functionally useful (for example, Sussman and Burchinal 1962; Litwak 1960a and 1960b; Adams 1968) and those who do not (see Parsons 1943; Pitts 1964). The debate largely grew from Parsons posing the issue in its extreme form: there is an isolated nuclear family system in the United States, which our society needs in order to fill its fluid occupational requirements. You may understand the ambiguity of this issue better if you ask yourself if you are part of an extended family or not. You could probably answer either way, depending on how you look at it. Even *"Ma Bell"* confuses the issue when we are told we are never more than a phone call away from our families.

The evidence accumulated by Sussman and Burchinal (1962), Litwak (1960a and 1960b), and Adams (1968), among others, made it clear that family relationships in America during the nineteenth century and earlier in this century often took the form of an extended family network, although not in its classical form. While three or more generations rarely lived in the same household, they often lived in reasonable proximity. More importantly, their lives were intimately intertwined in a network of rights and obligations that clearly separated them from strangers, casual acquaintances, and even close friends. Legally, in fact, the concept of extended family has gained an important recognition, although less precise than that of nuclear family (Robertshaw and Curtin 1977).

These ties even turned out to be useful for the socially and geographically mobile. Although we think of the extended family as living together or very near each other, as the size of the family expands so does its geographical range. In fact, not only has the extended family rarely been a millstone on the mobile person's neck, but often it has been just what is needed for immediate information and contacts in the new situations and new places that the mobile person has confronted. It remained only to relabel these ties across borders as a "modified extended family" to settle the debate for all but a few diehards.

Nowhere is the importance of kinship more evident than in the extended family. The essence of the extended family is based on the kinship bonds between parent and child and between siblings. In effect, these particular bonds make the extended family immortal: it continues generation after generation and, like the society as a whole, survives its individual members. In fact, a part of the fascination with *genealogy,* the tracing of one's family history as Alex Haley did in *Roots,* is that it shows us the extended family we were often not aware of.

Genealogy

Also, the size of the extended family provides potentially greater emotional, economic, political, and social support for its members than is pos-

*Polygamous families are not common in our culture, but they have some similarities with our nuclear and extended family forms:*

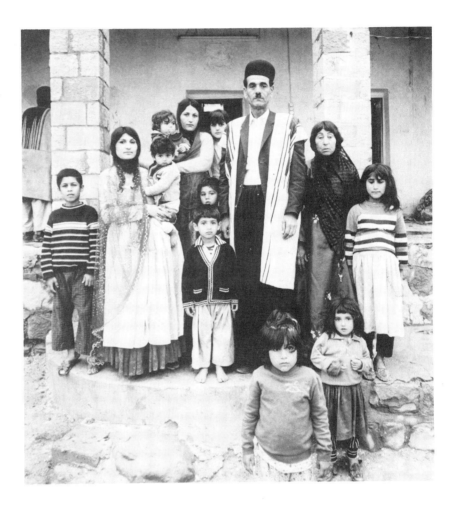

Cultural continuity

sible in the much smaller nuclear family. This combination of larger size and greater continuity gives the extended family a kind of strength and resiliency that is rarely found in the nuclear family structure. Such resiliency helps children socialize into adulthood with a sense of familial stability (Rae-Grant 1976). It also increases the likelihood of cultural continuity, that is, that ethnic, religious, or social customs will be maintained generation after generation (Stein 1978). On the other hand, the very fact of larger size and the emphasis on continuity are likely to minimize the importance of the unique and idiosyncratic needs, interests, and desires of the individual family members. Emphasis on the individual is one of the great potential strengths of the smaller nuclear family.

## The Polygamous Family

The *polygamous family* is a grouping of nuclear families bound by an extension of the husband-wife bond. The polygamous family is united through the presence of a common spouse. Thus, its tie is essentially conjugal rather than consanguineal.

As discussed in the preceding chapter, there are various forms of polygamy, with polygyny by far the most common. A colorful and entertaining example of polygynous family was evident in the excellent autobiographical book and film *Anna and the King of Siam,* which became the hit musical *The King and I.* There, the interplay of marital and kinship ties is beautifully illustrated, although the fact that the husband is a king introduces another element of complexity as well as of drama.

The larger number of members in a polygamous family, compared with a nuclear family, give it a strength and functional advantage similar to that mentioned in connection with the extended family. On the other hand, it is more nearly similar to the nuclear than to the extended family since it lacks the latter's continuity over generations. Just as the nuclear family tends to disintegrate with the loss of the parent members, so does the polygamous family evaporate with the loss of its common member.

## The Social Structure of Kinship

*Kinship* is perhaps the single most important principle of social organization in every known society and integral to our understanding of family form and organization. Kinship can be defined as ''a structured system of relationships, in which individuals are bound to one another by complex interlocking and ramifying ties'' (Murdock 1949, p. 92). Kinship is a social arrangement that delineates individuals' socially recognized relationships to each other. When I say Pete is my brother, Jack my stepbrother, Pauline my second cousin and Mr. Pearl my father-in-law—all of these reflect kinship designations, some consanguineal and some not.

There doesn't seem to be a society without a kinship system that plays an important role in its organization. But the most important thing to be understood about kinship is that, peculiar as it may seem, it is a social and not a biological concept. Brothers are brothers, sisters are sisters, and cousins are cousins—not to mention aunts, uncles, and in-laws—not because of biological reasons but because of social determinants! In fact, kinship serves to interpret blood relationships in a way that places them within the social context of the particular society.

The ties of person to person, their mutual rights and obligations, their inheritance, their place in the stratification system of society all require specification and social definition. No society leaves such fundamental is-

Figure 2.1
**Unilineal and Nonunilineal Descent Rules**

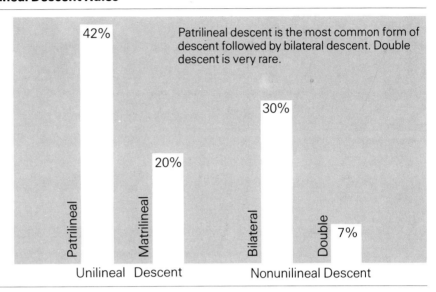

Source: Adapted from Murdock (1949).

sues to chance or to biology. The kinship system provides a major share of these necessary social definitions throughout life and, many societies believe, in the afterlife as well.

Kinship is extremely important in the organization of all societies. There are rules of lineage or descent, which define the link between successive generations, as well as rules of residence, defining the geographical distribution, and rules defining the structure of authority within the family. Together, these factors will help us understand the organization of the family unit more clearly.

## Rules of Descent

A social concept

As we said, kinship is more a social than a biological creation. It is the way in which a society establishes a network of reciprocal rights and obligations among its members. The variation among societies in how one traces descent and hence lineage testifies to its social character. There are two essential ways in which descent is reckoned: by unilineal or by nonunilineal descent rules (see figure 2.1).

Unilineal Descent   In *unilineal descent,* lineage is traced through only one specific descent line, the mother's or father's. These are more straightforward and less complex than nonunilineal descent systems. Stephens (1963) points out that unilineal kin groups, because they trace their heritage through a single line, tend to be more easily definable and have certain common attributes.

Table 2.1

**Most Common Surnames in the United States**

| Rank | Surname | Estimated no. of persons | Rank | Surname | Estimated no. of persons |
|---|---|---|---|---|---|
| 1 | Smith | 2,238,400 | 26 | Nelson | 401,400 |
| 2 | Johnson | 1,684,300 | 27 | Wright | 401,000 |
| 3 | Williams | 1,348,000 | 28 | Baker | 388,000 |
| 4 | Brown | 1,268,400 | 29 | Hill | 386,200 |
| 5 | Jones | 1,230,500 | 30 | Scott | 378,800 |
| 6 | Miller | 1,076,100 | 31 | Adams | 378,700 |
| 7 | Davis | 972,500 | 32 | Green | 375,800 |
| 8 | Wilson | 737,300 | 33 | Lee | 361,300 |
| 9 | Anderson | 712,500 | 34 | Roberts | 350,300 |
| 10 | Taylor | 648,400 | 35 | Mitchell | 345,300 |
| 11 | Moore | 646,900 | 36 | Campbell | 339,000 |
| 12 | Thomas | 632,800 | 37 | Phillips | 337,400 |
| 13 | Martin | 603,400 | 38 | Carter | 322,500 |
| 14 | Thompson | 594,500 | 39 | Evans | 316,100 |
| 15 | White | 592,200 | 40 | Turner | 305,800 |
| 16 | Harris | 587,800 | 41 | Collins | 301,700 |
| 17 | Jackson | 576,500 | 42 | Parker | 299,800 |
| 18 | Clark | 513,600 | 43 | Murphy | 297,900 |
| 19 | Lewis | 457,900 | 44 | Rodriguez | 292,600 |
| 20 | Walker | 450,900 | 45 | Edwards | 289,900 |
| 21 | Hall | 437,600 | 46 | Morris | 285,530 |
| 22 | Robinson | 429,000 | 47 | Peterson | 282,300 |
| 23 | Allen | 426,700 | 48 | Cook | 279,800 |
| 24 | Young | 423,800 | 49 | Rogers | 278,400 |
| 25 | King | 404,900 | 50 | Stewart | 273,100 |

Source: Elsdon C. Smith, *American Surnames.* Philadelphia: Chilton Book Company, 1964.

Family names

In most cases, they have a special name, a label for the line, that symbolizes the kin group and keeps its presence and importance ''on stage'': that is, before its members and the rest of society. ''We are the Smiths, and don't you forget it!'' Frequently the name is taken from some phenomenon of nature, such as animals, plants, or cosmic elements, or from an occupation; but they may also be corruptions of other words. The

Table 2.1

**Most Common Surnames in the United States**

| Rank | Surname | Estimated no. of persons | Rank | Surname | Estimated no. of persons |
|---|---|---|---|---|---|
| 51 | Morgan | 254,800 | 76 | Foster | 206,400 |
| 52 | Cooper | 251,100 | 77 | Henderson | 203,900 |
| 53 | Reed | 249,200 | 78 | Sanders | 198,300 |
| 54 | Bell | 248,400 | 79 | Powell | 197,700 |
| 55 | Kelly | 246,400 | 80 | Perry | 196,900 |
| 56 | Wood | 245,600 | 81 | Butler | 196,200 |
| 57 | Bailey | 245,300 | 82 | James | 192,400 |
| 58 | Garcia | 242,000 | 83 | Jenkins | 192,100 |
| 59 | Ward | 241,300 | 84 | Barnes | 191,600 |
| 60 | Cox | 239,300 | 85 | Gonzalez | 189,600 |
| 61 | Griffin | 231,300 | 86 | Reynolds | 187,100 |
| 62 | Howard | 229,400 | 87 | Patterson | 185,400 |
| 63 | Bennett | 228,500 | 88 | Wallace | 181,600 |
| 64 | Brooks | 224,900 | 89 | Graham | 181,500 |
| 65 | Watson | 224,100 | 90 | Simmons | 180,200 |
| 66 | Gray | 223,500 | 91 | Coleman | 179,900 |
| 67 | Sullivan | 222,100 | 92 | Hamilton | 179,400 |
| 68 | Hughes | 218,100 | 93 | Lopez | 178,500 |
| 69 | Myers | 217,700 | 94 | Rivera | 176,500 |
| 70 | Ross | 217,300 | 95 | Murray | 175,500 |
| 71 | Long | 216,400 | 96 | Cole | 174,100 |
| 72 | Price | 211,000 | 97 | McDonald | 173,900 |
| 73 | Russell | 207,800 | 98 | Alexander | 172,900 |
| 74 | Richardson | 207,300 | 99 | West | 172,700 |
| 75 | Fisher | 207,000 | 100 | Hayes | 172,500 |

Source: Elsdon C. Smith, *American Surnames*. Philadelphia: Chilton Book Company, 1964.

names of the authors of this book are linguistic corruptions: squirrel in Russian (Belkin) and a good person in German (Goodman). Table 2.1 lists the 100 most common family names in the United States.

Unilineal kin groups tend to marry outside the immediate group (see chapter 6 for a discussion of exogamy). You know which members of your close and distant family you may or may not marry. Unilineal kin groups often have a common set of religious obligations and sometimes their own religion. They may also own property together. This ownership may be outright, or the residual rights to property held by individual members of the kin group may become the groups'. Perhaps more important, there are generally reciprocal rights and obligations of mutual aid and hospitality among members of the unilineal kin group that are not required of other members of society. We expect different things from our own kin than we do from others. Finally, the unilineal kin group may set up its own economic enterprise and government. In short, as a defined group in society, the unilineal kin group may and often does engage in activities that take advantage of this common identity and serve to bind them even more closely to each other.

Unilineal descent may be patrilineal or matrilineal, as shown in figure 2.2. In the case of *patrilineal,* descent is traced exclusively through the male line. At birth, each person is assigned a place in the kinship group of his or her father as reckoned through all the men in that line. Predominance is given to the ties from son to father to grandfather to great grandfather, and so on. Relationships with the mother's family in tracing lineage and probably in determining inheritance are essentially ignored in patrilineal descent.

**Patrilineal descent**

There is, of course, a recognition of the priority of claims for social obligations of the mother and her kin over strangers. Generally, patrilineal societies are not ignorant of the biological contributions of the mother and her kin to the child. However, they assert that kinship is a social relationship that is not strictly limited to biological inheritance in the defining of social structure, although it generally takes this inheritance into account.

In Murdock's sample (1949), those having a patrilineal descent system far outnumber all others. Specifically, 105 (42 percent) report such a tracing of lineage.

**Matrilineal descent**

The other type of unilineal descent system is called *matrilineal descent.* Matrilineal descent is traced through the mother and all the women in the lineage. However, the matrilineal system is not simply the mirror image of the patrilineal system. Actually, it is a more complex system permitting a wider array of residential possibilities for the new family and having different implications for paternity. For example, according to Jewish law, a Jew must be born from a Jewish mother; the religion of the father is extraneous.

Figure 2.2
**Bilateral Descent Family Tree***

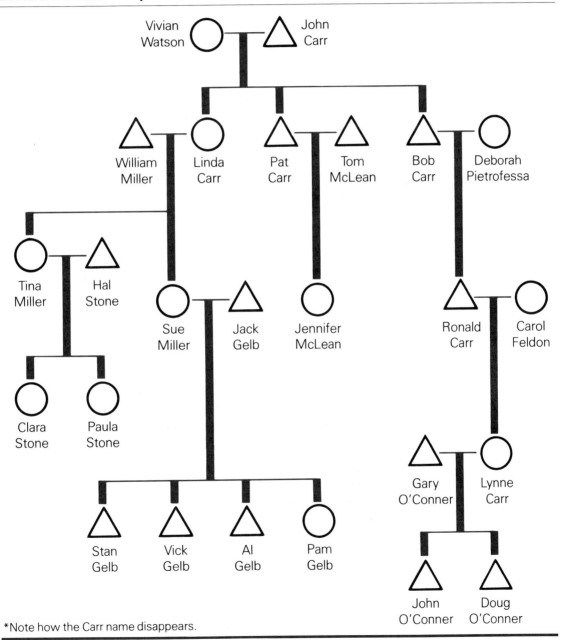

*Note how the Carr name disappears.

Matrilineal descent systems are much less frequent than patrilineal systems. In Murdock's sample (1949), only 20 percent of the societies report such lineage determination, a little less than half the number of societies having a patrilineage.

## Nonunilineal Descent
As the name implies, *nonunilineal descent* systems trace descent through more than one line, with each of the lines generally accorded equal kinship claims. Clearly, these systems are more complex than those just discussed. Since lineage is traced through more than one line, it is quite difficult, if not impossible, to constitute any recognizably continuous kin group with the collective attributes mentioned for unilineal kin groups. In fact, no two persons, other than siblings, belong to the same consanguineal kin group.

All relatives on each side

*Bilateral descent* is the second most common form of descent system found in Murdock's sample (1949). Seventy-five societies (30 percent) were reported to have bilateral descent. This particular mode of tracing kin is used in the United States and throughout most of the Western world. Here, lineage is traced equally through *both* the mother's and father's lines, in accordance with the laws of biology. Also, all relatives on each side (both men and women on the father's side and men and women on the mother's side) are counted. Thus, this system is not a simple combination of patrilineal and matrilineal descent.

The concept of close relatives

Strictly speaking, the number of kin reckoned in this way is quite large, almost beyond comprehension and certainly beyond mutual obligations. Consequently, the size of the functional kin group in bilateral descent systems is often reduced by restricting it to close relatives who are frequently but not always defined by those who are second cousins or closer. The definition of who is a close relative plays an important part in marriage and inheritance.

A relatively rare way of tracing descent is *double descent* which occurs in only 17 (7 percent) of Murdock's sample (1949). However, it is worth mentioning because it is illustrative of the possible complexities of kinship determination.

Double descent is actually a straight linear combination of patrilineal and matrilineal rules of descent. At birth, a child is assigned a place in *both* the father's patrilineal kin group and in the mother's matrilineal kin group. The father's maternal line and the mother's paternal line are excluded from the child's kinship determination. Thus, the child belongs to two different kin groups, with two different sets of rights and responsibilities.

And this is not even the most complex arrangement of kinship reckoning known! Murdock (1949) reports that among "the Buginese and Macassar of Celebes, the first, third, and odd-numbered offspring are affiliated with the mother, and even-numbered progeny with their father" (p. 45).

There are other societies that vary kinship for the sex of the child and the generation of birth. Clearly, there is more than biology involved in kinship. In fact, the determination of lineage is critical because it is often connected to the rules of how close a relative one might marry and the inheritance of property. In fact, the complexities of kinship determination often reveal structural elements of importance within the overall society.

## Rules of Residence

Related to the rules of descent and paralleling them in many respects are the rules of residence. There are wide and dramatic differences across the world in the rules that govern the establishing of residency by newly married couples. In fact, the familiar style in America, where the newlyweds set up their own home, is in a distinct minority worldwide. We shall briefly describe the different residence rules and then compare them with the rules of descent. We will also note, where applicable, how these rules affect the equality or inequality of the sexes.

### Patrilocal Residence
*Patrilocal residence* is by far the most common practice around the world (see figure 2.3). After marriage, the new couple live in the same dwelling or a dwelling adjacent to that of the husband's family. The woman packs her belongings, says goodbye to her family, and moves in with her husband's kin. Clearly, the result is that the woman is removed from her family's environment and any influence they may have on her is thereby weakened. In contrast, the authority of the groom's family is substantially increased. The frequency of this practice, 146 (58 percent) of Murdock's societies surveyed, exemplifies how much more power men have than women in societies around the world.

Matri-patrilocal residence

There is a slight variant of this form called the *matri-patrilocal residence*. In this practice, the newly married couple goes to stay initially with the wife's family for a specified period of time, usually about a year or until the first child is born, and then takes up permanent residence with the groom's family.

Quite possibly this variant is useful in allowing the woman's family (and particularly her mother) to help her plan for and deliver the first child, after which she and the rest of her nuclear family of procreation permanently come under the influence of her husband's family. This form was found in 22 cases (9 percent) of Murdock's sample (1949).

Figure 2.3
**Rules of Residence**

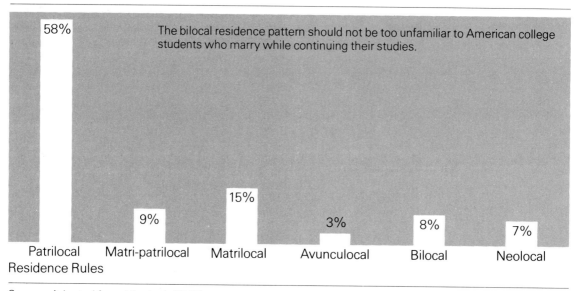

Source: Adapted from Murdock (1949).

Matrilocal Residence *Matrilocal residence* is the second most
frequently occurring rule of residence, reported in 38 (15 percent) of
Murdock's sample (1949), although it occurs considerably less frequently
than patrilocal residence. As the name implies, this rule specifies that
upon marriage the new couple take up residence with the wife's family.
There is a common variant of this rule called *avunculocal residence,*
where the new couple takes up residence with the maternal uncle of the
groom. It is grouped here with matrilocal residence since in both cases
residence in some way involves women and not solely men. This variant
occurs only in 8 (3 percent) of Murdock's sample.

Avunculocal residence

Bilocal Residence   This rule permits the couple to decide whether
they will live with the bride's family or with the groom's family. The
choice is put in the hands of the new couple, but it is restricted to one or
another of their family's residence. This pattern is found in 19 (8 percent)
of Murdock's sample (1949).
    This residence pattern should not seem too unfamiliar to college stu-
dents. Not infrequently, young married college students find that, at least

Living with either family

temporarily, they need to live with one or another set of parents. The choice of which set involves interpersonal relationships. Of equal importance, however, are the relative resources of the two sets of parents. Consideration must and is given to who has the most room and who can give the most help financially in this difficult economic period of many marriages. It is no different in the societies studied by Murdock. The same general factors were found to be influential in determining where the new couple would live.

## Neolocal Residence

*Neolocal residence* is the pattern familiar to most people in the United States. It means that the newly married couple chooses its own residence and sets up a new household. But the establishment of a new, independent household is in fact the least frequent form of residence rule across the world. Only 17 societies (7 percent) of Murdock's sample of 250 had such a residence rule (1949).

Kinship vs. marital ties

These figures are not surprising, given the view we have found all along about the relatively greater importance of kinship over marital ties in most societies around the world. Geographical proximity—and what is closer than being in the same dwelling?—is one effective way of maintaining influence, if not direct control, over the newly married couple. Permitting neolocal residence would strengthen the independence of this new nuclear family and give priority to marital over kinship bonds. Once more we see that one of our most cherished and expected practices is, from a worldwide perspective, distinctly a variant form.

## The Relationship between Rules of Descent and Rules of Residence

Since kinship ties are important in a society's social structure, we should expect to find some relationship between its rules of descent and residence. However, it should be pointed out that this relationship is likely to be complicated by another widespread tendency that we have discussed before, namely, the general granting of higher status and authority to men as compared with women.

In Murdock's sample (1949), 92 percent of the societies with a patrilineal descent system have either patrilocal or matri-patrilocal residence rules: the remaining 8 percent have either a bilocal or neolocal rule. Of those societies with a matrilineal system, 63 percent have a matrilocal or avunculocal residence rule, 29 percent a patrilocal or (matri-patrilocal) rule, and 8 percent a bilocal or neolocal rule. All but one of the societies with a double descent system have a patrilocal or matri-patrilocal resi-

dence rule, and that single case has a bilocal or neolocal rule. Of the societies with a bilateral descent rule, 31 percent also have either a bilocal
or neolocal residence rule, 52 percent have a patrilocal or matri-patrilocal
rule, and 17 percent have a matrilocal or avunculocal residence rule. In
short, 67 percent of all the societies have a patrilocal or matri-patrilocal
residence rule and 42 percent have a patrilineal descent system.

The above data make clear the positive relationship between rules of
descent and rules of residence. Moreover, when there are deviations from
this expected positive relationship, they are mostly in the direction of as-
signing greater weight to the man's family.

**Unequal distribution of status**

In short, this is another bit of evidence showing the unequal distribution of status and importance between men and women in societies
around the world. This evidence does not mean, and should not be interpreted to mean, that these differences are the "natural order of things,"
but it should not be overlooked by those interested in increasing the
equality between men and women.

## Rules of Authority

What constitutes authority in the family is not as clear-cut as it may seem.
Here we mean authority as a socially legitimate power and not as brute
force. Obviously a person who gives orders and expects to have them carried out may be said to have power. But many times these expectations
are so woven into the fabric of social life that orders need not be given. A
mild suggestion or a small request may be enough to accomplish a particular task. Or the orders might be anticipated and, therefore, never have
to be voiced.

Stephens (1963) has taken into account a variety of indicators of
power and authority, namely the according of privilege, the use of a
double standard especially in evaluating behavior, and the showing of
deference, or respect. We will use his data to examine the frequency of
occurrence of the different patterns of authority in the family.

### Patriarchy

**Family authority with the husband-father**

*Patriarchy* is by far the most frequently occurring pattern. Though this
type of finding has been suggested anecdotally for a long time,
Stephens's (1963) data allows us to characterize 66 percent of his ethnographic sample as exhibiting a patriarchal form of family authority with
the husband-father wielding mild to substantial control. In these societies, the husband-father is accorded the best resources and privileges

in the family and in society at large. These data appear to be in accord with a good deal of literature and descriptive reports that extend back to biblical times.

## Matriarchy

There exist exceedingly few *matriarchies:* societies where women are invested with power and authority over men. While there have been many fables and legends about them, such as the famous Amazon women, there seems to be little factual evidence of their existence as other than an extremely rare phenomenon.

*A rare phenomenon*

In Stephens's (1963) sample, they are present in only seven percent of the cases. And even in societies, such as matrilineal ones, that on the surface seem to accord higher status to women, power and authority is often vested in the male members of the female line, as in the maternal uncle in avunculocal residence rules. In most societies, "women's work" is generally less valued than is "men's work," women hold few positions of authority either in the family or in other parts of society, and they must give deference to their husband rather than receive it from him.

## Equalitarian Relationship

An *equalitarian relationship,* in which there is a relatively equal distribution of authority in the family between husband and wife, occurs more frequently than does a matriarchal family pattern. In Stephens's sample, 12 percent of the cases exhibited a general equalitarian pattern, and another 15 percent had the responsibilities and hence the authority divided into different spheres for husbands and wives. Thus, it seems that with but a few minor exceptions, men only occasionally share their power and authority with women.

*Authority divided between husbands and wives*

## The Nuclear Family: First among Equals?

In the discussions above, you may have noted the frequent reference, either explicitly or implicitly, to the nuclear family. It is the primary family form with all others being composites of it. It is also central to the discussion of residence rules, descent, authority, and mating. Thus, the nuclear family plays a central role in all discussions of kinship and the social institution we call the family.

Some have suggested that the nuclear family is one of the very few universal social facts. In this section we will delve into the basis of the claim and the evidence for the belief in the centrality and universality of the nuclear family. We will also look at its internal social structure, specifically the differentiation of the adult family roles.

## Is the Nuclear Family Universal?

Murdock's studies

All contemporary discussion of the universality of the nuclear family must start with George Peter Murdock. It has been Murdock's prodigious and encyclopedic efforts in this matter that have set the tone and direction of the debate on this question for the past several decades. It is for this reason that we cite his work so frequently in this chapter.

Murdock (1949, pp. 2–3) argues that the nuclear family "is a universal social grouping." He goes on to point out,

Either as the sole prevailing form of the family or as the basic unit from which more complex familial forms are compounded it exists as a distinct and strongly functional group in every known society. No exception, at least, has come to light in the 250 representative cultures surveyed for the present study.

But why should the nuclear family be universal? What is it about the nuclear family that gives it the resiliency to maintain itself despite the widely diverse social and cultural structures in which it is embedded?

Murdock (1949, p. 10) argues that the nuclear family is universal because it is a very special type of social group whose common residence provides the context for its efficient fulfillment of four fundamental societal needs. In his own words,

In the nuclear family or its constituent elements we thus see assembled four functions fundamental to human social life—the sexual, the economic, the reproductive, and the educational. Without provision for the first and third, society would become extinct; for the second, life itself would cease; for the fourth, culture would come to an end. The immense social utility of the nuclear family and the basic reason for its universality thus begin to emerge in strong relief.

Intimacy and sexual needs

A more contemporary rendering of these four important functions might label them slightly differently. What Murdock calls the "sexual" function is not in fact limited to (though it certainly does include) sexual intercourse. The main issue here is the higher degree of permissible "intimacy" with one another accorded to the marital couple that distinguishes them from others. They are permitted to and expected to be-

*Perhaps the nuclear family is universal because it is a special type of social group which fulfills fundamental needs.*

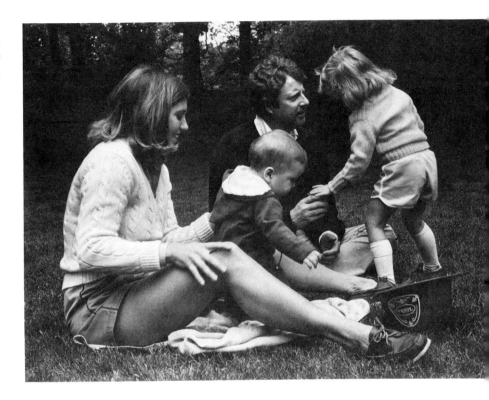

have and feel differently toward one another than they do toward others, outside the dyad. Weitman (1970) also points out that part of the development of intimacy between two people comes about by excluding others from the dyad. This intimacy, which in our culture we sometimes call love or loyalty, is socially acknowledged. For example, the law that a wife or husband cannot be made to testify against her or his spouse reflects this. In fact, the greater degree of permissible intimacy applies to all nuclear family members, children as well as adults, although the sexual facet is limited to the adults. We certainly accept as natural a parent kissing and touching his or her own child more than we would a stranger doing the same thing.

Economic needs

A contemporary view of the economic function might well include its larger context of a division of labor rather than solely the production and distribution of goods and services. The members of the nuclear family divide the necessary domestic tasks. This system is clearly more efficient than requiring each individual member of the family, including dependent and immature children, to meet his or her own needs separately, a clearly difficult and redundant procedure. The specialization of functions within groups and organizations has long been recognized for its efficiency and effectiveness, and the nuclear family is no exception (Durkheim 1893, Weber 1922).

The reproductive function needs no contemporary redefinition; it has had the same meaning from the dawn of time. However, the function of education is viewed today in its more sociological meaning of *socialization,* that process of transforming the biological organism into a functioning member of a particular society. The narrower definition in the sense of formal schooling is really only a small part of socialization.

Social reproduction

Socialization, as we view it, is the process of *social reproduction* and is as important for societal survival and continuity as is biological reproduction. Although socialization is carried out through a number of societal agencies, it is the nuclear family that provides the first, most potent, and most continuing socialization experiences for most people.

In sum, then, Murdock argues that the efficiency of the nuclear family as a common residential social group in carrying out four critical societal functions—sexual (intimacy), economic (division of necessary labor), reproductive, and educational (socialization)—has led to its evolution as a ''universal human social grouping.''

It should also be mentioned that Murdock believes that in many societies the nuclear family carries out additional functions as well. As a relatively stable social group, it often serves as the place for religious practices, recreation, security, and the care of the aged, sick, and infirm. However, it does not seem to perform these functions universally. There have been arguments raised against the presumed universality and permanence of the nuclear family, and it is to these that we now turn our attention.

## The Debate

Murdock's views, in short, have not been treated as revealed truth. There has been considerable debate and ferment in both the professional and lay media over the precise status of the nuclear family in the past, the present, and especially in the future. Stripped of its ideological content, much of the present-day argument against the universality of the nuclear family ultimately centers on whether it is the only, or even the most efficient, way in which a society can meet the four important functions discussed above. The question then is, How universal is the nuclear family?

Arguments against
Murdock's theory

Consistently, the argument against the universality of the nuclear family rests on two specific cases: the Nayar of India and the Israeli kibbutz. Occasional use is also made of the common-law practices on the islands of Jamaica, Mut'a marriage in parts of the Moslem countries in the Middle East and the Mokhthoditi marriages of the Toda of India. How-

*Division of domestic tasks among family members represents the economic function served by the nuclear family.*

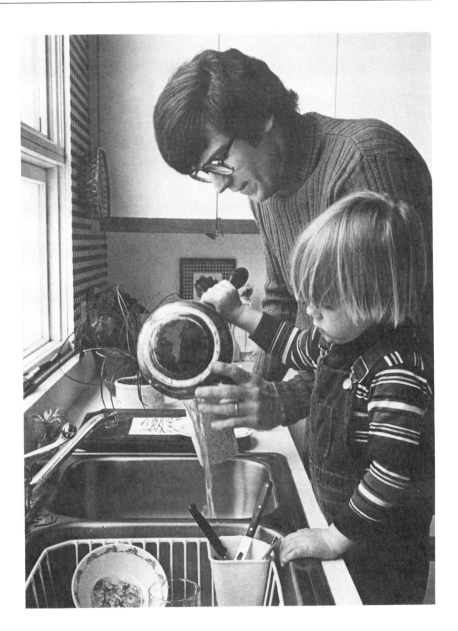

ever, each of these cases is a variant form practiced by a minority of members in a society that exhibits the nuclear family as its standard form.

The strongest case against Murdock's sweeping generalization is presumed to be the Nayar, a Hindu warrior subcaste living in the south of India (Gough 1959). The argument is that there are no nuclear families in

*Although socialization is carried out by many societal agents, the nuclear family provides the first and most continuing socialization for most people.*

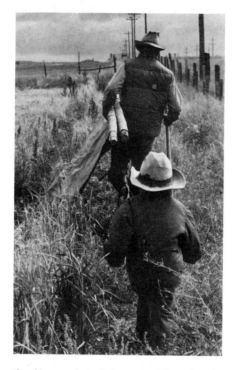

The Nayar

Ritual marriage

the Nayar since it is a matrilineal society in which a man lives in the house of his matrilineal kin. Sexual unions take place between a woman and her choice of a ''passing visitor'' or a ''visiting husband.'' The man arrives after supper and must leave before breakfast. Paternity is socially determined; one of the men publicly announces that he is the father and is required to do nothing else than to provide a small gift to the midwife. ''Visiting husbands'' present small gifts to the woman at the three main festivals a year.

The only wife-husband relation among the Nayar, as Murdock would define it, is the product of a ritual marriage at puberty, at which time the two young people stay together for a few days. After that, they separate and have no other special rights or obligations toward one another. However, the woman and all her children, no matter who the father, must perform a purification rite at the death of the ritual husband. Still, the ritual husband has no greater claim to sexual access than any other man. He does not live with his ritual wife other than the few days at puberty, necessarily call any of her children his own, play a required role in the socialization of the children, nor share any form of economic cooperation with her. In short, this case meets none of Murdock's requirements for a nuclear family: yet it exists as a viable system.

The second major example used to argue against the universality of the nuclear family is the Israeli kibbutz. Though it is clear that kibbutzim (plural for kibbutz) differ, most of the analysis is based on the work of Melford Spiro (1968) with one specific kibbutz, called *Kiryat Yedidim* in fiction. On the kibbutz, there is no formal marriage ceremony. A couple wishing to get married simply apply to the community's housing committee for a common room. They do not cooperate with each other economically, because finances are handled by the kibbutz as a whole. While the sexual and reproductive functions are localized in the married couple, their children live in a separate children's residence, not in the parents' room, and are taken care of and socialized by health and education specialists, hired and maintained by the kibbutz as a whole. In Murdock's terms, there is no common family residence and the nuclear family, such as it is on the kibbutz, does not cooperate economically for the needs of its members nor carry out the socialization of its children. Thus it does not appear to fall within Murdock's definition of the nuclear family.

## Toward a Resolution

Most informed opinion today tends to support the Murdock position on the nuclear family. One of the most important arguments for this view is that the two major cases against Murdock's thesis are both based on fragments of a society and not on really independent social groups. In essence, they are minority arrangements that are tolerated by the larger society, much as any society tolerates a variety of different social structures within its midst as long as they don't threaten the society as a whole. Moreover, in the case of the Nayar, the practices we described have been in the process of change for some time (Mencher 1965). And the residents of all the kibbutzim in Israel comprise only about 3.5 percent of the total population of the country.

Additional arguments can and have been made, even by Spiro himself, that the kibbutz case is not as strong as it looks at first. For example, despite the fact that children live in dormitories, when asked where their home is they tend to answer that it is their parents' room. Part of the reason for this answer is that they spend a considerable amount of time there with the parents, during which a good deal of socialization certainly takes place.

Also, although social cooperation in matters of health and education takes place at the level of the kibbutz and not at the nuclear family level, the ultimate responsibility for health care and education of children in the nuclear family rests with the parents. The parents play a part in the work assignments and distribution of the results of these economically cooperative activities and ultimately have the power to withdraw their participation completely if they do not like how things are being done. The same is even truer with respect to their children's socialization. The parents help hire the educational and health specialists and set the guiding philosophy for them. And, the parents retain the ultimate right to withdraw their children if they are not satisfied with the progress and care. Hence, the final responsibility for the socialization of the children and the necessary economic cooperation for the good of the nuclear family is in the hands of that family.

In closing this section, perhaps the best summary is from Stephens (1963, p. 29) who, after reviewing the published evidence on this matter and interviewing ethnographers from 53 social systems, concludes:

> Compared with this handful of borderline cases and possible exceptions, there are hundreds of societies that apparently *aren't* exceptions. Consider the fact that G. P. Murdock, with his encyclopedic knowledge of ethnographic literature, *could* conclude that the family *is* universal. Even if he was overly bold in coming to this conclusion, he never would have reached it if the societies that seem to have the family were not legion, and the societies that appear not to have the family were not few and inconspicuous. . . .
>
> I think we can tentatively conclude that, although the family may not be universal to all known societies, it is almost universal [italics in original].

## The Taboo Against Incest

*Incest,* which can be defined as socially prohibited sexual activity or marriage between two members of the same family or kinship group, has

A universal taboo

been banned in virtually every known society with a few exceptions. Murdock, in his classic study of 250 societies, found a universal taboo against incest in the nuclear family, with various incest rules changing from society to society outside the nuclear family (Murdock 1949). Many explanations for the universality of the incest taboo have been put forward, ranging from a biological to a psychological to the sociological position. We will see that, in fact, these merge.

The biological position

The biologically oriented explanation approaches the entire issue of kinship from a genetic perspective. It says that because incest is genetically dangerous and harmful to species survival it has not been able to prosper among societies. Many undesirable phenomena, such as retardation, birth deformities, and sickle-cell anemia, are carried as harmless recessive genes that only become apparent when an individual mates with another recessive carrier. Since people that are closely related biologically are much more likely to have the same recessive genes, inbreeding tends to produce a much higher incidence of these undesirable and dangerous qualities. Thus, the biological position is that incest has been banned as a natural means of protection.

The psychological position

The psychodynamic position, put forth by Sigmund Freud and his followers, argues that incest is a natural, strong desire in all people. It is even considered as innate, in the sense that the very young child wants to "consume" the parent. The parents, in turn, have incestuous desires toward their children. But the family members, in order to maintain intactness, either sublimate their incestuous feelings into nonsexual, loving relationships as we see in what we call parental love and filial love, or develop a "reaction formation," in which some type of psychological symptom is produced. An example of the latter would be the mother who will not allow her son to date girls for fear that he will be corrupted by them.

The sociological position

The sociological position is far broader than either the biological or psychological position and actually combines elements of both. Most social theories "explaining the widespread occurrence of exogamy—that is, taboo on marriage to certain kin—and the incest taboo, which forbids sexual relations between specified kin, state that these social rules were adapted due to the selective advantage they gave to those groups which observed them" (Schwartzman 1974, p. 171). This eclectic viewpoint relates the biological reality of inbreeding to the social rules. But sociologists have gone even further in fusing the psychological reality with the biological and social. They offer an explanation for the taboo that takes both into account.

The functional position

Talcott Parsons (1954), specifically, in explaining the prohibition in terms of his role theory argues that the taboo against nuclear incest is functional for the family and for society. He sees erotic drives as potentially disruptive forces within the nuclear family, forces that have to be controlled. The taboo serves this function.

In some cases not only the taboo but incest itself may be functional. According to Bagley (1969), functional incest can occur and has occurred under certain conditions. "There is evidence that individuals of normal intelligence and without mental pathology can contemplate and initiate incest when it seems to be a functional necessity for family survival" (p. 514). He cites several instances in which incest has served a productive purpose, either socially, economically, or in terms of holding the family together. In most instances, "the individuals who achieve this successfully appear to be dominant fathers whose life experience has been such that they are left with a relative detachment from the remaining social institutions of society" (p. 514).

For example, in Swedish prewar agricultural society father-daughter incest was not wholly uncommon. "In isolated farms," Bagley explains, "not part of any wider social system of communities, it appeared that the father would reassign the role of 'wife' to his daughter, when his own wife was incapable of filling that role." Bagley goes on (1969, p. 509) to interpret this:

> These isolated farms seemed to form communities or "societies" in themselves; they possessed Parsons's prerequisite of a society—long-term stability from within its own resources. The father's economic misfortune may well have accentuated the feeling of remoteness felt by the family from the wider community. In many of these cases, then, incest seemed to be morally sanctioned by the family, a micro-society.

Nonfunctional incest

Nonfunctional incest, "accidental" or "disorganized" incest, the kind we ordinarily think about when we hear the term, "occurs in communities which are in a state of social disorganization and which are highly overcrowded, two states which often coincide" (Bagley 1969, p. 512). This type is especially likely to occur at times of war, enemy invasion, or social catastrophe. In *pathological incest,* the type we are probably most familiar with, "one or both participants are mentally defective or psychotic. The mentally defective are 'extrasocietal' in the sense that they have been unable to internalize the moral rules prohibiting incest" (p. 513). Bagley's two final categories are incest through *object fixation* and *psychopathic* incest. Object fixation refers to an unhealthy sexual/emotional attachment to someone from the past, such as being overly attached to one's parent or sibling. Psychopathic incest is practiced by a person who lacks all feelings of guilt, conscience, and a sense of social propriety. Both result from severe psychological disturbances, where either one or both of the participants in the incest have not developed the social skills and emotional maturity that enable them to function outside the family. These types of incest have been investigated thoroughly by clinical psychologists, social workers, and psychiatrists (since victims often end up in the courts, hospitals, or clinics) and it is generally agreed that frequently there is a history of parental alcoholism, familial emotional disturbance, and incomplete socialization of the child-victim (Browning and Boatman 1977).

Pathological incest

Evaluation   How adequate are the explanations of the origin and universal application of the incest taboo? Do they explain why the incest taboo exists in every single society on record despite the great diversity of cultures and social structures particularly in relationship to the family?

And why does the taboo exist despite the lack of uniformity of who is included in the incest taboo beyond the members of the nuclear family?

Some of the explanations are patently wrong: it is difficult to believe, for example, that our ancient forbears possessed or even that many isolated contemporary societies possess the technical genetic knowledge that would make the biological position a possible explanation. Also, while ardent psychoanalysts might be able to make a case among themselves for their explanation of the incest taboo in modern Western society, it can hardly account for the vast numbers of other quite different societies around the world, as Malinowski (1927) demonstrated over half a century ago.

No single explanation

More than likely, there is no single explanation for the origin and universal application of the incest taboo. In fact, it is commonplace sociology to understand that the maintenance of a social practice may have an entirely different basis than its initiation.

Perhaps Murdock (1949, pp. 292–300) offers the best eclectic explanation. He believes that the sexually experienced members of the family (parents and older siblings), knowing the consequences of unregulated sexual behavior, discourage any such incipient actions on the part of the immature child early in life. Also, cultural norms stress the importance of mutually cooperative and supportive relationships in the family. These would be rent asunder by the pressure of sexual rivalry, with a resulting catastrophic confusion of family roles and authority.

Stimulus generation

Finally, Murdock attempted to explain the extension of the incest taboo beyond the members of the nuclear family in terms of the phenomenon of *stimulus generalization.* Those persons who are classified together in kinship terms with members of the nuclear family—for example, one's mother and her sister are likely to be included in the incest taboo. While this view attempts to synthesize explanations from anthropology, sociology, and behavioral psychology and is a decided improvement over the earlier attempts to explain the incest taboo on the basis of a single factor, it still cannot adequately explain the fundamental initiating cause. It is better utilized as an explanation of the historical and cross-cultural universality of the taboo.

## Victoria and David

A brother and sister, who had not seen each other for 20 years, have gotten married.

Now they have been arrested on incest charges by Massachusetts authorities—and face up to 20 years in prison.

Victoria Marie Pittorino, 23, found her brother, David

Goddu, 22, by painstakingly going through birth certificate records in Lawrence, Massachusetts.

They had both been given up for adoption as babies.

The two recently confronted their natural mother, who said she was "horrified" to learn of their marriage last month.

"They know they are brother and sister," she told the *Lawrence Eagle Tribune.* "But I guess they think they're in love and I know they don't think this is wrong."

The mother, whose name was withheld by the paper, said she thought Victoria married David "because she didn't want to let go of her brother and thought she could hold on to him this way.

"I don't think she knew marrying her brother was against the law. Neither did he."

The mother told the Lawrence newspaper she had been assured when she gave up her children for adoption that "no way" would they ever find her or would she ever find them again.

"If I had known this would happen, I would never have put them up for adoption," she said.

"I wish they had never found me," she added.

According to the paper, Victoria looked up her mother's name in the city hall records.

Then she sought out her brother.

The paper reported that the Lawrence birth records were easily obtainable—and clearly state the names of the natural and adoptive parents.

"They came here together the Saturday before Easter," the mother said.

"We talked all day."

Later they stayed in her home for a week.

"They came crying to me and said the other mothers had kicked them out. I think the other mothers began to suspect something was going on."

She told the paper she thought the two were now staying with David's adoptive parents.

But the Goddus denied the young couple was at their Holyoke home.

"We knew nothing of it [the marriage]," said Eileen Goddu. "We are just tired and fraught with anxiety."

Her husband, James, said Victoria had come to visit the family "a few months ago to find out where David lived.

"But we never would have approved of it [the marriage]," he said. "They aren't staying with us."

Victoria and David were released on their own recognizance pending a July 25 court date.

The natural mother said she gave her son and daughter up for adoption after her marriage broke down. Victoria was three years old, she said, and David was 18 months.

The mother said she was in the process of moving out of her home.

"I'm very glad I'm moving," she said. "And I'm not going to tell Vicky and David where I'm going.

"I've kept this quiet all my life. People wouldn't understand. I'd lose my job."

## Summary

1. Most of us encounter two types of nuclear families during our lifetime: the nuclear family of orientation and the nuclear family of procreation. The extended family and the polygamous family each consist of a number of nuclear families.

2. Kinship is a very important principle of organization. It is a social, not a biological, concept.

3. There are many kinship regulations, which have practical implications in terms of descent, residence, and family authority. Rules of descent, through which our line of relatives is established, is either unilineal or nonunilineal. There are various possibilities of descent: from the mother's side, from the father's side, or from both sides of the family. Rules of residence affect where a newly married couple lives, and rules of authority state who heads the family.

4. Whether or not the nuclear family is truly universal is a perennial issue. Although there is disagreement, there is strong support for its universality, especially in light of the fact that it provides the context for some basic human and societal needs.

5. There are many explanations for the universal taboo against incest. The biological position rests on the genetic damage done by incestuous relations. The psychoanalytic position examines incest in terms of its unconscious motivation. Parsons's functional argument combines these, suggesting that the incest taboo allows the family to remain intact. Murdock provides a useful framework for integrating anthropological and sociological findings into an eclectic explanation.

## Key Terms

The following terms were introduced and defined in this chapter. Definitions also appear in the glossary.

avunculocal residence
bilateral descent
double descent
equalitarian relationship
extended family
family
genealogy
incest
kinship
matriarchy
matrilineal descent
matrilocal residence
matri-patrilocal residence
neolocal residence

nonfunctional incest
nonunilineal descent
nuclear family
nuclear family of orientation
nuclear family of procreation
pathological incest
patriarchy
patrilineal descent
patrilocal residence
polygamous family
socialization
social reproduction
stimulus generalization
unilineal descent

## Discussion Questions

1. In your growing up, how did you personally experience the impact of a nuclear family? Are you familiar with the single-parent family structure? With the extended family? In what ways has your experience affected your socialization?

2. Using standards of kinship in our society, construct a three-generation

family tree, showing all persons that would be considered your kin and putting next to each name what the kinship designation for that person is; for example aunt, second cousin, great grandfather.

3. What do you personally believe is the basis for the taboo against incest? How would you defend your position with evidence cited in this or the preceding chapter? From your personal experiences?

4. Conduct an informal survey of five or six of your married friends or classmates to obtain the following information. When they married, where did they reside in relation to their families? What networks, if any, were established between the pair and their two nuclear families of orientation? Which marital partner, if either, would be considered by both the authority for the new family? Now interpret your findings.

5. From your reading of this chapter, what arguments would you give to support or refute the idea that the nuclear family is a universal form?

## Suggested Readings

1. Meyer Nimkoff. *Comparative Family Systems.* Boston: Houghton-Mifflin, 1965.

An extensive review and analysis of the literature on comparative studies of the family and the diversity of family forms provides the backdrop for an examination of the relationship between the family and other aspects of society, and family trends as seen by a respected sociologist in the early 1960's. In addition, there are detailed descriptions of life in 12 different societies around the world.

2. Stuart A. Queen and Robert Habenstein. *The Family in Various Cultures* (4th ed.). Philadelphia: Lippincott, 1974.

A book that draws upon both comparative and historical perspectives in the study of the family to focus on family arrangements in selected specific societies.

3. Edward Shorter. *The Making of the Modern Family.* New York: Basic Books, 1975.

A psychohistorical view of the factors that lead to the establishment of the modern family, particularly maternal sentiment, demographic changes, and industrialization.

4. Ruth Nanda Anshen (Ed.). *The Family: Its Function and Destiny* (revised ed.). New York: Harper and Row, 1959.

With contributions by leading investigators and writers in the field, this book offers a cross-cultural examination of family functions and structures. Part One examines family patterns in different cultures. Part Two focuses on family structure and the role of the contemporary family.

# Chapter 3

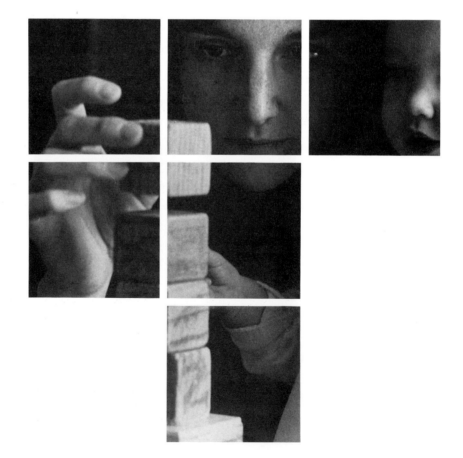

# Socialization and the Family

## Chapter Aims

1. To define and explain the functions of socialization, delineating the components of the socialization process, particularly in terms of status and role.

2. To differentiate further between the nuclear family of orientation and the nuclear family of procreation.

3. To show the importance of these types of nuclear families in terms of identity development and other aspects of socialization.

## Overview

The process by which you learn who you are in relationship to society goes on throughout your lifetime. Of primary importance in this learning process are both the family in which you are a child and the one in which you are a parent.

You come to understand your position in the social group and how you are expected to behave in this position, particularly as it pertains to your being a man or a woman. To the individual, this lifelong learning process is critical to the development of a personal identity.

# The Importance of Socialization

Socialization

In order to understand the way in which the family serves as an agent of socialization, we will begin by considering what socialization means and why it is such an important concept in understanding the individual and the family in relation to society. Socialization has been an object of intensive study. Anthropologists, psychiatrists, psychologists, sociologists, and even some social historians have viewed socialization as a legitimate and important area of investigation. These disciplines approach the study of socialization in different manners. In keeping with the general perspective of this book, we will approach socialization and its role in the family from a social psychological viewpoint, blending the insights of clinical psychology with the conceptual analyses and empirical data of sociology.

# What Is Socialization?

It is important to start with a working definition of socialization. However, we wish to remind the reader that all definitions are merely devices used in learning and discovery. They are neither right nor wrong, but merely useful for the purpose at hand. Definitions should not be invested with any mystical qualities; they are merely means to an end, and it is that end that is ultimately important.

With this concept in mind, *socialization* may be viewed as a lifelong process by means of which a human being becomes and continues to be a more or less adequately functioning and contributing member of a particular social group (including society). Socialization is a learning process. It needs to be understood that socialization is also an interactive process of mutual, although not necessarily equal, influence between the individual and the social group to which he or she belongs. The process of socialization is influenced by the people being socialized.

# The Functions of Socialization

It is through the process of socialization that a group is able to transmit its values, customs, and beliefs—in short, its culture—from one generation to another. In this respect, socialization permits a society to transcend the mortality of its individual members. Socialization, then, provides for a group's social reproduction, that is, the transmission of social values from one generation to the next.

Socialization, especially as it pertains to the family, is also a road to individual growth and development. "Clearly," Cole (1979, p. 102) points out, "the family is the most important agent for socialization of young children. As children grow older and attend school and make friends, the peer group and schools become important agents of socialization. One important function of socialization, then, is to provide the child, who is initially totally dependent upon and influenced by the nuclear family, an opportunity to become an individual, socially functioning person.

Learning to conform

Socialization has another important function within society. Through socialization members of a society are encouraged to conform to the ways of the group by making the group's norms and values their own. In effect, the members internalize the culture of the group to which they belong through the process of socialization. Without this internalization, social order would require each member's behavior to be constantly monitored and supervised by a personal guard. And who would guard the guards? Thus, socialization may also be viewed as a mechanism of social control.

Imagine if we had to learn all the ways of a group, all of its culture, in small bits and pieces. The information would be so complicated, so out of any context, and so disorganized that it would probably be meaningless to us. Fortunately, socialization does not take place in this way.

Social position

Role

The bulk of socialization involves the learning of statuses and roles. These include the following: *social statuses or positions,* specific locations within social networks of relationships; *role prescriptions,* the behavior, values, and beliefs expected of the occupant of a particular status; and *role performance,* the actual enactment of role-relevant behavior of a status occupant. For example, a minister, a physician, a bus driver, or a handicapped person all have social positions. Each of these individuals holds a certain position, a relationship, with respect to the larger social group. Examples of role prescriptions are the competent so-called professional behavior we expect of a physician or minister, the polite, trip-directed, unobtrusive behavior of the bus driver, or the presumed dependent behavior of a young child. These are not natural behaviors, but are learned, rehearsed, and practiced in social situations. The physician and minister are taught how to act like physicians and ministers just as the young child is taught to be dependent. As we will see later, if people do not conform to their expected roles—for example, if the young child is able to function well without help—others may become uncomfortable since they expect different behaviors with these roles.

Through socialization we learn how to perceive ourselves and others in the social hierarchy, we learn what kinds of behaviors are expected from us and by us, and we are given an opportunity to practice these behaviors.

These three functions of socialization are particularly important for learning to live in a social group. From the point of view of the individual, however, perhaps the most important function of socialization is the formation, development, maintenance, and transformation of *identity*. Who we were, are, and will be emerges from the experience of socialization. It is through my interaction with others, their responses to me, and my interpretation of their reactions that I come to see myself in a certain way that I define as "ME." Consequently, identity is another, and from the individual's perspective perhaps *the* important, function of the socialization process.

Looked at carefully, the learning of social positions, role prescriptions, role performance, and identity reveals that socialization is a crucial link between the individual and his or her group(s). The interests of the individual and the group(s) meet in the socialization process.

This arena of human experience, it should be emphasized, is neither the turbulent battleground of the individual and society as portrayed in orthodox psychoanalytic theory, nor the mythical "best of all possible worlds." For most of us the relative smoothness or roughness of the socialization process is influenced by our own unique characteristics and by social forces such as war, inflation, and prejudice.

## The Family as an Agent of Socialization

Socialization is not a random process. The social contexts within which socialization takes place are themselves socially ordered. They comprise some of the major social institutions and organizations, such as the family, the media, the church, and the school, all of which play an important continuous part in the life of the individual. It is within these recognizable social contexts that the agents of society make their values known to us.

The various agencies of socialization are not all of equal influence; nor are they of equal salience throughout all phases of the individual's life. For example, the nuclear family of orientation, the school, the peer group, and the media of mass communication are the most important

*(margin note: Identity)*

*(margin note: Agents of socialization)*

agencies through which socialization occurs during infancy and childhood (Denzin 1977). On the other hand, adult socialization, while still influenced by the nuclear family of orientation and the peer group, is also greatly affected by two new socialization agents: the nuclear family of procreation and the workplace. Since this is a book about the family, we shall focus exclusively on the two types of nuclear families and their roles in the socialization process during childhood and adulthood.

## The Nuclear Family of Orientation

Continuous interaction

The nuclear family of orientation is the family in which a person is raised. One's kin are traditionally the first, most important, and most continuous agents of socialization. In our modern industrial society, this is particularly true of one's nuclear families, especially the nuclear family of orientation. However, even here there is some socially structured variation. For example, members of the working class have traditionally had stronger extended family ties than those of the middle class. These stronger ties have been explained by several factors, including educational level, the economic need to remain in the parents' home for a longer period, and more authoritarian upbringing. Recently, however, some sociologists have questioned whether or not this pattern is still true and if it ever were true (Pitts 1964; Clayton 1975).

With the exception of the maternity ward of the hospital during the first few days of life, for most infants the nuclear family of orientation is the major if not sole social context within which they experience the extra-uterine environment. The family thus provides the infant with its first perception of the world and its introduction into the nature of social life.

## Bases of the Family's Importance

Most agents of socialization, aside from the family, serve some other ostensible purposes: the media to entertain, inform, and sell and the church to attend to our spiritual needs, for example. But for the family, socialization is an intentional and recognized function. The nuclear family of orientation has the manifest function of socializing the infant and child. But the importance of the family in the socialization process has several other bases as well.

First, socialization within the nuclear family of orientation takes place while the child is very young and thus especially dependent upon family

*Human beings have the longest period of youth and dependency of any species.*

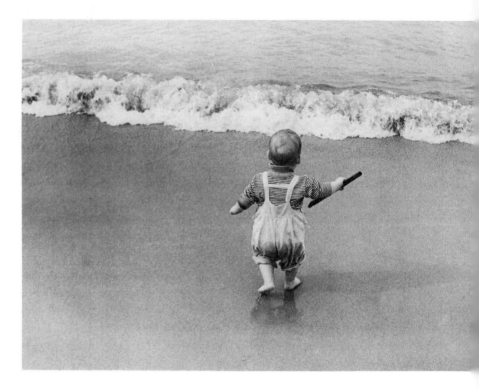

members for the satisfaction of practically all basic needs. Human beings have the longest period of youth and dependency of any species (Bronowski 1973). This fact of life renders the human offspring susceptible to the influence of others, especially his or her earliest socializers, the nuclear family of orientation, for a relatively long period of time. And this lengthy period of dependency serves to increase the potency of these early and continuous socializing agents.

A second important basis of family influence stems from the intimate emotional nature of family interaction. While being cared for by his or her family and receiving love, warmth, and nurturing, the child is imbibing the values, beliefs, and norms of the family. Moreover, the family is where the child first learns about the meaning of authority, the expression of emotions, and the nature of social relationships. Some of the learned emotional attitudes and behaviors we take for granted are actually a direct result of what we learned through our family experiences (Kemper 1978). How much feeling are we allowed to express in public? How much tolerance should we show to others who are different? Is crying a sign of strength or of weakness? Is it permissible to be physically affectionate to same-sex nuclear family members? We learn our own individual answers to these questions within our family context.

The family is truly a microcosm of society, a model of the whole of social life. In the family, the child gains experience in hierarchical (parent-child) and in equalitarian (sibling) relationships. By viewing interactions between members of the same and opposite sex, the child begins to learn sex roles. In observing the subtle interplay of power and feeling, the child begins to gain a perspective that he or she will carry throughout life. In short, the young child receives his or her most elemental and important lessons in the nature of role interaction and sex-role identification.

The importance of the family in identity formation is an important additional base. Practically all of the major theoretical perspectives used to study socialization or personality development recognize the centrality of the family in the formation and development of identity, self-image, and self-esteem (Anthony and Chiland 1978). The professional literature in psychiatry, psychology, and sociology testifies to the importance of the family in this realm. Even those perspectives that stress the importance of later life in identity maintenance and identity change do not deny the critical nature of childhood and the family.

These first three bases are essentially social psychological in nature; that is, they combine insights from clinical psychology with sociological research. The fourth and most sociological basis of the importance of the nuclear family of orientation is its function in locating the newborn infant in the social structure. This social placement of the child in terms of the ascribed characteristics of social class, religion, and race serve to channel the child's life into a particular style and to structure his or her probable life chances with respect to health, education, and work. The very fact of being born into a specific family exposes the individual to a particular socialization context and a probable set of life experiences. In addition, these ascribed statuses will play an important role in the formation and development of the individual's identity. The child born to the President of the United States and his wife will have different chances in life than the child born to a third-generation welfare mother. It is important to note, however, that important as these initially ascribed characteristics are, they need not completely determine a person's future life. People are socially mobile, do change religions, and are capable of altering these initial contingencies of life experience.

## The Role of the Mother, the Father, and Siblings in Socialization

Since children are born without the capacity to survive on their own and

Parental role behavior

Caretaking styles

without a knowledge of social conventions, the perceived role of the mother and father during the child's infancy are critical in determining how the child ultimately develops. Parental role behavior is learned. To some degree, parents follow explicit conventions and to some degree they differ from them. The research, in fact, suggests a clear discrepancy between "official" childrearing advice, as provided by manuals, and the actual behavior of parents. Parents do not always listen to the official sources. Machling (1976, p. 49) points out that the styles of parenting depend more on *primary* socialization (which takes place through the nuclear family of orientation) than on *secondary* socialization (which takes place through other social relationships and institutions, such as peer groups, the schools, the media, etc.). In short,

> persons in a culture learn the role of parent and the entire constellation of childrearing customs associated with that role primarily through interaction with their parents. . . . Any later-life learning of the parent role becomes a modification of the role as it was originally internalized.

He points out that despite secondary socializing influences, this early parental model remains predominant.

Although there are major differences in patterns of childhood socialization during the early years, generally three things can be said to be true from culture to culture, although there are some important variations:

1. The mother is usually the primary caretaker.
2. The child is generally made aware that he or she is a member of a nuclear family unit.
3. Pressures are brought to bear on the family, or on whoever is responsible for the child's socialization, that the child exhibit socially acceptable, conforming behaviors, consistent with the status of child.

We will see as we look at different childrearing practices in chapter 10 how these three motifs prevail. We now focus on the roles the mother, father, and siblings have in the socialization of an individual.

## Maternal Environment and the Origins of Socialization

Culture is transmitted from mother to child through the mother's behavior in the maternal relationship. William A. Caudill, a pioneer in investigating cross-cultural analyses of infant-mother interactions, found evidence of this early cultural transmission affecting the differences between cultures. He showed, for example, significant differences between Japanese and American infants, differences that were a result of the mothers in the two cultures engaging in different styles of caretaking (Caudill and Schooler 1973). In this section, we will consider some of the specific influences that maternal environment has on early social development.

It is generally acknowledged that the most significant single factor in early emotional development is the emotional, physical, and nurturing environment provided by the mother, or the "mothering one," as Harry Stack Sullivan calls the child's primary caretaker. The mother (or "mothering one"—that is, the person primarily responsible for the child's daily care) is primarily responsible for protecting the child from dangers, for providing nourishment, and for stimulating the child into emotional maturity. One of the most important things provided by the mother to the child is her touch: the way she physically handles the child, which becomes the catalyst for early stimulation and the precursor to later social involvements. "To be deprived of enough touch," psychologist Arthur Janov (1973) argues, "is not to be loved, no matter how loudly the parents protest to the contrary." This need for physical contact has been borne out consistently by the research. Klatskin, Jackson, and Wilkin (1956) investigated the effects of childrearing practices and maternal care on the child's early behavior. They concluded that "child behavior

*The mother has traditionally been the most socializing member of the nuclear family of orientation.*

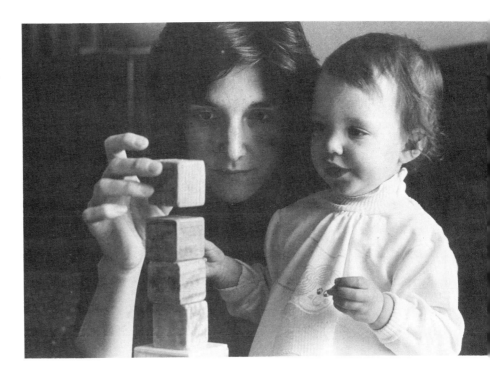

during the first three years is more consistently influenced by maternal handling than by other environmental factors."

Some of the most important research in this area has been conducted by Harry F. Harlow. In Harlow's landmark experiments, baby monkeys were separated at birth from their natural mothers and were provided with surrogate mothers. The monkeys were divided into two groups, each of which was provided with a different type of surrogate mother: one made of wire mesh, with a wooden block at the head position and the other of the same size and shape, but covered with a soft terry cloth, backed by sponge rubber, with its head painted and glued with false features. Both mothers contained a hole through which the nipple of a nursing bottle protruded at feeding time. Each mother was a source of food for the monkeys assigned to it, but Harlow found that between feedings all the monkeys preferred to cuddle up to the cloth mother, even those who were fed by the wire mother. And when a fearful object was placed near them, all the monkeys clung only to the cloth mother as a security base. The wire mother was never used in this way. This led Harlow to conclude that the warmth and comfort of the mother is just as important as the fact that she is the source of food.

## Some Effects on Socialization

The implications of this behavior in terms of socialization and subsequent bonding have also been examined. In follow-up research on the monkeys, Harlow (1971) found that monkeys raised in isolation, or deprived of maternal warmth, showed little or no interest in normal sexual behavior as adults. For example, the male monkeys raised in isolation were unable to copulate at maturity with female monkeys, although they were able to masturbate to ejaculation (as normally raised monkeys do). When the females were mated without wanting to and became mothers, they failed to show any maternal behavior. However, the monkeys that were given an opportunity to interact with other young monkeys during childhood, as well as maternal contact, showed normal heterosexual adjustment as adults.

In a similar study, Ruppenthal et al. (1974) investigated the development of firstborn infant monkeys who were reared in a nuclear family setting for the first three years of their lives. They found that these monkeys, who were allowed close proximity to the family, developed "sophisticated patterns of social behavior seldom observed in laboratory-reared monkeys and maintained levels of interactive play longer chronologically than has been reported for feral-raised [in the wilds] monkeys" (p. 670). These results again support the thesis that the nuclear family situation facilitates socialization and that the premature separation from the parents may be a factor that impedes appropriate socialization.

*One of the most important things provided by a mother to her child is her touch.*

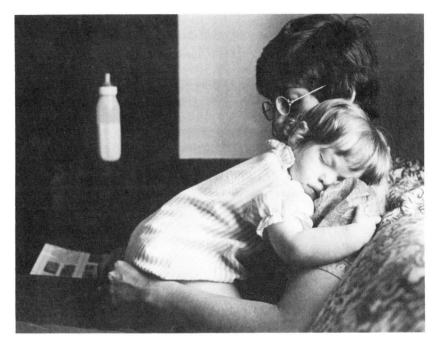

Other studies, using human subjects, have also attempted to investigate the relationship among family intactness, maternal behavior, and different aspects of socialization. This investigation is important insofar as childrearing practices are undergoing changes in response to the expanding role of women in our society. Korner (1975), in expressing the general conclusions of all these studies, points out that the mother's role is especially important during the first eighteen months of life, but that it has not been clearly determined which aspects of her role can be surrogated. Bowlby (1958, 1960, 1969), in a landmark series of studies on attachment and separation, concluded, like Harlow, that close physical contact between child and mother is essential for the well-being of the infant and for its subsequent development and normal adjustment in later childhood, adolescence, and adulthood. Spitz (1975) has also found that children who were deprived of adequate care during this early stage of life suffered serious and long-lasting aberrations in development. This finding has been supported by many other experiments and longitudinal studies (Papalia and Olds 1979).

### The Father's Role

Despite the almost universal attention that has been given to the mother's role in childrearing, several investigators (Nash 1973; Hamilton 1977) have recently focused attention on the father's role. This growing concern with the role of the father coincides with the movement for equality between men and women. The increasing drive for equality between men and women, in fact, is gradually reducing the disparity of parental influence. As more women work and more men take an active part in childrearing, the traditionally wide differences in their relative influence in early childhood socialization is slowly, if grudgingly in some homes, narrowing. Lamb (1977), for example, found that by the mid-1970s children between the ages of one and two were showing an increased desire to be with their fathers. Fathers too were showing an increased interest in their children, especially if the child was a boy. By two years of age, most children were equally attached to both parents.

As one might expect, the change is more visible among the most recent generation of fathers. It is they who have taken increasing responsibility for the traditionally defined ''feminine'' tasks of bathing, feeding, and dressing the infant and have played a part in meeting the social needs of older children.

Siblings and Family Size   It is sometimes forgotten in analyses of socialization within the family that parents are not the only societal agents. Most families, at one point or another in their histories, are likely to contain two or more children. Thus, a child's siblings must also be seen as potential socializers within the nuclear family of orientation. Essman (1977), for instance, has found that older siblings role behavior towards younger children influence the child's socialization into the parental role. Children, it was found, learn parenting behaviors from their siblings as well as from their parents.

Brim (1958) demonstrated that different sibling configurations of five and six year olds were associated with different behavioral styles as seen by the children's teachers. More recently, in reviewing all the literature of the past 30 years, Sutton-Smith and Rosenberg (1970) have confirmed that the child's relationships with siblings influence almost all facets of socialization. Family size is also an important variable in socialization. In several of their writings, Bossard and Boll (for example, 1966) point out differences between large and small families. Although these differences cannot automatically be attributed to the number of siblings, neither can the role of siblings in creating these differences be ignored.

Zajonc and Marcus (1976), in an impressive research effort, spanning several years, have linked family size to intellectual development. They found that as the size of the family increases, the average IQ of the children tends to decrease. This is partly accounted for, according to their theory, because in larger families children tend to be more heavily in-

Reducing disparity of parental roles

Intellectual development

As men take a more ac-
tive role in childrearing,
studies show that small
children desire to be with
their fathers more.

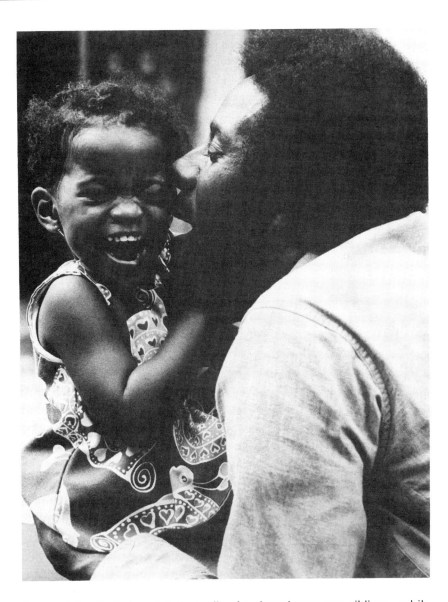

Birth order

fluenced by their less intellectually developed younger siblings, while
children in small families have more contact with adults or with older siblings. Some of these ideas will be explored further in chapter 10, where
we look at the effects of birth order on personality and socialization. Here,
we can say simply that in different ways and through different members,
the nuclear family of orientation plays a critical role in the socialization of
the infant and child.

## Effects of Social Structure in Socialization

Clearly, not all families socialize their children in the same way. Obviously, there are profound differences among families. Your mother is not the same person my mother is. But since we both call a person that is very important to us "mother," there must be some similarity in what they do. That is to say, in sociological terms, they both have the same social status, both the same role expectations.

**Family differences**

However, the role prescriptions attached to particular social statuses often vary for different social, cultural, religious, ethnic, racial, and educational groups (DiRenzo 1977). There have been countless studies of differences in childrearing among families differing in religion, in race, and in social class. All of these studies point to the way in which families differing on major social variables tend to structure socialization experiences differently for their children.

To take a classic example, sociologist Melvin Kohn (1969) found that working-class parents were more likely than their middle-class counterparts to use physical punishment in childrearing. This particular form of discipline has been shown to be associated with the development of such traits as obedience, neatness, and respect. Middle-class parents, on the other hand, are more likely to avoid physical punishments in favor of verbal and psychological ones, such as threats of the withdrawal of love and the use of sarcasm, with the result that they are more likely to inculcate self-control in their children.

**Class differences**

Perhaps the more important part of this study by Kohn is his analysis of the association between the traits inculcated in working- and middle-class children and the requirements of those jobs that they are most likely to hold as adults. The working-class individual is likely to find himself in a job where following orders of a supervisor is of central importance. Thus, the early instillation of obedience and respect accords well with this likely occupational requirement. On the other hand, middle-class individuals are more likely to find themselves in occupations, such as supervisory positions and the professions, where self-control and initiative are more highly valued than simple obedience. Thus, their upbringing prepares them for this internal control and responsibility.

Although Kohn's work has shown the clear relationship between early socialization and later occupational requirements, rarely—as a detailed reading of Kohn's work makes clear—is the relationship between activities in early childhood and later adulthood simple, straightforward, and direct. Such findings should not be used to justify a rigid and unyielding class structure in which social mobility is seen as an exception.

Studies of this kind are primarily useful in demonstrating the importance of social variables in the socialization process carried out by the nuclear family of orientation and in attempting to specify the nature of the uncovered associations. Still, it should be pointed out that other studies have continued to support the different socialization capacities and intellectual development of the middle-class compared to lower-class children in school and in other settings, not only in the United States but in such diverse cultures as French Canada (Chiland 1976) and India (Srivastava 1977).

## Socialization as a Reciprocal Process

So far, in common with practically all treatments of the role of the nuclear family in the socialization process, we have seen that parents influence their children and that siblings influence other siblings. The issue of whether the parents are also influenced, that is, socialized, by their children is usually ignored. Let us say as clearly as possible that socialization is a reciprocal process. Infants and children socialize their parents as well as being socialized by them!

Reciprocal socialization

How to be a mother, much less a good mother, is never learned completely in the abstract. One learns to be a mother, father, brother, or sister in large measure by actually playing these parts and by having to consider and respond to an infant, child, or sibling. In other words, social interaction is involved.

The infant or young child may initiate activities that require a response by the parent or sibling. The responses of the parent or sibling then require a further response from the initiator. Thus, socialization is a two-way street. The more obvious flow of influence from the older to the younger members of the family should not blind us to the reciprocal nature of socialization. For example, adolescents have been noted to contribute to the socialization of their parents in various ways (Baranowski 1978). The parents of an adolescent may take on some of the adolescent's values especially if there is mutual respect between them.

If one is open to it, it is easy to see the reciprocal nature of the socialization that takes place within the nuclear family of orientation. Why do new parents typically completely rearrange their former lifestyles with the arrival of a child? Why do parents get up at such peculiar hours of the night, sometimes even when a cry is just starting, to provide the bottle or the breast? Why do parents treat their different children in quite different ways, both as infants and as young children?

The answer to these and countless similar questions is that socialization is a reciprocal process and we must recognize the role of children in structuring their parents' and siblings' behavior.

Parents rearrange their preparental lifestyles to take into account new additions to their intimate circle. They get up at ungodly hours to provide the nourishment and care that they have learned from their parents, from books, from classes, from friends, and from the children themselves. The child actually teaches, that is, socializes, the parents by showing them his or her needs and how to satisfy them. And parents certainly do not act identically with each of their children: most parents learn from their experiences with prior children as well as take the unique characteristics of the new child into account.

Young children and adolescents especially are also potent socializers of parental behavior. Many parents are concerned with how they are perceived by their children, and this concern motivates changes in behavior. The older the child, the greater the concern is likely to be. This attempt to please can be quite humorous. How often has the parent of an adolescent made a vain attempt to be "cool" or "relevant" or, worse yet, "hip"!

Parental behavior is modified by actions, or by the anticipated actions, of their children. While it is certainly understandable that some incidents, for example, marital infidelity, are likely to be hidden from the children as well as the spouse, breaches of business and social ethics are likely to be hidden only from the children. While one's spouse is permitted to see one in a variety of situations and hence able to put together a balanced assessment, the same is not generally true of one's children. Hence, children are often "protected" from the seamier side of parental behavior. Parents modify their behaviors because of their roles as parents. In truth, there could be no better admission of the importance we attach to our children's view of us and thus of their role in our socialization.

## Socialization in the Nuclear Family of Procreation

The advent of adulthood does not eliminate our family of origin as an important agent of socialization. Even after we marry, our nuclear family of orientation remains influential, and sometimes too much so! Why else would there be so many "in-law jokes" if there were not some potential source of conflict.

In addition, however, the other nuclear family that many of us belong to or will belong to—the nuclear family of procreation—emerges as a forceful agent in the continuing process of socialization. In fact, a number of the difficulties in married life can be traced to the occasional conflicting

*Young children and adolescents are also potent socializers of parental behavior.*

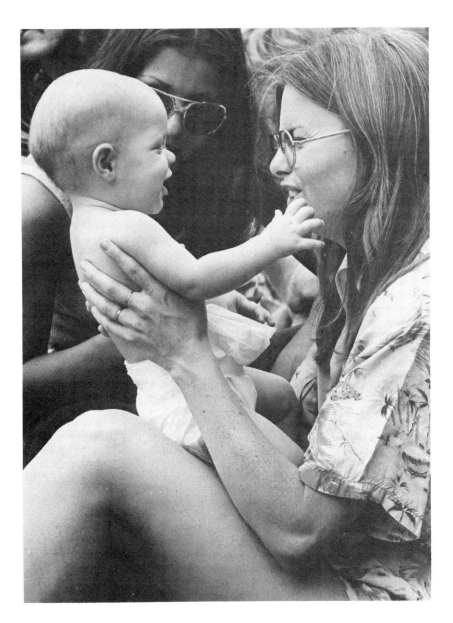

demands made on a person by his or her nuclear families of orientation and procreation. The conflict between husband and wife—''What do you mean your mother wants you to help her today. I need you here now!''—is an example of this.

Anticipatory
socialization vs. actual
role behavior

In the nuclear family of procreation, the focal members are the parents and the new family they have created. However, the prior discussion of the reciprocal, albeit unequal, influence of parents and children is especially relevant here. Recall that we pointed out that a person only really learns to become a parent by actually being a parent, that is, by playing the role of parent. It is true that a good deal of *anticipatory socialization* takes place in childhood or adolescence. This is the process by which a person learns about and rehearses the behaviors, values, and norms of a particular role or group as a preliminary to possible entry into that group. However, the nuances and the range of any role can only be learned by playing it. It is not enough to simply play house as a young child or to have deep, philosophical discussions with one's girlfriend or boyfriend about how children should be raised. One can only truly understand what it means to be a parent by being a parent. Both the anticipatory socialization and the actual role playing are necessary.

The same point may be made about the role of spouse. Anticipatory socialization within the nuclear family of orientation and through the media of mass communication takes us only to a point in learning to be a husband or wife. The rest, and perhaps the most interesting, exciting, and difficult part, must be learned ''on the job'' because the role requirements for the social status of spouse allow room for the individuality of both members of the couple. What pleases one particular wife or husband may not please another. What is expected of one may not be expected of another. Each spouse must learn how to express his or her feelings and expectations to the other person so that some reasonable and satisfactory understanding of what each wants from the other and what each is willing to give to the other can be worked out.

Communication and Roles The admonition that communication in the family is important is based on the sound principle that agreement can only take place through some form of discussion between or among the parties. And, in the case of the couple, agreement is important in defining roles. A lack of communication averts the possibility of adjusting different views of the role of spouse and parent, views that were learned in the nuclear family of orientation. Also, communication is necessary for ''fine tuning'' the general picture of spouse given by society to the specific desires of the individuals concerned. Thus, husbands and wives play an extremely important role in socializing each other into the role of spouse. And they do so within the context of the nuclear family of procreation.

# Socialization in Identity Development

The family provides socialization opportunities in the important area of *identity development.* By identity development, we mean not only the formation of self-image and status identity but sex-role identity as well.

Significant others

Practically all major theoretical perspectives, with Freudian psychoanalysis as the major exception, view identity development as not unalterably set in childhood but as constantly being developed, modified, and even transformed throughout life. This relative fluidity of identity depends on interaction with *significant others,* those persons who have great influence on our behaviors as well as on our attitudes, values, and norms. The term was first used by the psychiatrist Harry Stack Sullivan to refer to the importance of family members in the development of a sense of self. For most adults, the most significant others are their spouses and children, that is, their nuclear families of procreation. These family members constitute the major cast of characters with whom the person is involved in a broad range of important concerns over a considerable period of time.

## Gender-Role Learning in the Nuclear Family

Gender roles

One of the most important aspects of socialization in the nuclear family is the learning of *gender roles,* also called *sex roles.* Gender roles can be defined as a set of expected social behaviors specifically associated with one sex or the other. There are masculine and feminine sex-role behaviors. If you look at the following list, for example, and force yourself to say the first word that comes to mind—*male* or *female*—even though you probably realize that the activity is applicable to members of either sex, you have probably been socialized to associate it more with one sex than with the other:

- Cooking dinner
- Wants to have sex
- Cleans the house
- Does the laundry
- Driving a taxi
- Wants to get married
- Washes the car
- Is very athletic

Although research during the past decade has focused on the large

number of interactive factors that contribute to our gender-role socialization, and particularly to sex-role stereotyping, we still recognize that
the nuclear family of orientation is of prime importance. The learning of
gender roles begins very early in life. As King (1973) points out, ''If
young children are highly aware of the social life that goes on in their

Table 3.1

**Comparative Data on the Division of
Labor by Sex**

| Activity | Number of Societies in Which: | | | | |
|---|---|---|---|---|---|
| | Men always do it | Men usually do it | Either sex may do it | Women usually do it | Women always do it |
| Metal working | 78 | 0 | 0 | 0 | 0 |
| Weapon making | 121 | 1 | 0 | 0 | 0 |
| Pursuit of sea mammals | 34 | 1 | 0 | 0 | 0 |
| Hunting | 166 | 13 | 0 | 0 | 0 |
| Manufacture of musical instruments | 45 | 2 | 0 | 0 | 1 |
| Boat building | 91 | 4 | 4 | 0 | 1 |
| Mining and quarrying | 35 | 1 | 1 | 0 | 1 |
| Work in wood and bark | 113 | 9 | 5 | 1 | 1 |
| Work in stone | 68 | 3 | 2 | 0 | 2 |
| Trapping or catching of small animals | 128 | 13 | 4 | 1 | 2 |
| Lumbering | 104 | 4 | 3 | 1 | 6 |
| Work in bone, horn, and shell | 67 | 4 | 3 | 0 | 3 |
| Fishing | 98 | 34 | 19 | 3 | 4 |
| Manufacture of ceremonial objects | 37 | 1 | 13 | 0 | 1 |
| Herding | 38 | 8 | 4 | 0 | 5 |
| House building | 86 | 32 | 25 | 3 | 14 |
| Clearing of land for agriculture | 73 | 22 | 17 | 5 | 13 |
| Net making | 44 | 6 | 4 | 2 | 11 |
| Trade | 51 | 28 | 20 | 8 | 7 |
| Dairy operations | 17 | 4 | 3 | 1 | 13 |
| Manufacture of ornaments | 24 | 3 | 40 | 6 | 18 |
| Agriculture: soil preparation and planting | 31 | 23 | 33 | 20 | 37 |
| Manufacture of leather products | 29 | 3 | 9 | 3 | 32 |

Source: Adapted from Murdock, 1937 (Zelditch, 1955, p. 57).

midst, then they are certainly cognizant of the sex-role behavior that is appropriate in the culture" (p. 67). Earlier we noted the division of labor within the nuclear family as one of its key elements. Beginning with this idea of a socially cooperative relationship, we can gain some insight into how gender-role socialization takes place in the nuclear family.

Table 3.1

**Comparative Data on the Division of Labor by Sex**

| Activity | Number of Societies in Which: | | | | |
|---|---|---|---|---|---|
| | Men always do it | Men usually do it | Either sex may do it | Women usually do it | Women always do it |
| Body mutilations, for example, tattooing | 16 | 14 | 44 | 22 | 20 |
| Erection and dismantling of shelter | 14 | 2 | 5 | 6 | 22 |
| Hide preparation | 31 | 2 | 4 | 4 | 49 |
| Tending of fowls and small animals | 21 | 4 | 8 | 1 | 39 |
| Agriculture: crop tending and harvesting | 10 | 15 | 35 | 39 | 44 |
| Gathering of shellfish | 9 | 4 | 8 | 7 | 25 |
| Manufacture of nontextile fabrics | 14 | 0 | 9 | 2 | 32 |
| Fire making and tending | 18 | 6 | 25 | 22 | 62 |
| Burden bearing | 12 | 6 | 35 | 20 | 57 |
| Preparation of drinks and narcotics | 20 | 1 | 13 | 8 | 57 |
| Manufacture of thread and cordage | 23 | 2 | 11 | 10 | 73 |
| Basket making | 25 | 3 | 10 | 6 | 82 |
| Mat making | 16 | 2 | 6 | 4 | 61 |
| Weaving | 19 | 2 | 2 | 6 | 67 |
| Gathering of fruits, berries, and nuts | 12 | 3 | 15 | 13 | 63 |
| Fuel gathering | 22 | 1 | 10 | 19 | 89 |
| Pottery making | 13 | 2 | 6 | 8 | 77 |
| Preservation of meat and fish | 8 | 2 | 10 | 14 | 74 |
| Manufacture and repair of clothing | 12 | 3 | 8 | 9 | 95 |
| Gathering of herbs, roots, and seeds | 8 | 1 | 11 | 7 | 74 |
| Cooking | 5 | 1 | 9 | 28 | 158 |
| Water carrying | 7 | 0 | 5 | 7 | 119 |
| Grain grinding | 2 | 4 | 5 | 13 | 114 |

Source: Adapted from Murdock, 1937 (Zelditch, 1955, p. 57).

## Zelditch's Study

In a classic and still relevant paper, Zelditch (1955) examined gender-role socialization on a cross-cultural basis. Drawing on the exciting research then going on at Harvard, where he was, Zelditch conceived of the family as a small social system or group that should exhibit the same formal characteristics as all other small groups. Specifically, he argued, the roles of the adult members should be differentiated into *instrumental roles* and *expressive roles.* The primary concern in an instrumental role is to provide the family with the means of subsistence and physical security; specifically, to deal with the environment external to the family. In expressive roles the focus of attention is within the family itself, its harmony and solidarity.

Zelditch (1955) examined these theoretical expectations in light of data from a sample of 56 societies. In brief, he found that all but 5 of them separated the responsibilities of the parents into instrumental and expressive roles. Thus, while this specific form of role differentiation was not universal, it did seem to be a fairly widespread phenomenon.

Zelditch (1955) also addressed the more important question of whether there was any consistent association between the sex of the parent and the specific role played in the nuclear family. He reasoned that the man's greater selective physical strength (stronger muscles, arms, shoulders, chest, and legs) and greater mobility (due to freedom from childbearing and breast-feeding) made it more effective and efficient for him to deal with the relatively harsh external environment. In short, the man seemed to be better suited biologically to play the instrumental role in the family. On the other hand, the fact that women gave birth to children and were required to nurse them seriously restricted their mobility and thus their utility in dealing with the external environment (other than local agriculture in near proximity to the family dwelling).

Coupled with the issue of selective physical strength, Zelditch (1955) argued, these characteristics seem to suggest a greater efficiency in having women play the expressive role in the family. In many respects, the breast feeding and nurturance of the infant is an example par excellence of the expressive role and, Zelditch argued, it would be quite inefficient to have the women switch from this to the instrumental role. Though "anatomy is destiny" may be an oversimplification, it did seem to have some implications for efficient role playing in the family.

Zelditch also examined the data on the original 51 societies in his sample that had shown a differentiation of family roles into instrumental and expressive to ascertain whether these were related to the sex of the parent (see table 3.1). Again, he found a clear relationship: in 48 societies the father played the instrumental role and the mother the expressive role. Moreover, these figures coincide with Murdock's (1949) delineation of the division of labor in society by sex.

Instrumental role

Expressive role

Zelditch's analysis has been attacked by a number of investigators (see Aronoff and Crano 1975, for example), and most vigorously by those subscribing to a conflict theory of society, that is, those who view society as a collection of antagonistic groups or social classes who compete with each other for control. The conflict theorists tend to define role differentiation in the family and between the two sexes generally in terms of a "class war" between men and women rather than as efficient functional specialization. In this "battle between the sexes," the generally greater physical superiority of men, it is argued, has led to the subjugation of women.

However, a careful analysis of the conflict theory view in the light of available anthropological evidence (Gough 1971) generally supports Zelditch (1955). One can trace the division of labor back to the dawn of hunting among our predecessors, the early hominids, when pregnant mothers were unable to keep pace and travel far from home with their men. Stephens, a noted researcher on the family in different cultures, examining the roles of husbands and wives across the world, puts it this way (1963, pp. 304–5):

> Zelditch's generalization regarding the universal attributes of husband-wife roles needs some qualification. It is probably too much to claim that there is a certain type of role differentiation that is universal to all families. I feel sure Zelditch would agree to this. It would be safer to claim universality on a societal level (thus allowing for exceptional families within societies), and even this is a bit rash.
>
> Still, making allowance for these qualifications, I think there is some validity to Zelditch's statement. There are extraordinary cross-cultural regularities in husband-wife roles. . . . Murdock's and my data support him (that is, support the general drift of his argument). Perhaps there are no universal marital-role attributes. But there do seem to be some near-universals . . . of husband-wife roles:
>
> 1. A standard division of labor by sex.
> 2. The "essential femininity" of some tasks, such as child care, and the "essential masculinity" of other tasks, such as fishing.
> 3. Power and privilege: the husband's status is either equal to or higher than the wife's; matriarchies are rare.

It must be emphasized that Zelditch (1955), Gough (1971), Stephens (1963), and Murdock (1937, 1949) were analyzing cross-cultural regularities in husband-wife roles and possible reasons for their origin and continuance. None of them, to our knowledge, has argued that such a division of labor is a necessary and inherent facet of social life. It seems eminently clear that if Zelditch and Gough are correct, then the basis for the traditional and widespread division of labor between men and women no longer exists, certainly not in modern, technologically advanced societies. Babies are now fed by bottle as well as breast, and the tremendous advances in relations between women and men make most role assignments irrelevant. In short, a division of labor by sex is supported by the attitudes, values, and power systems in society and not by the biological differences between sexes (Goodman and Marx 1978).

We will examine sex-role stereotyping and the changing roles of men and women in greater detail in later chapters.

## Summary

1. Socialization is the lifelong learning process by means of which a person becomes a functioning and contributing member of society. Through the process of socialization a group is able to transmit its culture from one generation to another.

2. Socialization has several functions. From the point of view of the society, the primary function is the social reproduction function; namely, the transmission of culture from one generation to the next. It also provides for the general conformity of most individuals to the society's norms and values, which is known as the social control function.

3. Socialization also involves the learning of statuses and roles, the social learning function. A status is an individual's position in relation to others in the social hierarchy or group. A role is a set of behavioral expectations that accompany a status.

4. Whereas these functions serve important societal interests, from the point of view of the individual, the most important function of socialization is the formation, development, maintenance and transformation of identity: the identity formation function.

5. The two types of nuclear families have important roles in the socialization process. The nuclear family of orientation provides the child

with his or her first perception of the world and an introduction into the nature of social life. The family is a microcosm of society. By observing the subtle interplay of power and emotion, the child begins to gain a perspective that he or she will carry through life. The nuclear family of procreation is also a forceful agent in the continuing process of socialization and may change in many ways patterns of earlier socialization.

6. Not all families socialize their children in the same ways. The role prescriptions attached to particular social statuses often differ for different social groups, although to varying degrees. A classic study found that working-class parents were more likely than their middle-class counterparts to use physical punishments in childrearing. The consequences of the types of punishment administered seem to be related to later life behavior and occupational requirements.

7. Socialization is a reciprocal process, in which parental behavior is also modified by the actions of children.

8. One of the most important aspects of socialization in the nuclear family is the learning of gender roles, as a set of expected social behaviors specifically associated with one sex or the other. Research during the past decade has focused on the large number of interactive factors that contribute to our gender-role socialization, and particularly to our sex-role stereotyping. However, the nuclear family of orientation is still of prime importance in one's perceptions of gender roles.

**Key Terms**

The following terms have been introduced and defined in this chapter. Definitions also appear in the glossary.

anticipatory socialization
expressive role
gender role
identity
identity development
instrumental role
role

role performance
role prescription
sex role
significant others
socialization
social position
social status

**Discussion Questions**

1. Think about your present attitudes, values, behaviors, and perceptions. Jot down on a piece of paper the five or six that you consider most significant in your life now. How, specifically, would you say you were socialized so that the end product is what you have just jotted down? What are some of the factors, such as social class, family structure, and the like, that you think have contributed substantially to your socialization?

2. What significant values of yours differ from those of your family? What secondary agents of socialization have influenced the formation of those values?

3. Can you think of any ways that you or your siblings influenced your parents' attitudes or behaviors? Was this influence a result of your actions or your parents' anticipations?

4. How would you describe your perception of gender roles? Are you prone to sex-role stereotyping, and would you say you learned your attitudes from your nuclear family of orientation?

5. Define the following terms as they are used in this chapter: primary socialization; secondary socialization; social group; status; role; reciprocal socialization; gender-role; instrumental role; expressive role.

6. Briefly summarize Zelditch's classic study, indicating its importance for our understanding of family roles, both in the anthropological and contemporary perspectives.

**Suggested Readings**

1. Urie Bronfenbrenner. "Socialization and Social Class Through Time and Space." In Eleanor Maccoby, et al. (Eds.). *Readings in Social Psychology* (3rd ed.). New York: Holt, 1961 (pp. 400–425).

An insightful analysis of the changing nature of childrearing advice as a consequence of social processes.

2. John A. Clausen (Ed.). *Socialization and Society.* Boston: Little, Brown, 1968.

A collection of excellent papers resulting from a major conference of the Social Science Research Council on socialization by some of the most renowned psychologists and sociologists in this field.

3. Kurt Danziger. *Socialization.* Middlesex, England: Penguin, 1971.

A short, incisive review of much of the work in socialization by a British social psychologist who takes a critical stance toward the emphasis on studies in the laboratory as opposed to natural settings, and to the over concern with the static outcome of what is essentially viewed as the impact of parents on passive, receptive children.

4. Frederick Elkin and Gerald Handel. *The Child and Society: The Process of Socialization* (2nd ed.). New York: Random House, 1972.

A useful, well written introduction to a sociological analysis of the process of socialization and its social structural concomitants.

5. Melvin Kohn. *Class and Conformity: A Study in Values.* Homewood, Ill.: Dorsey, 1969.

An important book that reports on the results of three empirical studies (two in the U.S. and one in Italy) of the relationship of social class background to parental childrearing values and practices.

6. Brian Sutton-Smith and B.G. Rosenberg. *The Sibling.* New York: Holt, 1970.

A carefully thought out analysis of the effects of siblings on one another in the family, richly endowed with solid empirical evidence.

7. Michael E. Lamb (Ed.). *The Role of the Father in Child Development.* New York: Wiley, 1976.

The sorely neglected area of how important the father is in the child's socialization and social psychological development finally comes into its own. This reader is a fine beginning. Topics covered include the fatherless home, and psychological and cultural elements of the father-child relationship.

8. Erik Erikson. *Childhood and Society.* New York: Norton, 1963.

This landmark work outlines the "Eight Ages of Man" as well as reformulating Freud's basic developmental theory to include the monumental importance of society in individual development.

9. William Damon. *The Social World of the Child.* San Francisco: Jossey-Bass, 1977.

This book offers a detailed analysis of how the child develops the basic social skills, emphasizing how the child perceives his or her social relationships and interpersonal interactions.

Intimate Relationships

In the first part of this book we noted several times that the concepts of romantic love and courtship play a relatively small part, cross-culturally, in the establishment of marriages and families. In our own culture of conjugal courtship, however, love and romance are of prime importance. While in many societies marriage is a fairly impersonal arrangement, based solely on practical considerations, in our culture marriage and the establishment of a family is usually the culmination of a process that begins with the attraction of two people for each other, undergoes a period of courtship and developing intimacy, and culminates in marriage or in some other living-together arrangement.

In this part of the book we will explore in depth how and why we become intimate with another person, how love blossoms, and how we finally decide on our mate.

We will begin in chapter 4, ''Intimacy, Sexual Attraction, and Love,'' by discussing sexual attraction, the differences between liking and loving, and the process of falling in love. Some of the questions we will attempt to answer are:

- Is physical attractiveness the same as being sexually attractive? Can a physically unattractive person still be considered ''sexy''?
- When we develop an intimate relationship with another person, what factors determine whether we like the person as a friend or fall in love? What is romantic love, and how does it differ from other forms of love?

- What are the physical and psychological signs of being in love, and how does our society recognize romantic love?

After completing this discussion, we will take a broader view of a wide range of sexual activity outside the marital relationship. Some of the questions to which we will address ourselves in chapter 5, "Nonmarital Sex," are:

- What are the trends in our culture regarding premarital sexual activity? Is there, in fact, a sexual revolution?
- How are young people today making decisions about abstinence vs. permissiveness? Do males and females react differently in dating situations, and have different expectations about sex? What is the social purpose of dating?
- Is the double standard of sexual behavior still in effect, or has it become obsolete?
- What is the current thinking about masturbation? About petting? About nonnormative behaviors, such as voyeurism and fetishism?

Finally, in chapter 6, we will look at how a person chooses a mate: a permanent partner, presumably for marriage. We will see that there are many social factors that limit our choices, some of which we may not be aware of. We will also note that the choice itself is an interaction of social and psychological variables, most of which have been identified and studied. And we will answer such questions as, Do people marry likes or opposites? How does the society, overtly and covertly, tell us who we can and cannot consider as acceptable marriage partners? Who influences our choice of a mate: parents, friends, or others?

# Chapter 4

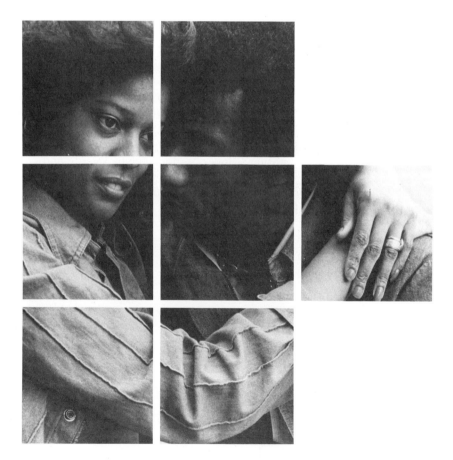

# Intimacy, Sexual Attraction, and Love

## Chapter Aims

1. To show how intimacy develops between two people and how intimacy can be the forerunner of either liking in the sense of friendship or of romantic love.

2. To discuss the social psychological dynamics and processes of interpersonal attraction and to indicate the relationship between physical attractiveness and sexual attraction.

3. To consider the meaning of romantic love and look at some of the theories of why we fall in love.

4. To examine the dating process as a part of the development of intimate relationships.

## Overview

In addition to relationships in which you had no choice, such as the relationship to your parents, there are relationships made by choice and to which both parties agree. These range from acquaintance to friendship to love. You may be attracted to people because they are physically attractive. Others may draw you through nonphysical qualities that cause you to fantasize.

This sexual attraction may bring you together and you may eventually find that you are also comfortable with each other and signs of being in love will appear. By being together, as in dating in our culture, the mystery of love may occur.

## Social Relationships

A recent discussion between two high school girls in the cafeteria of a Long Island High School went something like this:

"I don't want him to get the idea, we're 'going out' or anything. I mean we're just friends, you know. That's all. I hope he realizes that."

"But you're always going everyplace together. And neither of you is seeing anyone else."

"Yeah, I know, and I really like being with him. We have a lot of laughs together. But just as a friend, you know. I mean I could never really think of him as a boyfriend. He doesn't turn me on physically or anything. Not Ron."

Here we see an example of a male-female relationship being defined by the components of liking, friendship, and probably some degree of closeness, or intimacy. At the same time, according to what we have overheard, the relationship specifically excludes any romantic and passionate dimensions. And, this exclusion makes an important difference in defining what the boundaries of the relationship are, what the expectations of the participants should be.

Defining boundaries

Social relationships between people can assume various forms. The relationship between a parent and a child is different from the relationship between a boss and an employee, which in turn is different from the relationship between two friends. Yet they all have something in common since they are all defined as social relationships. In general, there are two things that characterize all social relationships: (1) each person in the relationship takes "into account the other in orienting significant aspects of their behavior" (Hoult 1974, p. 303) and (2) each party in the relationship can predict the behavior of the other with a fairly high degree of accuracy. A *social relationship* is an organized way of interacting between

Social relationships

the participants. Moreover, it serves important social and personal purposes, as Rose (1976, p. 85) points out:

> From the viewpoint of the interacting persons, a relationship exists when each party can accurately predict what kind of act is likely to be forthcoming from each other person. A husband knows, for example, that if he makes certain praising comments to his wife, she will respond in certain predictable ways. Without this ability to predict the response of those with whom we interact, we should find ourselves in a psychologically intolerable situation.

**Consensual relationship**

In this chapter we are going to look at consensual relationships between men and women. A *consensual relationship* is one we enter out of choice as opposed to the relationship we have with our parents and siblings, for example, or with our bosses at work. Consensual relationships include all kinds of social relationships from casual friendship to deep friendship to an intimate relationship of passionate love and romance.

A few of the questions for which we will be seeking answers in this chapter are:

1. Why are we attracted to some people and not to others?
2. Is there a difference between liking a person very much and really loving someone? How does that difference affect the social relationship?
3. What is the connection between sex and love? Does being sexually attracted to someone cause you to fall in love, or is it the other way around?
4. Is physical attractiveness a socially recognized trait? Are there ways to make oneself more attractive to others (without plastic surgery!)? What social effects does being physically attractive or unattractive have on others?
5. When we meet someone we find attractive, how do we go about developing an intimate relationship? What does intimacy actually mean in terms of how two people behave toward each other?

## Interpersonal Attraction

What attracts us to others? What are some personal qualities that contribute to social attractiveness? How important are physical chracteristics in attractiveness? Why are some physically unattractive individuals so socially successful? Are there differences between what men look for in women and what women look for in men?

These are some of the questions that have fascinated philosophers,

*Generally our culture pre-fers thin to fat, tall to short, hair to bald, and muscular to emaciated.*

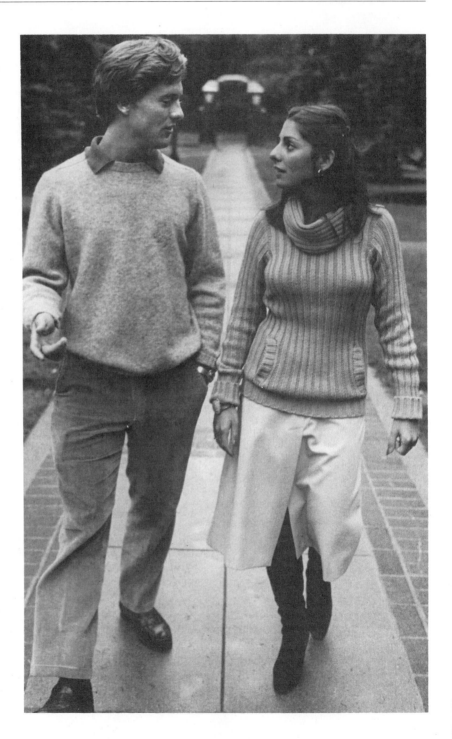

pychologists, poets, and social scientists for centuries. We now have some answers, although not all of them, to be sure, and we are on the verge of understanding the social psychological components of interpersonal attraction and how it affects social interaction.

Paired relationship

One of the more important considerations of initial interpersonal attraction, especially if it is to lead to a *paired relationship,* in which two individuals begin to function as a couple, is whether or not it is accompanied by sexual feelings. We know that we can be attracted to people in other than a sexual way. But, in the kind of paired relationships we are discussing in this book, sexual attraction is an integral component of interpersonal attraction. Sexual attraction may begin as physical attraction, but more is added to this feeling as we get to know the person, as intimacy develops. Let us consider the total process of attraction to

Sexual Stimulus Value

intimacy, along with the idea that each person has a distinct *sexual stimulus value,* that is, a quality of being able to arouse others sexually.

## Physical Attractiveness and Its Social Meaning

Although each of us is unique in the kinds of individuals we personally find attractive, evidence suggests that there are certain social norms by which physical attractiveness is judged. Given a jury of average raters looking at pictures of people, there is likely to be general agreement about who is physically attractive and who is physically unattractive. Of course, many of the subjects would fall in the middle, rated attractive by some and not attractive by others. But generally, our culture prefers thin to fat, tall to short, hair to no hair, and muscular to emaciated. There are some notable exceptions, however.

Attractiveness = status

The way we perceive others in terms of their attractiveness deeply affects the way we behave toward them, the amount of social attention we give them, and even the way we feel about them as people (Bersheid and Walster 1977). We have probably seen examples of this hundreds of times and don't need scientific studies to convince us, but research does help us understand the subtle ways that one's physical appearance affects one's social standing. Evidence generally indicates that physical attractiveness offers the individual a special social status, higher than he or she would otherwise have, whereas physical unattractiveness is a stigma that actually lowers one's social status. Some of the manifestations of this phenomenon may be surprising.

Research has shown, for example, that physical attractiveness is related to almost every facet of how we are treated by others, including social institutions as well as individuals. In one study, people who were unattractive were more likely to be perceived by clinicians as mentally disturbed than were people who were physically attractive and acting in the same way as the unattractive ones (Jones, Hansson, and Phillips 1978). In another study it was found that in simulated court cases attractive defendants fared far better with the jury than did unattractive defendants (Stephen and Tully 1977), and in the case of mock civil suits they were awarded higher sums than their unattractive counterparts. Even in traffic court, physically attractive defendants received more lenient treatment than the unattractive did (Piehl 1977). Other studies have shown that a person's status is affected by the attractiveness of the company he or she keeps: college women were rated more positively by their peers when they were seen with an attractive male partner than with an unattractive male date (Strane and Watts 1977).

So, we see the social advantages of being physically attractive or, if that is not possible, at least of being seen with someone who is. These examples help us understand why we prefer partners who are objectively physically attractive in our paired relationships to objectively physically unattractive ones. Such partners add to our own value socially. Berscheid and Walster (1974), who have conducted extensive research, suggest ''that a 'physical attractiveness' stereotype exists'' and that its content is ''What is beautiful is good'' (p. 171). This cultural stereotype, they suggest, influences our judgment and perception in several key ways.

First, we have internalized the widespread belief that only physically attractive people can be romantic and sexy. For many years, this cultural value was promulgated through movies, where heroes and heroines were always beautiful people. In recent years this has undergone dramatic change. Still, if we look through advertisements in magazines, we rarely find a Plain Jane or Plain John enticing us to buy the advertiser's product. We have come to believe that to have certain romantic feelings about someone, that person should be physically attractive.

Second, we prefer dating attractive partners because it increases our social prestige. Part of our own social status is determined by the person we are with. And to the degree that that person is viewed as physically attractive, we benefit from the association: that is, our own status increases.

There is a third important factor at work also. It is related to the other two. Physically attractive people of both sexes are expected to be more likely to possess almost every socially desirable personality trait. For example, attractive people were perceived in a study by Dion, Berscheid, and Walster (1972) to be more likely to be ''sexually warm, and responsive, sensitive, kind, interesting, strong, poised, modest, sociable and outgoing'' (p. 285) than less attractive persons. They were also expected to be more exciting dates and to have better characters than persons of

Social advantages

Beautiful = good

Attractive partners = prestige

*Physically attractive people are expected to possess almost every socially desirable personality trait.*

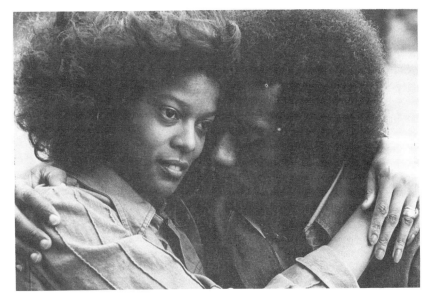

less attractiveness. Subjects also predicted that the occupations of physically attractive people would be more prestigious and that they would have happier marriages and would tend to lead more fulfilling lives in general than less attractive people. In short, when we select a physically attractive person we are, by implication, expecting to find a host of social traits that are deemed desirable.

## Sexual Stimulus Value

Sexually attractive vs. physically attractive

Physical attractiveness and sexual attraction, although related, are not exactly the same things. Some very sexually attractive people are not physically attractive. Rather, there is something about their social presence, in the way they act or cause others to feel, that makes them sexually attractive to others.

Sexual attraction, in the sense we think of it, is a unique phenomenon in the animal kingdom. Our attraction is not purely physical or chemical, although these words are sometimes used to describe a strong attraction. Rather, our attraction to others is a complex interaction of a variety of physical and psychological processes. We can better speak of sexual attraction and its relationship to the development of intimate relationships if we understand that any given person is not sexually attractive or sexually repugnant per se but holds a specific Sexual Stimulus Value (SSV) for someone else. Sexiness, like beauty, is truly in the eye of the beholder.

Sexual arousal and
fantasy

Let's begin by defining *sexual attraction* separately from physical attractiveness. We can say that sexual attraction is a bodily feeling of arousal that prompts fantasy. The type of fantasies and bodily feelings it encourages differ from person to person, from situation to situation.

Dr. Robert J. Stoller (1977), a psychiatrist at the UCLA School of Medicine, has developed a fascinating psychodynamic theory of sexual arousal that helps us better understand why we are sexually attracted to certain persons over others. Stoller says that sexual excitement is the reawakening of a scenario that has been in one's mind since childhood. This scenario allows a person to convert painful feelings to pleasureable ones, thereby resolving a psychological conflict from childhood. For example, a man may be primarily attracted to timid women, who recoil at his sexual advances. This type of woman may turn on the man because of his unconscious fear of sexually adventurous women: a fear that goes back to his childhood. The "scenario" of frightening a woman through his sexual boldness gives pleasure and produces excitement whereas the fear of an aggressive woman only brings pain.

Using Stoller's theory as a basis, we can say that a person with a high SSV is one who allows another to fantasize this scenario. Even if we examine such a fundamental phenomenon as physical attractiveness, we find that many people we consider physically attractive (as well as sexually attractive) are those who "trigger off" in our minds the most sexual fantasies, because we have been conditioned to associate physical attractiveness with sexual arousal by our cultural stereotypes. The real difference between physical attractiveness and sexiness, then, is that the former is a condition of the body, measured strictly against a cultural ideal, while the latter is an expression of the personality. A superstar may not be physically attractive but can still be very sexy.

Of course physical attractiveness can be an important element of sexiness, and to this extent sexual attraction is culturally determined. The tribesmen of Western Africa find the women with stretched protruding lips erotic, and the Nigerian women adore men whose faces have been intentionally scarred by knives. These features would probably repel a Westerner, who might not be able to find such markings sexually exciting no matter what the individual's personality. In our culture, certain types of body shapes and appearances are considered more attractive than others. Lavarakes (1975), for example, found that among American women "the medium physique is preferred over the thin upper trunk. . . or the broad lower trunk" (p. 237). In other cultures, however, the reverse is true; hefty men or broad-bottomed women are the ideal.

Sexual Stimulus Value varies in quantity; it can be manipulated by a variety of factors. Realistically, at different times different people may

Cultural norms

stimulate us with different degrees of arousal. When we care about a person, we may try to cue them about how to increase their SSV for us.

## Elaine and Andy

Elaine loves Andy, her boyfriend, and at times really gets aroused by his wavy hair and his wide, muscular shoulders. At other times she finds herself unequivocally turned on by his small bottom, which is accentuated in the tight jeans she bought him for Christmas. Once at a party, Elaine found herself turned on to Burt, the husband of one of Andy's coworkers. Burt was talking to Andy, and Elaine had a spontaneous fantasy of going to bed with him. At that moment, Andy lost his Sexual Stimulus Value for Elaine and Burt gained it.

Later that evening, Elaine noticed Burt's moustache and was turned on. As they were driving home, she asked Andy, "Why don't you grow a moustache? You would look really nice with one." Elaine was trying to increase Andy's Sexual Stimulus Value for her by adding to him some quality she found stimulating in another.

We might also say that Elaine, by encouraging Andy to change his physical appearance, was trying to increase his fantasy value for her. As Andy became more of an object for her fantasies, his Sexual Stimulus Value would become greater *for her.*

SSV = total effect

When we understand that an individual's Sexual Stimulus Value is his or her ability to prompt fantasies in another, we can see why certain people are sexually attracted to others. We tend at times to think of sexiness as an objective quality, with which all people would agree, and yet it is not objective. SSV is more than just good looks, although it includes physical appearance. It is the total effect of one person on another. Thus, we can change our SSV by changing or controlling certain things about ourselves and about the way we relate to others. With this idea in mind, let us look at five key elements that contribute to the Social Stimulus Value. Understanding these elements may help you better understand why you are attracted to certain people and why certain people are attracted to you.

Self-Confidence   Confidence is the first characteristic of Sexual Stimulus Value. Even though in the movies the shy and diffident outcast may sometimes win, in life self-confidence is usually a prerequisite for sexiness. Recently, an actress on a talk show was asked what she most liked about a leading statesman, a man she had dated before his marriage. "His confidence," she replied immediately. "Henry was always sure of what he was doing. That's a very appealing quality in a man."

*Every person is not sexually attractive or repugnant per se, but holds a specific sexual stimulus value for someone else.*

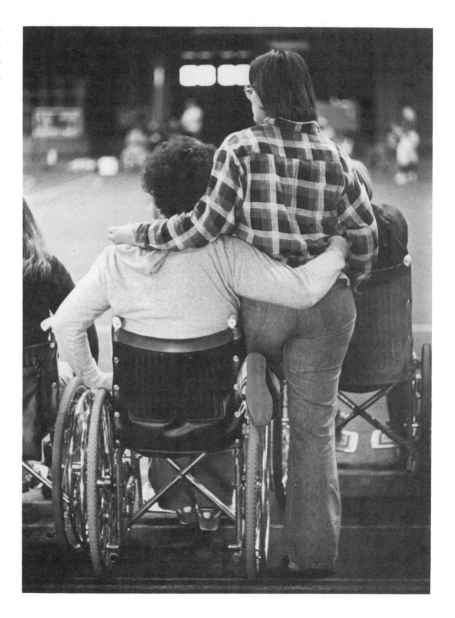

While our society emphasizes this quality in the man, confidence is just as appealing in a woman. Women express their confidence through their demeanor, through the way they relate to men and to other women. Traditionally, our culture has encouraged women to express their sexual confidence in a crude form: the "Whatever Lola Wants, Lola Gets" attitude. The pinup girl, with her confident, sexy, and smug smile, is the most debasing example of this attitude. But in recent years, as the role of women has begun to change, the way men and women express self-confidence is beginning to find a common expression.

Confidence vs. conceit

It is important to know the difference between confidence and conceit. Confidence says, in a genuine way, "I am pleased with the way I am. I am the person I want to be." Conceit, on the other hand, says, "I am better than anyone else." Confidence reveals an appreciation of self; conceit shows a disdain for others.

Power   Power, the second element of SSV, is closely related to confidence. People in higher-status positions generally enjoy a higher level of SSV than they would ordinarily have. Whatever people's physical endowments, they become much more attractive when placed in seats of power. The politician, the teacher, the boss—all of these derive as much SSV from their positions when dealing with lower-status individuals as they do from their personal presence. Just as SSV gives a person power, power gives a person SSV. The two are reciprocal.

An aphrodisiac

Public Recognition   Public recognition is the third important element. Fame is an aphrodisiac. Almost anyone recognized by the public will attract a following of sexually attracted admirers. This "celebrity complex" manifests in many strange ways. Mass murderer Richard Speck, a celebrity sociopath, has received dozens of marriage proposals in jail while serving a life sentence for the killing of eight student nurses in Chicago. Charles Manson reportedly receives more fan mail from teen-age admirers than all of the other convicts in the penitentiary put together.

Or consider Tiny Tim, the eccentric singer, as the perfect example. According to his biographer, Harry Stein (1976), this strange-looking and pathetic creature had been the butt of jokes throughout his life. Despite his strong crushes on pretty girls, he never had a single date; so repugnant was he that no one would go out with him. Then, with the sudden confirmation of celebrity status, ardent female admirers began to swarm around him with a passion. He did not change physically, he didn't have much confidence, and his power was questionable. But he was a celebrity, and that was enough. At the height of his fame, he had to hire two bodyguards to keep his women fans out of his dressing room. Such is the power of public recognition.

Because confidence, power, and public recognition are not things we ordinarily associate with sexiness, we may not be aware of why we are attracted to another person. And we may not even know that we are attracted if that person does not appear physically attractive on the surface. This lack of awareness can be a source of confusion:

**Lack of awareness**

### Jane and Jerry

Jane can't figure out her interest in Jerry, her boss, who is twenty years her senior. She's always liked him at the office—he was a good boss and the only one who treated her with respect—but she never thought of herself as the slightest bit physically attracted to him. He just wasn't her type. When Sal, her boyfriend, acted jealous about Jerry, that is, about "Mr. Vincent" as she coyly referred to him, she would laugh and say, "C'mon, Sal; he's old enough to be my father." And, she almost believed it.

But now, after they've had lunch together a few times—just friendly, she assured herself—she finds that she is experiencing feelings for him that are different from her feelings about Sal. She can't understand exactly what she is feeling and is tempted not to go out for lunch with him anymore because she is confused. In fact, Jane is experiencing a kind of sexual arousal that is far different from what she is used to experiencing with the fellows she dates. Because this feeling is new and different, it is frightening to her. What Jane doesn't recognize is that she is attracted to Jerry not because of his looks and not because they like the same music or have the same interests. She is attracted to him because of his social position as the boss, his confidence in himself, and the realization that others in the office are enviously following what's going on, or at least what they think is going on, and that attention makes Jane feel very important. Jane is attracted to the Confidence-Power-Recognition triad that Jerry offers.

If these first three elements of SSV—confidence, power, and public recognition—help us better understand why we are attracted to someone, the next two elements will help us see how we can be more attractive to others.

Showing Interest  Being an attentive, interested, responsive listener is an important part of SSV. Since sexiness means that the other person will fantasize freely and since the ability to listen contributes to this fantasizing, listening is a part of being sexy. Sexually stimulating people, especially those who are not gifted with physical attractiveness, intuitively know this. They have learned to "socially seduce" others with a quality called *empathy*. Empathy means listening to others and experiencing their feelings with them. It is seeing things from the other person's frame of reference. Since we can learn to listen to others, showing interest is one way of increasing our SSV. It is based on the simple principle that we find people we can talk to freely attractive and interesting (Belser 1977):

*Empathy*

### Peggy

Peggy is having trouble with Dick, her fiancé. As the wedding date approaches, they are both getting the jitters, and neither is really sure if they should go through with it. At work, Peggy has been talking to Vern about her feelings. Vern is always willing to listen to her, and she finds that she is beginning to express things to him that she can't talk to Dick about. Through her talks with Vern she begins to better understand the way she is feeling. The other night she had a very erotic dream about Vern and couldn't help giggling when she saw him at work. When he asked what was funny she told him, since he was her confidante, and that set the process in motion by which they ultimately became lovers. Vern's ability to listen enabled Peggy to discover how sexually attractive she found him and, at the same time, to find out that she was almost going to marry the wrong man.

Gentleness  Gentleness, a quality often ignored in our culture, is also a key part of SSV. No matter what one's public image is, no matter how rough and tough one comes across, the quality of gentleness shows strength and confidence: it shows the willingness to give to another. It takes a strong person to be gentle. And, when we encounter gentleness in another, it may actually produce a physical effect, a tenderness that recalls primitive feelings about mother-love.

*Gentleness = strength*

# From Attraction to Love

Of course, being physically and sexually attracted to someone doesn't mean that we will fall in love with them. Sexual attraction is only one part of what moves us into loving relationships. Many other factors come into play when we speak about what love means and examine how and why love develops.

First, we should recognize at the outset that romantic love and friendship are culturally defined *roles* which are learned through the socialization process. Whatever the biological and psychological bases for love and friendship are, it is the culture that defines the roles through which these bases are expressed socially. In other words, we learn to interpret our feelings and perceptions about someone as *romance* or as *friendship;* as *love* or as *liking.* In fact, many cultures have no word equivalents for our "romance" or "friendship" because they do not ascribe to such roles; that is, individuals do not interpret their feelings as romantic. In our contemporary culture, however, the very opposite is true. Elaine Walster (1976) points out, "In America . . . individuals are encouraged to interpret many emotional as well as sexual feelings as love" (p. 83).

The concept of romantic love has evolved through many different definitions. A matrix of social and economic factors has been shown to influence how love is defined culturally. It has been suggested that the concept of romantic love flourishes in modern, industrialized societies, where residential migration and promising financial prospects make romance a useful invention (Theodorson 1965). For the Ancient Greeks, on the other hand, love was largely homosexual, serving an important purpose militarily. For clarity, we will focus our discussion on romantic love as compared to liking and friendship. An appropriate place to begin is with the work of Zick Rubin.

# Rubin's Studies

One of the more interesting investigations of what romantic love is, how it relates to attraction, and how it differs from liking was undertaken by Zick Rubin (1973), who investigated the differences between romantic love and liking. According to Rubin, *romantic love* is an attitude a person holds toward a particular other individual and it has three components: *attachment,* or needing; *caring,* or giving; and *intimacy,* a close bond or link between two people. *Liking* has two fundamental dimensions: *affection,* experienced as emotional warmth and closeness, and *respect,* which is liking based on another person's admirable characteristics, such as intelligence, competence, and trustworthiness.

Rubin's self-report scales

Rubin devised two 13-item self-report scales to measure the concepts of romantic love and liking and predicted that there would be at least a moderate correlation between them. His love scale included such items as "If I were lonely, my first thought would be to seek _____ out''; "I would do almost anything for _____''; and "I feel I can confide in _____ about virtually anything.'' The liking scale includes such items as: "I have great confidence in _____'s good judgment'' and "I feel that _____ is an extremely intelligent person'' (p. 216).

Rubin administered these two scales to 182 dating couples at the University of Michigan. The subjects were asked not to sit near their partners and to answer both scales, first with respect to their dating partner and later with respect to a close friend of the same sex as they were. For each item, the respondents were to indicate how much they agreed or disagreed by placing a check on a scale ranging from "not at all sure; disagree completely'' through "moderately true; agree to some extent'' to "definitely true; agree completely.''

As predicted, there was a moderate correlation between the love and liking scores. It was also found that, whereas the average love scores of men for their girlfriends and women for their boyfriends were almost identical, women *liked* their boyfriends significantly more than they were liked in return.

To no one's surprise, the students reported loving their partners much more than their friends. As table 4.1 shows, men and women had almost identical scores for liking same-sex friends, but women reported greater love toward same-sex friends than did men. Rubin points out that this difference is consistent with our cultural stereotype that women express more love toward each other than men do.

Table 4.1
**Average Love and Liking Scores for Dating Partners and Same-Sex Friends**

|                     | Women | Men   |
|---------------------|-------|-------|
| Love for partner    | 90.57 | 90.44 |
| Liking for partner  | 89.10 | 85.30 |
| Love for friend     | 64.79 | 54.47 |
| Liking for friend   | 80.21 | 78.38 |

Source: *Liking and Loving: An Invitation to Social Psychology* by Zick Rubin; p. 221. Copyright © 1973 by Holt, Rinehart and Winston, Inc. Reprinted by permission of Holt, Rinehart and Winston.

Women's friendships

Evidence from surveys suggests that women's friendships tend to be more intimate, involving more spontaneous joint activities and exchanging of confidences than do men's. The man's role in our culture may limit the ability to love. "Loving for men may often be channeled into a single opposite-sex relationship, whereas women may be more able to experience and express attachment, caring, and intimacy in other relationships as well" (Rubin 1973, p. 221).

Rubin's work has been duplicated often, and the results generally borne out, especially the validity of his scale (Dion and Dion, 1977). These studies help us understand better how love differs from liking, but they still do not fully answer two basic questions: what love is and why we make the transition from sexual attraction to love?

## The Signs of Love

Being in love

We all recognize that being in love can cause even the most stable, predictable, and logical person to act strangely. Love has its own internal "language": its own way of inspiring us, of motivating us, of changing the predictable course of our behavior. Literature is full of examples of lovers whose behavior ranged from the bizarre to the fantastic—all because of the intense feelings of love they experienced. And, from our own experiences, we probably realize the effect that being in love has upon us personally.

Physical signs

Much has been written on the different signs of being in love. Love affects us in many ways. We know that it can, and usually does, have a physical effect as well as a psychological one. "Some of the physical signs," Freid (1975, p. 4) points out, "include: changes in equilibrium and body language; flying sensations and mild dizziness; increased anxiety; preoccupations with fantasy, often at the expense of what is happening in the "real world."

Some people can't eat when they fall in love; they lose their appetites. Others become absolutely gluttonous, eating as never before. Specific physical changes in heartbeat, blood pressure, pulse, respiration, and perspiration level have also been recorded in the presence of the one we love or while thinking about that person. Stanley Schachter and J. E. Singer (Schachter and Singer, 1962) have proposed a two-factor theory of emotion, which Walster and Berscheid think may be helpful in explaining passionate love and its effects upon us. It is also helpful in understanding why we think of a certain state as the state of being in love.

This theory says that whenever we experience an emotion, two factors determine our reaction: our physiological arousal and the way in which we label the emotional state. In other words, if we are given a drug secretly in a cigarette we are smoking and it makes us feel slightly dizzy and unable to think clearly, this is a marked physical change. Now somebody says to us, ''I just slipped some wonderful marijuana in your cigarette and you are experiencing a high.'' You might then interpret these physical feelings as pleasant and high. But if someone says, ''I think you just smoked some contaminated tobacco,'' these very same physical feelings might be iterpreted in an opposite way: ''Help, I'm sick.''

### Two-factor Theory of Love

What does this theory have to do with love? Walster and Berscheid suggest that the same two components are necessary for a passionate experience: arousal and interpretation. They suggest, for example, that negative experiences are effective in inducing love because they intensify one's physiological arousal; that is, they cause such reactions as rapid breathing, heart palpitations, nervous tremors, and flushing. Jealousy, anxiety, guilt, loneliness, hatred, fear, and confusion all increase one's physiological arousal and thus intensify one's emotional experience. If, because of particular circumstances, the person attributes his or her agitated state to passionate love, he or she will then experience love.

In other words, any factor that increases one's level of physiological arousal or one's tendency to label one's arousal as love would intensify the amount of passion one experiences. This idea received some support in a study in which experimenters told male subjects they would receive painful electric shocks, thus arousing fear in them. Those subjects were more attracted to a young girl whom they were subsequently introduced to than were men in the control condition who were not told to expect shocks and who were, therefore, not aroused (Brehm et al. 1974). The experimenters concluded that fear, although irrelevant to the emotion of liking, facilitated the attraction that could ultimately lead to love.

### Eye Contact and Body Language

Zick Rubin's findings, along with much other evidence, indicate that eye contact and body language speak boldly of our feelings of love, liking, and sexual attraction. To check the validity of his love scale, Rubin measured the amount of time the couples spent looking into each other's eyes, since eye contact has been shown to provide a channel through which intimate feelings can be directly expressed (Goffman 1963). He invited dating couples who had previously completed the questionnaire to take part in a laboratory experiment. While they sat across a table from one another waiting for the experiment to begin, they were observed through a one-way mirror. Rubin tested only those couples in which, based on their test scores, both partners were rated as ''strong lovers'' or in which both were rated as "weak lovers." The results clearly indicated that the strong lovers made significantly more eye contact than did the weak lovers. Moreover, they were much more likely to look at one another simultaneously and to gaze romantically into each others' eyes.

In addition to eye contact, many other forms of body language have been shown to be related to the expression of liking, love, and intimacy. Fast (1977) has pointed out a wide range of body signals that members of pairs send to each other. He uses the term *courting signal* to describe the body language messages sent out by members of the pair as feelings of intimacy begin to develop. The term *gender signal* differentiates between body language more common to the man and body language more common to the woman. The term *courting gender signals* describes how each sex approaches the other. These body signals are so specific, according to Fast (pp. 19–20), that they can actually communicate the type of relationship expected: liking, friendship, or romantic love.

**Courting gender signals**

> The most obvious gesture for a woman is the lifted hand that pushes back the hair from the face or rearranges it above the ears. It's a flirtatious gesture, and it spells femininity. The equivalent in the man is the unconscious adjustment of the tie. Watch a man who has just been introduced to an attractive woman. Within the first five minutes, you can often count three of four preening gestures: touching the tie or the jacket lapels, straightening the creases in the pants. . . .
>
> Showing the palm of the hand is a feminine gesture, usually associated with courting, but like any courting gesture, showing the palm can also be used when sex is not involved. Qualifiers turn off the sexual implication and leave only the "I want to be friends" impact.
>
> The qualifiers that turn off a courting signal, that modify or contradict it, can be gestures as simple as twisting a wedding ring. Or the context of the courting gesture can alter its meaning. Watch any woman in politics as she gives a speech; chances are you'll see her show her palms to "court" the audience in body language.

We see then that there are clear physical signs of love and liking both internal and external, and that these signs help the individual and the other member of the pair understand messages that are perhaps more easily spoken without words. Cultural influences play an important part in the development of a "language of love," by cueing us on how to translate the signals another person sends us. We see this not only in sexual signals, but in other messages (aggression, caution) that have no sexual meanings.

Studies by Walster and Berscheid (1971) ''demonstrate that physical arousal is a crucial component of love, and that fear, pain, frustration, delight and sexual gratification can all deepen the passionate experience under certain conditions'' (p. 62). What are these conditions? What causes us to label these feelings as love? Walster and Bersheid show that our culture encourages people to interpret a wide variety of feelings as love. If we are emotionally aroused and the romantic cues are there, we are likely to call these feelings love. This propensity may account for the

Summer romances

large number of summer romances that bloom under a full moon in a beautiful country setting, in which love is the socially acceptable feeling only to fade when the romantic cues are gone and one is back in one's everyday surroundings. Then, too, individuals who think of themselves as romantic are more likely to label their feelings as love than would an unromantic hard-to-catch bachelor, for example.

### Romeo and Juliet Effect

The Romeo and Juliet theory that emotional arousal can intensify feelings of love may help to explain why parental opposition to a romance often succeeds in fanning the flames of

Parental interference

love. Driscoll, Davis, and Lipetz (1972) set out to see whether parental opposition may increase a couple's love for each other. They termed this the *Romeo and Juliet effect* after Shakespeare's famous play, in which a family feud forces the lovers to choose between family loyalty and love, a dilemma that serves only to intensify the lovers' feelings for one another. The investigators gave dating couples in Boulder, Colorado, a questionnaire that measured the intensity of their love for each other and the amount of parental interference they had experienced. Parental interference, as perceived by the partners, was correlated with the intensity of love reported by the dating couples on a scale similar to the Rubin scale. This finding supports what many have long suspected: that parental attempts to break up a romance may only succeed in intensifying it.

### Conceptions of Love

Philosophers, poets, theologians, psychologists, sociologists, as well as almost everyone, has at one time or another pondered the meaning of love, particularly if one has experienced some of the feelings described above, that is, if one has felt ''in love.'' Philosophers constructed elaborate systems to differentiate love from the other feelings and to place it in a perspective. Social scientists have concerned themselves more with trying to put together all the evidence in order to arrive at a functional definition of love, which would help us understand its social purpose, and an interactional definition, which would describe it in terms of the symbolic behaviors of the participants.

The ancient Greeks, a passionate people, were obsessed with love: in their theatre, in their poetry, in their philosophy, and in their religion. They named one of their three basic gods *Eros,* the word for love, indicating the fundamentalness of love in life. Much of their writing about Eros reflects their belief that ''love leads men to doom,'' underlying their theory of tragedy. From its very beginnings, Greek culture has used language to differentiate among different types of love. They distinguished, for instance, between homosexual passionate love and heterosexual passionate love, between love in friendships and love for family members, between love of country and love of knowledge. They used the term *Eros* to refer to all the passionate, romantic types of love and the word *Philia* for the loves based on fondness, friendship, or respect. These would be roughly equivalent to our distinction between loving and liking.

Contemporary commentators have gone well beyond making simple philosophical distinctions, but still primary is the difference between passionate or romantic love and other forms of love such as friendship or love for brothers and sisters or parental love. In other words, we still recognize that a key element in defining love is whether or not passion is a part of it.

Reiss (1971), among others, uses the term *courtship love* to differentiate what the Greeks called *Eros* from what they called *Philia.* Courtship love, he points out, is ''an intense emotional feeling developing from a primary relationship involving a single male and female and consisting of rights and duties similar to husband and wife.'' The key here is (1) that there is an intense emotional feeling and (2) that courtship love is a marriage-directed paired relationship. Most other sociologists and psychologists, although they may differ on details, would go along with this. Romantic love involves intense feelings and fantasies of a permanent relationship.

**Courtship love**

## Why Do We Fall in Love?

**Need fulfillment and love**

We may intuitively recognize that an important part of why we become involved in a paired relation is that we are looking to the other person to fulfill many of our needs. When the other person is able to perform that function, we find a satisfying relationship; when the other person is not, we find ourselves in a frustrating relationship. But in trying to understand what needs are being satisfied and how we go about satisfying them, there are differences among theories about why and how we fall in love. In order to maintain a balanced perspective, let us survey briefly the concepts of need-fulfillment and love from three theoretical viewpoints.

## The Psychoanalytic Position

We mentioned in the preceding chapter that our first socializing experience in life is with our mother, by whom our original needs are satisfied. Psychoanalysts, especially, look back on that relationship in trying to understand how we go about finding someone to satisfy our needs and why we choose the people that we do. Their theory (with variations, of course) is this: *we repeat our early experiences throughout life.* If we had a satisfying relationship with our mother, we develop satisfying relationships with others later in life. But if our early relationship was disappointing and frustrating, we tend to repeat this disappointment and frustration throughout life. This phenomenon is called the *repetition compulsion.*

Repetition compulsion

The psychoanalytic viewpoint attempts to account for the unhealthy aspects of why we fall in love as well as the healthy reasons. As Dr. Edrita Freid (1975) points out, it is recognized by psychotherapists that many neurotic people constantly seek relationships "that gradually fill them with depression, despair, and a sense of doom." She goes on to point out (p. 173),

Unhealthy aspects

> In particular, they get sexually and emotionally entangled again and again in identical or similar problem situations. Such episodes usually have similar beginnings, middles, and endings; first, there is considerable infatuation with a partner who appears very special and from whom extraordinary satisfactions are expected. Gradually, dissatisfaction and hostility creep into the relationship, and eventually there are either fantasies of a more ideal mate or actual separation. . . . Sooner or later, a new infatuation will arise with full intensity.

If this pattern looks familiar to you, there is an explanation for it. According to Dr. Freid and the psychoanalysts, it is caused by the repetition of unsatisfying childhood experiences. "One of the chief problems," she explains, "that propels such persons into ruts in sexuality and love is their extraordinary impoverishment as far as their feelings, thoughts, defenses, [and] sexual excitations are concerned. *They run always to the same type of mate and type of love because such a choice represents the only one that the[ir] impoverished psyche permits*" (Freid 1975, p. 206, italics in original).

## The Humanistic Position

Of course, there are other, more positive, ways of looking at our needs and specifically how we seek the fulfillment of these needs through falling in love. The psychoanalytic position emphasizes only the early-life needs and even those on a rather basic level. On the other hand, what we call the humanistic position presents a more diversified view of needs and will perhaps serve us better in understanding why we fall in love and what needs are being met by doing so.

Self-actualization

Its main emphasis is on *self-actualization,* the complete fulfillment of our potentiality, a fulfillment accompanied by a feeling of satisfaction and personal self-worth. The humanist says that we fall in love with people who help us self-actualize. The two main proponents of this humanistic position are Carl R. Rogers and Abraham H. Maslow.

## Rogers' View

Rogers says that there are two universal needs: the need for *positive regard* and the need for *self-regard.* The need for positive regard develops as awareness of the self emerges early in an individual's life. This need leads the individual to desire acceptance and love from the important people in his or her life. They may accept him or her conditionally ("I will love you only if you do this or that . . ."), or they may accept the person unconditionally ("I will love you no matter

Figure 4.1
**Maslow's Hierarchy of Needs**

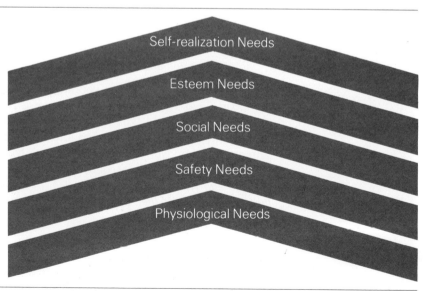

Source: Abraham H. Maslow, "A theory of motivation," in Motivation and Personality, 2nd ed. (New York: Harper and Row, 1970).

what.''), as he or she is, offering what Rogers calls *unconditional positive regard*. The person needs positive regard not only from others but from himself or herself as well.

The need for self-regard develops out of self-experiences associated with the satisfaction of, or frustration of, the need for positive regard. If a person experiences only unconditional positive regard, his or her self-regard would also be unconditional. Such a state represents genuine psychological adjustment and full functioning.

Most people, unfortunately, do not achieve such ideal adjustment. Inevitably, the child's need to retain the love of his or her parents conflicts with his or her individual needs. When this conflict occurs, according to Rogers, children begin to avoid or to deny completely the experiences that they have learned are not worthy of positive regard and try to be what they think the parents want them to be. This reaction can then affect the kind of people we fall in love with later in life.

## Betty

Betty's problem is that no matter whom she falls in love with, she always feels unworthy of the person. She reasons that the lover will tire of her and reject her eventually, so she provokes this. Relationships never work out for her because she is jealous, possessive, and untrusting of men. She cannot believe that anyone she loves can love her in return. This is because she doesn't feel worthy of love; she has a poor (inaccurate) self-image.

Rogers believes that defenses result in rigid and inaccurate perceptions, and, thus, serve as crippling restrictions on self-actualization. They prevent us from truly knowing ourselves and expressing our complete potential.

Maslow's View   Maslow believed that in every individual there is an innate will toward health, an impulse toward growth or toward the actualization of human potential. Our behavior is goal-directed. Human nature is essentially good; whenever we are unhappy or neurotic, it is because we have distorted our thinking.

Maslow suggests that human beings have different kinds of needs that are ordered in a hierarchy (see figure 4.1), with certain basic needs that must be satisfied before other, higher-level, needs can emerge. At the bottom of the hierarchy are the basic physiological drives that must be gratified in order for the person to survive. When these needs are met, the need for safety and security emerges. Once we feel safe and secure in

Impulse toward
growth

our surroundings, we try to satisfy the need for love and belonging; for affectionate relations with people; for being with our own group, our home, our family. The need for esteem comes next, the need for a stable, firm, positive evaluation of ourselves, a need for self-respect, achievement, adequacy, and mastery. Then, at the top of the list is self-actualization, the highest goal of all. This represents the need to be all that we can be, to be true to our nature, to accept ourselves as we are. When all our lower needs are met, we can satisfy our aesthetic needs: for justice, goodness, beauty, order, unity. These needs are called *metaneeds,* and when they are met, Maslow says, we rejoice in the experience of living; we have made the most of our abilities and have become all we are capable of being.

**Metaneeds**

The humanistic view offers some valuable insights about why we fall in love with one person rather than another. According to this view, ideally we find partners who help us self-actualize, who help us fulfill our potential in life. This view also helps account for some of the differences in individual and social-class variation. A very poor person may fall in love with someone who brings home a weekly paycheck because this meets the basic security needs, near the bottom of the hierarchy. But someone who is at a self-actualizing state may seek a person who meets needs of a much higher level, such as the need for goodness and order, because that is the level of need functioning this person is trying to achieve. In other words, we seek individuals who meet the needs at the level at which we personally are functioning.

## Social Psychological Positions

Sociologists and social psychologists have proposed many valuable insights into why we fall in love. Albert Bandura (1969) suggests that loving is a *modeled behavior;* that is, we are behaviorally and emotionally following the examples of significant others early in our lives. We learn, from our very early years, that being in love is an accepted symbol of adulthood (or, at first, of adolescence) and therefore fall in love partly because it is expected of us and partly because it confers a higher status on us. Whenever we repeatedly observe such behaviors in others, even if there is no reinforcement or reward associated with the behaviors, these observed behaviors become ''a potent source for social learning'' (Brody, Lahey, and Combs 1978).

**Modeled behavior**

Moreover, according to the modeling viewpoint, the very process of falling into love, the stages and signs, can be modeled after what we have seen at home, in the movies, and in all our surroundings (Ryan 1977). The behaviors we exhibit, as well as the feelings we experience, are learned by observing others going through the same process. So, we not only fall in love because of modeling, but modeling also explains why we experience what we do when we fall in love.

## Lydia

Lydia sits at the dinner table, stares blankly into her plate, thoughtlessly mushes her food with her fork, and thinks intently of Jose, the boy she is in love with. "Eat or you'll be a skeleton," her concerned mother tells her, while her older sister, Joy, tries to talk to her to find out about what she and Jose have been "up to." Lydia doesn't remember, but four years earlier Joy was in love for the first time and did the same things at the dinner table. In fact, during the past five years Lydia has had countless opportunities to watch Joy as she fell in and out of love with one boy after another, so by this point Lydia not only knows what it means to be in love but she also has an idea of how one acts when one is in love.

Wheel theory of love

Another social psychological theory that has enjoyed much attention is Ira Reiss's (1960) *wheel theory of falling in love,* as shown in figure 4.2. This is a developmental theory that conceptualizes the process of falling in love as a number of connected stages. It conceives the wheel of falling in love as a circular process, which can wind either way: that is, you can fall in love or out of love, in each case going through the same developmental stages, but in different directions.

At first, the dating couple experiences rapport, a feeling of being at ease, of being able to speak freely to each other, of empathic understanding. They are now experiencing something more than just attraction; they are comfortable with each other. If rapport is not there, they feel awkward and uncomfortable, and the wheel on which the relationship is driven is not likely to turn for them. But if rapport does exist, the relationship takes an important turn and the couple enters the next phase, self-revelation, where they are more open with each other, telling each other more intimate details of their lives, their private feelings, and more honestly how they feel about one another and what they expect from the relationship. This phase of self-revelation is accompanied by new feelings of trust and intimacy, which are the beginnings of love.

As they begin to spend more time with each other, the come to depend on each other more: for support, for companionship, even for verification of their perceptions of others and themselves. This mutual dependence upon one another facilitates the creation of an atmosphere in

Figure 4.2
**Reiss's Wheel Theory of the Development of Love**

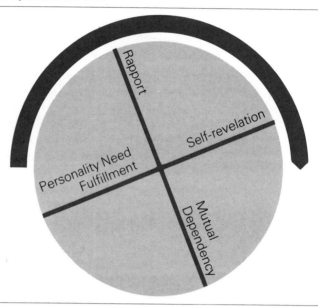

Source: Reiss (1960).

**Need fulfillment**

which they learn to fulfill each other's needs, both similar and divergent. It is at this point, on Reiss's wheel, that their feelings of rapport have now fully blossomed into love.

## Inclusion and Exclusion

One last point, not included in Bandura's or Reiss's formulations, may help us better understand an important social aspect of falling in love. This is part of a theory of intimacy as social exclusion developed by Sasha R. Weitman (1976). It is based on the premise that in the process of falling in love we include one other person more in our world as we exclude others. The paired love relationship is an isolating relationship in the sense that it says to others, ''We two exist more closely, more intimately *together* than we do with anyone else in the world.''

**Intimacy as social exclusion**

Weitman (1976, pp. 221–22) cites this implicit message as the reason that expressions of intimacy are universally concealed from others:

> The fundamental reason for this universal tendency on the part of human beings to hide in order to give rein to their intense affection is out of a deep recognition that one unmistakable meaning

of intimacies to those who witness them but are not privileged to partake in them is that they are excluded from the bond of affection being cultivated in their presence. . . . Public intimacies, then, are best understood not only as acts of gratification of the love between two people but also as gestures of exclusion unequivocally (even if unintentionally) communicated to all those present.

As two people in the process of developing a paired relationship become more intimate with each other, there are social pressures to express this intimacy privately rather than in public. These pressures move their romantic-bound behavior forward by forcing them into closer private proximity to each other.

Social prelude to mate selection

The process through which the two individuals develop this intimate, paired relationship, in which others become excluded from their intimate dyad, is called *dating*. Dating behavior is primarily defined by the culture. It almost always reflects recreational activities and natural affiliations among the young and what are viewed as necessary conditions for developing the intimacy that leads to permanent attachments. Let us examine the dating process in greater detail to see how dating serves to facilitate intimate, loving relationships in our contemporary American society.

## Dating

Dating comprises conventions that allow the individual to attract, interact with, and possibly initiate sexual relations with persons of the opposite sex. Dating, which allows the progression from liking to loving, is the social prelude to mate selection. The choice of a dating partner, moreover, is a clear instance of how the individual is affected by a host of social forces. If we begin by looking at how we choose *whom* to date it will help us better understand the entire dating process.

### How Do We Choose Whom to Date?

What, in addition to physical attractiveness and sexual attraction, influences our initial choice of whom to date? In a classic study of the dating preferences of college students in the 1930s, Willard Waller proposed a model that is still widely used today. His model, which is called the *rating and dating complex*, suggests that people make choices of whom to date based on external, prestige factors, such as physical attractiveness, wealth, ownership of a car, social popularity, or other status objects, such as fashionable clothing or knowing how to dance.

Rating and dating complex

While subsequent studies have challenged the exclusivity of Waller's scheme, it is generally true that prestige factors are important when people make decisions about whom to date. Hansen (1977), for example, in a recent study, found that students still perceived these prestige characteristics as most important, at least on a questionnaire. When it came down to selecting their own dates, personality characteristics assumed importance too. Hansen also found a racial difference in dating preferences. "White students, in general, placed more value on internal or personality characteristics of an individual; whereas black students place more value on external characteristics" (p. 137). The reason for this difference is not clearly understood and needs to be investigated further. It may well be related to Kohn's (1969) study of social-class differences in childrearing (see Chapter 10), with Hansen's white students appearing similar to Kohn's middle-class youth and Hansen's black students aligned with Kohn's working-class subjects.

Other important principles of date selection will be discussed in detail in chapter 6, "Mate Selection," where we will explore the complex of factors that affect our choice of a permanent partner.

## What Does Dating Accomplish?

Dating serves the multiple functions of recreation, socialization of cross-gender relationships, status enhancement, and potential mate selection.

Gender-role identity

Another major function of the dating process and of many specific dating behaviors is the further development and clarification of one's gender-role identity. Previously learned gender identities, from the nuclear family of orientation, take on new importance when boys and girls begin to assume adult social roles through dating.

Stereotyped role differences

Because these gender roles have been (and still are) often narrowly and stereotypically defined and viewed as mutually exclusive, there arise a number of problems during the adolescent years. For example, until recently girls have not generally been allowed the socially permissible outlets, such as boxing or football, for expressing aggression that are opened more readily to boys. Although the basis of this difference in aggressive behavior is cultural—that is, it is learned and not inborn—it holds true throughout almost all societies. In extensive cross-cultural research, Rohner (1976) found that "young boys the world over tend to be somewhat more aggressive than the same-aged girls," although this difference tends to decrease as children reach adolescence. Rohner emphasizes that the level of aggressive behavior displayed by both sexes is not innate, but the result "of experience, especially [socially learned] pressures shared by children within individual social systems around the world (p. 61).

*A major issue for girls in gender role identity is finding socially acceptable outlets for aggression.*

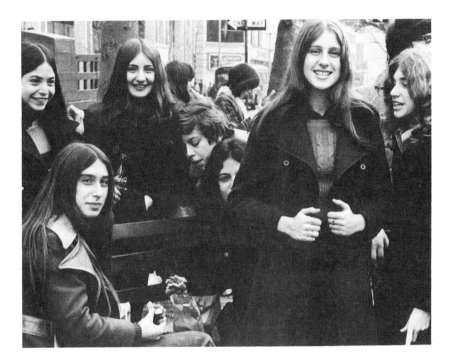

Still, the difference may cause problems. For instance, it reinforces stereotyped role differences. "The problem for the girl," Konopka (1966, p. 121) points out "is the fact that since aggression in itself is considered bad, it is forbidden to her." She goes on to suggest that, "the ideal image of the girl is still 'sugar and spice'." The process of gender-role identification for the boy may also lead to a variety of conflicts, different than the girl's but just as severe. For example, boys are exposed to more social pressure against openly expressing many of the feelings that girls are allowed to express freely. Specifically, it is expected that boys will not display publicly their "softer" side, such as the overt expression of love, sorrow, or pity, which are considered feminine feelings. Boys are discouraged from crying in public. This reticence of expression may have serious consequences in dating and in the development of intimate attachments, where the boy may be less able to express intimate and tender feelings than can his girlfriend.

It could be argued that successful dating helps young boys and girls, who are separated by these role expectations, come to understand each other better. This process can be explained by *social exchange theory*. This theory says that people maintain social relationships when the rewards are greater than what they have to forfeit, when the benefits are greater than the costs. In dating, boys and girls may each have to give

Social exchange theory

Figure 4.3
**Adolescent Dating Intimacy**

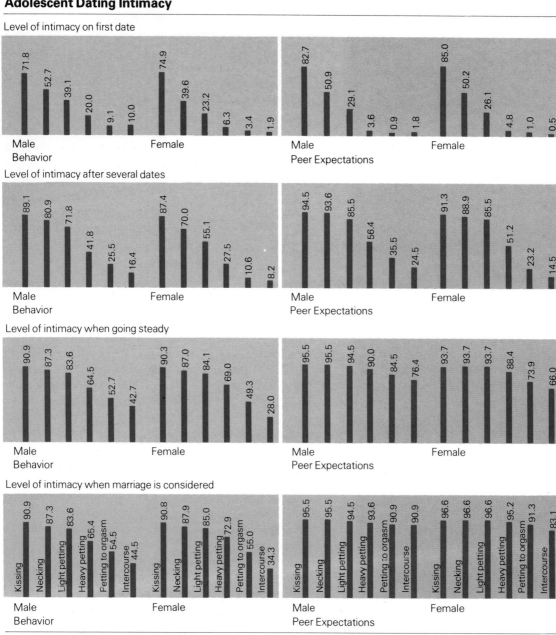

Level of intimacy on first date

Level of intimacy after several dates

Level of intimacy when going steady

Level of intimacy when marriage is considered

Source: Collins (1974, p. 321, Table 1)

something up, but they each gain something at the same time. For instance, in one interesting study, Collins (1974) shed some light on how dating works and we can see how this relates to social exchange theory (see figure 4.3). Collins found that through the dating process, boys and girls tried to reach some compromise between their different perspectives at the time they began to date. They each gave something up but received something in return. Boys, according to Collins's study, approach "the relationship from a pronounced psychobiological orientation," meaning simply that their minds are focused very much on satisfying their sexual needs. The boy goes into the relationship with sex in the front of his mind. Girls, on the other hand, begin "from an initial psycho-affectional position," meaning that they are seeking affection, love, intimacy, and rapport. She is looking for something deeper than simply a physical relationship. Through the dating sequence, if it is successful, they reach a point where the needs of both are satisfied. The boy develops affectionate feelings for the girl and she in turn engages in sexual activity with him. They have made an exchange in which both benefit and find pleasure.

## Summary

1. Interpersonal attraction consists of more than just physical attractiveness. In our society physically attractive people enjoy greater prestige and more social privileges than do unattractive people. However, a more important quality in paired interpersonal relationships is the Sexual Stimulus Value one individual holds for another.

2. Sexual attraction involves both the physical feeling of arousal and a psychological stimulation to fantasize. The Sexual Stimulus Value (SSV) one person holds for another is determined by the ability of that person to initiate physical and psychological arousal in the other person. There are various components of SSV: self-confidence, social power, public recognition, interest in the other person's world (empathy), and gentleness.

3. Sexual attraction may instigate a relationship but is not in itself enough to transform a relationship into the dimensions of intimacy and love. Zick Rubin investigated the differences between liking and romantic love and found that the latter involves attachment, caring, and intimacy, while the former comprises mostly affection and respect. Using specially constructed scales, he found that liking could be clearly differentiated from romantic love and that there were significant gender-related differences between college men and women who were respondents in this study.

4. When we are ''in love,'' there are demonstrable physical signs. Changes in appetite, interest, and in many areas of biological functioning may occur. We tend to have more direct eye contact with the person we love, and our body language changes noticeably with that person. Stanley Schachter and J. E. Singer's two factor theory suggests that some of these physical changes tell us we are in love, as we learn through our socialization to interpret them that way.

5. Sometimes parental pressure against a developing relationship can actually have the effect of making us feel that we love the other person more. This is known as the Romeo and Juliet effect.

6. There are several theories on why we fall in love. The psychoanalytic position emphasizes the repetition of early-life emotional experiences. The humanistic position views love as part of our pattern of need-fulfillment and suggests that as we love we are self-actualizing, developing ourselves to our fullest potential. Love has also been conceptualized as modeled behavior. Reiss's ''wheel theory'' sees falling in or out of love as a series of connected stages.

7. The dating process is a socially defined path for developing an intimate relationship. Dating allows boys and girls, who may have sharply different attitudes, to find a common ground for mutual respect and love.

8. Dating serves several functions, among which are recreation, socialization of cross-gender relationships, status enhancement, and potential mate selection.

## Key Terms

The following terms have been introduced and defined in this chapter. Definitions also appear in the glossary.

consensual relationship
courtship love
dating
empathy
Eros
liking
metaneed
modeled behavior
paired relationship
Philia
positive regard
rating and dating complex
repetition compulsion

romantic love
Romeo and Juliet Effect
self-actualization
self-regard
sexual attraction
Sexual Stimulus Value
social exchange theory
social relationship
unconditional positive regard
wheel theory of falling in love

## Discussion Questions

1. How important has your interpersonal attractiveness been to you. Think of some specific examples of where your being perceived as either attractive or unattractive acted as a help or hindrance in some social interaction.

2. The concept of Social Stimulus Value considerably expands our limited view of attractiveness as being a purely physical attribute. What *nonphysical* qualities of yours and of those to whom you are attracted would best illustrate the broad concept of SSV? Particularly, do you see some of your nonphysical qualities as contributing to your sexiness?

3. Using Rubin's distinction between loving and liking and some of the signs of love we discussed, describe your own "love reaction." Then consider if you had any difficulty distinguishing between whether you liked or really loved someone. Was it difficult to know whether the feelings were romantic and sexual or nonsexual and platonic?

4. Do you know of anyone whose romantic relationship was influenced by the Romeo and Juliet effect? What ultimately happened to the couple, and how important do you think the parental interference proved? How would you feel and act if your parents insisted you stop dating someone you felt you loved?

5. What is love? This is a question that has puzzled philosophers, poets, and social scientists from the beginnings of time. Try to outline how you personally define love. What are some different types of love *you* have experienced, such as friendship, parental love, or romantic love, and how do they differ from each other? Which theory of why we fall in love discussed in the chapter would best account for your personal experiences?

6. From your reading of this chapter, how would you describe the social dimension of physical attractiveness? What, specifically, has the research indicated about the status and role of physically attractive people and how they are perceived by others?

**Suggested Readings**

1. Ellen Berscheid and Elaine Walster. *Interpersonal Attraction.* Reading, Mass.: Addison-Wesley, 1969.

An interesting book on the social psychological concomitants of interpersonal attraction in a variety of contexts.

2. Hugo G. Biegel. "Romantic Love," *American Sociological Review,* No. 16 (June 1951), pp. 326–334.

A detailed, historical review of the concept of love from ancient times to the present.

3. William J. Goode. "The Theoretical Importance of Love," *American Sociological Review,* No. 24 (February, 1959), pp. 38–47.

An incisive analysis of the widespread view of love as potentially disruptive of society's social structure and of the varying ways that different societies have evolved to deal with this issue.

4. Ira L. Reiss. "Toward a Sociology of the Heterosexual Love Relationship," *Marriage and Family Living,* No. 22 (May 1960), pp. 139–145.

An interesting conception of the social psychological process of falling in love in terms of the spinning of a wheel that has had a major impact on this facet of family study since its publication.

5. Zick Rubin. *Liking and Loving.* New York: Holt, 1973.

A nice blending of conceptual analyses and empirical data to study the important concepts of liking and loving.

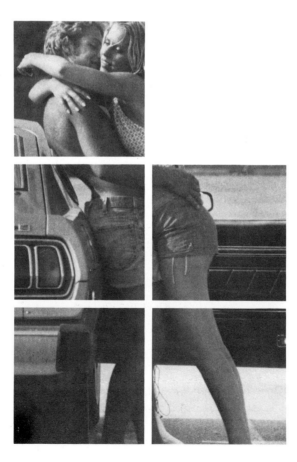

# Nonmarital Sex

## Chapter Aims

1. To survey the changing premarital sexual standards, attitudes, and behaviors and attempt to understand the double standard of sexual behavior.

2. To look at the range of normatively accepted sexual behaviors from abstinence to permissiveness, including masturbation, petting and nonmarital pregnancy.

3. To differentiate between the normative and deviant, and to look at some nonnormative sexual practices, such as voyeurism, exhibitionism, and fetishism.

## Overview

The way in which adolescents and young adults view sex outside of marriage for themselves and others has changed in recent years. The family, media, and one's peer group influence the way one expects men and women to approach sex, and the expectations of each sex are different.

Sociologists and psychologists generally agree that certain sexual behaviors are considered acceptable by most people, such as intercourse between two married adults, and that others are not considered acceptable in themselves, such as extreme forms of voyeurism.

## Sex and the Adolescent

**New social roles**

During the adolescent years, as the young person begins to establish his or her own identity outside the nuclear family of orientation, dramatic new social roles are explored. These roles are increasingly, though not exclusively, defined by the peer group (Goodman 1969, among others) for an important reason. The adolescent's search for identity, for "who I am," which is the major developmental task of adolescence, is complicated by the fact that the adult world does not place much value on what the adolescent is doing. Moreover, it is in the peer group that adolescents find those who share many of their circumstances and problems. Thus, it is quite reasonable for the adolescent to seek approval there. As Ruth Lyell (1973, pp. 85–86) aptly points out,

> The "who he is," or his sense of identity, is disturbed at adolescence because the "what he does" is not culturally valued. What the adolescent does is looked down on; his confusion and identity problems follow from this. His elders are generally indifferent to what he thinks and does; his approval and acceptance are rarely sought by adults; he is ignored or merely tolerated in their

*Many adolescent activities are directly related to the adolescent's new sexual awareness and interests.*

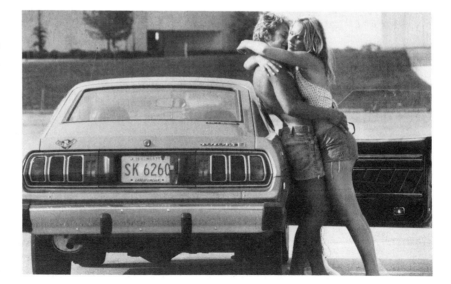

face-to-face interaction; he is taken seriously only by his peers—all because the *activities* of adolescents are not culturally valued.

Many of these activities are directly related to the adolescent's new sexual awareness and interests. Most people have their first homosexual or heterosexual experiences, although not necessarily intercourse, during their adolescent years. These experiences constitute an important part of adolescent socialization. As we look at adolescent sexual socialization, we should pay special attention to the way new roles are learned, the interaction between the family and the peer group as socializing agents, and how new sexual attitudes, roles, and behaviors are developed.

## Biosocial Basis of Adolescent Sexual Socialization

Puberty

The biological changes that characterize the beginning of adolescence, or *puberty* interact with cultural factors to form the basis of adolescent sexual socialization (Aubrey 1975). In many cultures, the attainment of puberty is marked by rites and rituals, which signal the beginnings of adulthood. According to their law, for example, Jewish boys are required to celebrate the puberty rite of bar mitzvah, in which the privileges of adulthood are conferred on the 13 year-old. Other cultures initiate the boy or girl into adulthood with their own rituals, such as practical tests of hunting ability or of the ability to survive under harsh conditions. Although our society does not generally accord to the pubescent the full rights of adulthood, biologically the pubescent is capable of all the activities of the adult.

There is no specific age that clearly marks the beginning of puberty, although some general norms have been established. For boys, the onset of puberty has traditionally been considered to be between the ages of 12 and 14½, while girls are generally thought to reach puberty slightly earlier, between 10 and 13 years of age. If we consider the hallmark of puberty to be "full sexual development," then these figures are basically accurate. *Menarche,* the first menstruation, signals the girl's entrance into puberty; *sexual potency,* the presence of sperm in the semen, signals the boy's entrance. Even more important in terms of social and psychological development is the appearance of *secondary sex characteristics.*

Secondary sex characteristics are physical characteristics that differentiate boys from girls but that are not directly related to the reproductive process. They include for the boy such characteristics as pubic hair, facial hair, deepening of the voice, heavy muscular development, and angular body build. For the girl, the secondary sex characteristics are enlargement of the breasts, triangular pattern of pubic hair, and more subcutaneous

Menarche

Sexual potency

Secondary sex
characteristics

*Biological changes as well as cultural factors form the basis of adolescent sexual socialization.*

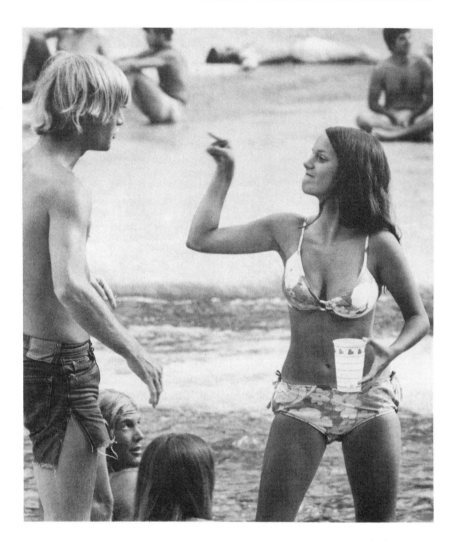

fat giving a rounded body contour. These changes in the body are the clearest signs of the onset of puberty. And, more importantly socially and psychologically, some are signs that are readily visible to others.

The physical changes of puberty are accompanied by changes in attitude and interests, which are either the direct or indirect result of the rapid sexual maturity. Many of the responses from the peer group are responses to the manifestations of these secondary sex characteristics. The size of a girl's breasts may help or hinder her popularity with the boys. Her breast size may make her an object of jokes, an outcast, or an object of admiration, respect, and lust to be pursued by the socially prestigious older boys. Likewise, a boy's lack of facial and body hair may place him at a disadvantage in comparison with boys who have more facial and body hair by peers who equate this characteristic with virility. There is an important but sometimes subtle relationship between the pubescent's physical maturity, social standing, and the resultant behavior and performance with his or her peers. While we would not suggest that it is only the physical reality of this period that exerts a profound influence, it is a highly significant part of the early adolescent's experience and must be recognized as such.

## Premarital Sexual Attitudes and Behaviors

Kinsey Studies

In the late 1940s Professor Alfred C. Kinsey (a zoologist by training) and his associates published a landmark volume, called *Sexual Behavior in the Human Male*. Five years later they published *Sexual Behavior in the Human Female*. Together, these two works, based on over 18,000 personal interviews, provided the first comprehensive survey of sexual attitudes, standards, and behaviors in the United States. In effect, they brought sex out of the closet and let the public know what people were thinking and doing in the privacy of their bedrooms.

Even though these studies are now over 30 years old and have been roundly criticized for a variety of methodological flaws, ''they are still the most complete inventory of American sex behavior that we have'' (Rose 1976). They are especially valuable in providing a baseline against which we can measure changes in sexual attitudes and behaviors, as indicated in more recent surveys.

Kinsey's data revealed two important points about nonmarital, including premarital, sexual behavior. First, there were significant differences between boys' and girls' expectations and standards of acceptable behavior. For instance, although boys expected to marry girls who were virgins, they did not expect to remain virgins themselves. This attitude re-

Double standard

flects what we call the *double standard*. Second, Kinsey found some notable social class differences, indicating that the so-called *middle-class morality* was not always applicable to members of the lower socioeconomic class.

Over the next 30 years, particularly during the 1960s and 1970s, several other large-scale surveys were conducted, and comparison of these with Kinsey's data allows us to measure social changes with a fair degree of accuracy. An important study with respect to adolescent sexual behavior was published in 1973 and is called *Adolescent Sexuality in*

Table 5.1

**"Two people shouldn't have to get married just because they want to live together."**

|  | Agree | Not sure | Disagree | Total |
|---|---|---|---|---|
| All adolescents | 72% | 0% | 28% | 100% |
| Boys | 76% | 1% | 23% | 100% |
| Ages 13–15 | 63 | 2 | 35 | 100 |
| Ages 16–19 | 87 | 1 | 12 | 100 |
| Girls | 67% | 0% | 33% | 100% |
| Ages 13–15 | 66 | 0 | 34 | 100 |
| Ages 16–19 | 67 | 0 | 33 | 100 |
| Virgins | 64% | 0% | 36% | 100% |
| Inexperienced | 55 | 0 | 45 | 100 |
| Beginners | 71 | 0 | 29 | 100 |
| Nonvirgins | 78% | 1% | 21% | 100% |
| Monogamists | 80 | 0 | 20 | 100 |
| Adventurers | 78 | 2 | 20 | 100 |

Source: *Adolescent Sexuality in Contemporary America* by Robert C. Sorensen. Copyright © 1973 by Robert C. Sorensen, by permission of Harry N. Abrams, Inc.

*Contemporary America* (Sorenson 1973). This detailed and comprehensive study sampled the sexual attitudes of hundreds of 13- to 19-year-olds who represented a cross sample of the country's adolescent population in terms of race, family income, geographical location, and the like. Thus, even though the sample is much smaller than Kinsey's, it is a more statistically controlled representation and is probably as accurate.

Respondents were given a series of statements and asked to agree, disagree, or state if they were not sure. The data, as shown in tables 5.1, 5.2, 5.3, and 5.4, indicate that, in general, young people are more willing than the people in Kinsey's sample to experiment sexually, to have sexual relations before marriage, and to be more open in discussing sex with their peers and sometimes even with their parents. Most young

Sexual
experimentation

### Table 5.2
### "I wouldn't want to have sex with someone only for the physical enjoyment of doing it, and nothing else."

|  | True | Not sure | False | Total |
|---|---|---|---|---|
| All adolescents | 57% | 4% | 39% | 100% |
| Boys | 49% | 4% | 47% | 100% |
|     Ages 13–15 | 52 | 6 | 42 | 100 |
|     Ages 16–19 | 46 | 2 | 52 | 100 |
| Girls | 65% | 5% | 30% | 100% |
|     Ages 13–15 | 60 | 6 | 34 | 100 |
|     Ages 16–19 | 71 | 3 | 26 | 100 |
| Virgins | 60% | 6% | 34% | 100% |
|     Inexperienced | 60 | 2 | 38 | 100 |
|     Beginners | 62 | 6 | 32 | 100 |
| Nonvirgins | 54% | 3% | 43% | 100% |
|     Monogamists | 62 | 3 | 35 | 100 |
|     Adventurers | 56 | 2 | 42 | 100 |

Source: *Adolescent Sexuality in Contemporary America* by Robert C. Sorensen. Copyright © 1973 by Robert C. Sorensen, by permission of Harry N. Abrams, Inc.

people were willing to have sexual intercourse with partners with whom they had a serious loving relationship but would avoid the casual sexual encounter, commonly, although apparently erroneously thought to be part of the typical teenage experience. To these young people, the intensity of love and its seriousness are more important than its duration, and the key ingredient is being able to relate to another person on a deep and loving level. Love is seen as a truly fulfilling relationship.

Conflict with parents

We also see that many adolescents are in conflict with their parents about sexual attitudes. Apparently, parents do not change as quickly as the times do. The young people feel that their parents have given them too little information about sex. Moreover, the report also indicates that as adolescents grow older, into late adolescence, their opinions differ

Table 5.3

**"When it comes to sex, my attitudes and my parents' attitudes are pretty much the same."**

|  | True | Not sure | False | Total |
|---|---|---|---|---|
| All adolescents | 36% | 4% | 60% | 100% |
| Boys | 28% | 6% | 66% | 100% |
|   Ages 13–15 | 38 | 3 | 59 | 100 |
|   Ages 16–19 | 20 | 7 | 73 | 100 |
| Girls | 44% | 2% | 54% | 100% |
|   Ages 13–15 | 38 | 4 | 58 | 100 |
|   Ages 16–19 | 50 | 0 | 50 | 100 |
| Virgins | 46% | 3% | 51% | 100% |
|   Inexperienced | 49 | 3 | 48 | 100 |
|   Beginners | 44 | 2 | 54 | 100 |
| Nonvirgins | 27% | 5% | 68% | 100% |
|   Monogamists | 39 | 1 | 60 | 100 |
|   Adventurers | 15 | 13 | 72 | 100 |

Source: *Adolescent Sexuality in Contemporary America* by Robert C. Sorensen. Copyright © 1973 by Robert C. Sorensen, by permission of Harry N. Abrams, Inc.

even more from those of their parents. This increasing difference seems to coincide with the increase in sexual experience as the adolescent grows older.

## Is There a Sexual Revolution?

The evidence from those surveys seems to indicate that although there have been many dramatic changes in adolescent sexual attitudes and behaviors, the change can hardly be characterized as a revolution, at least not in the sense of a sudden, violent upheaval. Perhaps it would be more accurate to say that there is an evolving new sexual awareness. Berg (1975) lends credence to this belief by supporting with evidence the posi-

Awareness

Table 5.4

**"I have a lot of respect for my parents' ideas and opinions about sex."**

|  | True | Not sure | False | Total |
|---|---|---|---|---|
| All adolescents | 65% | 6% | 29% | 100% |
| Boys | 56% | 8% | 36% | 100% |
|   Ages 13–15 | 66 | 7 | 27 | 100 |
|   Ages 16–19 | 47 | 9 | 44 | 100 |
| Girls | 75% | 3% | 22% | 100% |
|   Ages 13–15 | 80 | 3 | 17 | 100 |
|   Ages 16–19 | 70 | 3 | 27 | 100 |
| Virgins | 74% | 6% | 20% | 100% |
|   Inexperienced | 80 | 4 | 16 | 100 |
|   Beginners | 72 | 5 | 23 | 100 |
| Nonvirgins | 56% | 6% | 38% | 100% |
|   Monogamists | 70 | 2 | 28 | 100 |
|   Adventurers | 38 | 12 | 50 | 100 |

Source: *Adolescent Sexuality in Contemporary America* by Robert C. Sorensen. Copyright © 1973 by Robert C. Sorensen, by permission of Harry N. Abrams, Inc.

Changes in behavior and attitude

tion that the concept of a sexual revolution is something of a myth; that, in fact, men's and women's perspectives have remained relatively unchanged over the past two decades. Specifically, he found that men continue to stress the physical attributes of women in assessing sexual attraction, while women still gauge masculine appeal according to men's dress and sexuality. In another study, it was found that high school students' attitudes about sex have changed considerably more than their actual sexual behavior has. Although there is a greater permissiveness in attitude, this has not directly affected the way individuals behave in making decisions about sex (Godenne 1974).

There is some evidence in the other direction too, that there is a revolution of sorts, and much depends on how we interpret the evidence, which is fairly consistent from survey to survey. One study has shown there is an increasing interest in sexual intercourse, which is a primary concern for both boys and girls during this period (Rubenstein et al. 1976). Hopkins (1977) compared dozens of surveys of adolescent sexual behavior from the 1930s through the 1970s and arrived at three key conclusions about what changes in sexual behavior have taken place. These three conclusions seem to be consistent with most other research:

1. A larger number of older adolescents (in college years) are more sexually experienced now than they were in earlier generations.
2. There has been a greater incidence of premarital intercourse for females than males, although most surveys still report a higher absolute incidence for males.
3. While data for younger adolescents are not as clear, they suggest a trend toward earlier sexual experience for both males and females.

Important studies by Kaats and Davis (1970), illustrated in table 5.5, and Bell and Chaskes (1970), among others, also indicate significant changes in premarital sexual behavior as well as in attitude.

Table 5.5

**Mean Scores[a] and Percentages Agreeing with Items Assessing Acceptance of Premarital Intercourse under Four Types of Relationships**

| Type of relationship | Means and percentage agreeing with item | | | |
| --- | --- | --- | --- | --- |
| | | | Males (N = 239) | Females (M = 319) |
| I believe that full sexual relations are acceptable for the (male) (female) before marriage when (he) (she): | Ratings for males % | Ratings for females % | Ratings for males % | Ratings for females % |
| is not particularly affectionate toward (his) (her) partner | 55 | 37 | 37 | 14 |
| feels strong affection for (his) (her) partner | 73 | 68 | 53 | 34 |
| is in love | 81 | 76 | 68 | 57 |
| is engaged to be married | 80 | 78 | 71 | 61 |

[a] Based on a forced-choice scaling of 1–6 where 1 = strongly disagree and 6 = strongly agree.
Source: Kaats and Davis, The dynamics of sexual behavior of college students. *Journal of Marriage and the Family,* 1970, 32, 390–399.

One recent survey compared data from questionnaires completed by undergraduate women at a southern university over a ten-year period, from 1965 to 1975. It was found, "that the premarital sexual revolution which was reported to have begun during the late 1960s has actually accelerated during the 1970s" (King, Balswick, and Robinson 1977). Specifically, what their data suggest is that women, even more than men, have changed their attitudes and behavior in regard to premarital intercourse. But still, it must be emphasized, women tend to be interested in one-partner rather than multiple-partner relationships. They have not become more promiscuous.

What can we conclude from these data? The most prudent conclusion at this period of time is that it is unclear whether or not there is a sexual revolution. However, there have been significant and important changes in adolescent and young adult sexual behavior and attitudes. These changes have occurred particularly in premarital activity.

## Contemporary Sexual Standards and Practices

In this section, we will look in greater detail at some specific sexual standards and behaviors, trying to determine how they evolve, seeing what influence they have on the individual and society, and attempting to understand them in a contemporary perspective.

Agents of socialization

These standards, or values, are influenced by the interaction of several agents of adolescent sexual socialization. The chief agents include the influence of the nuclear family of orientation, the separate influences of siblings and parents, the values of the peer group, and the influence of the media, especially films and television. The latter often serve as sexually stimulating forces in the adolescent's immediate environment, initiating fantasies and defining role models with which the young person can easily identify. From these role models the adolescent may learn sexually relevant role behaviors. For example, such films as *Saturday Night Fever* and *Grease,* cue the young viewer on ways to act with same- and opposite-sex peers. Within months after *Saturday Night Fever* was released, there was an entire line of John Travolta clothing for young men who, we would assume, identified with the person he played in the film.

Media influences

The media also provides important information about expected behaviors and values to the young person. This information may agree with or conflict with other information and values. The average adolescent spends more time watching TV than in the performance of any other single activity. Sebald (1968) has pointed out correctly that "televised models are important sources of social behavior" (p. 177) and that with the parents and peers they contribute to the total perspective of values. Hines (1976) has found the media an important agent, along with parents and peers in socializing young people for marital roles. However, the bulk of evidence indicates that the more important the value, the less influential the media is. Television and the other media seem to have greater influence on our "frill" values, the superficial facades we present to others, such as dress and colloquialisms. It has also been suggested

that some of the sexual fears and conflicts of this stage of development can be viewed as a result of the mixed messages conveyed to the adolescent. The adolescent may get one message from the family, a different one from the peer group, another from the media, and still other conflicting messages from different cultural forces. Sometimes, multiple and conflicting messages emanate from the same source. In any event, a lack of ambiguity and confusion in this sphere of adolescent life is relatively rare (Giuffra 1975).

An important question raised by this entire issue is whether the media present a reasonably accurate representation of what is happening in the adolescent subculture. Or, are the realities of adolescent life being distorted to suggest an environment that in fact does not exist? For instance, are class differences realistically represented on television and in films, or are they primarily geared to middle-class values? With these questions in mind, let us examine some specific contemporary sexual standards.

## Abstinence versus Permissiveness

*Abstinence* means refraining from sexual activity. There are varying degrees of abstinence, ranging from no contact at all with the opposite sex to some physical contact, such as kissing, without heavy petting. *Permissiveness* refers to an open sexual standard. As with abstinence, there are varying degrees of permissiveness, ranging from engaging in sexual relations only with one steady partner to a completely open sexual lifestyle, with many partners. The latter is sometimes called *promiscuity*.

What are some of the factors that determine whether a person will chose abstinence or permissiveness? Religious factors play an important

part, especially where the church is an integral part of the individual's social life (McGowan 1977). Religious restrictions against nonmarital sexual activity may inhibit a person's tendencies toward more permissive behaviors. Psychological factors may play a role too. The person who will feel a strong sense of guilt from engaging in nonmarital sex is more likely to abstain. There are also several "risk" factors associated with a permissive sexual standard. Biological factors such as the risk of venereal disease and accidental pregnancy and social factors such as the risk of exclusion and ridicule act to discourage permissiveness and encourage abstinence.

In the 1950s Ira Reiss conducted important research on abstinence and permissiveness. Reiss pointed out—and this was some 25 years ago!—that

> Abstinence has lost adherents because its ancient supports have been greatly weakened, e.g., the risk of pregnancy, venereal disease, social condemnation, and guilt feelings are quite different in present-day society. . . . This sort of change in abstinence is what one would expect to occur in a society which has become much more open in its attitude towards sexual behavior and was also becoming freer and more equalitarian in its treatment of young people. (Reiss, 1960)

In other words, there was, and is, a trend away from abstinence and toward more permissiveness.

**Affectionate vs. nonaffectionate permissiveness**

Reiss differentiated between "permissiveness with affection" and nonaffectionate permissiveness. The former, he suggested, is an integral part of healthy adult sexual functioning, while the latter may be a sign of disturbance. For instance, very permissive men whose orientation was nonaffectionate tended to feel disgusted and let down after sex.

Recently Libby, Gray, and White (1978) retested Reiss's work on a college population. They found that Reiss's theory could only be partly supported and that other factors, played a part in determining self-permissiveness. For instance, a person's "closeness to [his or her] mother's sexual standards was considerably more predictive of self-permissiveness than was obvious in Reiss's theory," which placed more emphasis on friends' and peers' standards. These results suggest that permissiveness is a complex trait, combining social and psychological factors.

**Socioeconomic differences**

There have also been noted socioeconomic class differences in reported levels of permissiveness. Zelnik and Kantner (1972), for example, found that adolescents from lower socioeconomic groups tended to become sexually active at a younger age. They also found that black teenage girls tended to have premarital sexual experiences earlier than their Caucasian counterparts. This tendency can be explained in part by the fact that blacks are disproportionately represented in the lower class.

## The Double Standard of Sexual Behavior

A *double standard* of sexual behavior has been reported from the time of Kinsey's survey through the present.

Although the situation is changing, there are still some marked differences in the expectations of attitudes about sex between boys and girls. It is expected that boys will be more oriented initially toward having sex while girls will be motivated more toward seeking affection and love as an integral part of their sexual needs. Many studies support the existence of this attitude. McBride and Ender (1977) found, for example, that men would engage in more personal intimate physical contact without affection toward their partner or without a sense of commitment to the relationship. Women, on the other hand, required both a sense of commitment and a feeling of affection to enjoy sexual intimacy. The study also revealed that more college-age men than women reported experiencing petting, intercourse, oral sex, and group sex. McBride and Ender did find similarities in some attitudes; namely, that there were no significant differences between men and women in their attitudes toward responsibility for initiating sexual activity, for birth control, or for sexual satisfaction. Other studies have emphasized gender-related differences. Peplau, Rubin, and Hill (1977) found, for example, in surveying college-age dating couples that despite ''generally permissive and egalitarian attitudes, traditional sexual role playing in which the man encourages intercourse and the woman limits the couple's sexual intimacy was common'' (p. 86). The stereotypical scene of the man insisting and the woman protesting does apparently have some basis in fact.

When we examine the underlying reasons for this persistent double standard, it becomes evident that social norms exert pressures on boys and girls to conform to different stereotyped behaviors. These are trans-

*Peer pressures*

mitted by the peer group, among other socializing agents, which may tell the individual what the culture expects. For instance, a boy who admits that he doesn't ''score'' may not gain the admiration of his peers. Likewise, a girl who is promiscuous may find herself shunned by other girls. Of course, what the boy or girl believes the peer group thinks is not always accurate. Collins (1974), in fact, found that typically what boys and girls think their peers expect of them is not always realistic. It takes little imagination to realize the confusion this misinterpretation can cause a young person—when he or she thinks that friends have expectations, which in fact are almost impossible to fulfill.

## Sexual Variations

Unlike lower animals, for whom the purpose of sexual behavior is clearly entwined with the reproductive functions and whose form is basically dictated by nature, the human being displays an imaginative variety of sexual preferences, many of them clearly unrelated to procreation. Human

*Despite the increase in the amount of nonmarital sex in our society, a loving relationship is still desired.*

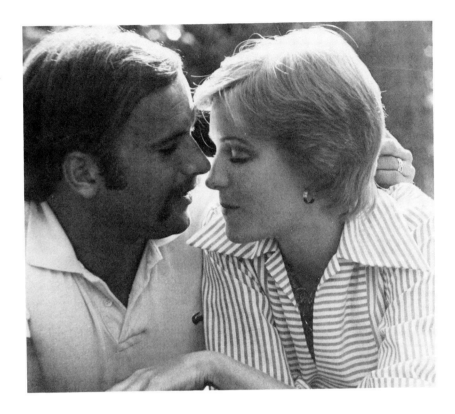

beings are capable of choosing from a wide range of sexual behaviors and exhibit many individual preferences in the ways they attain sexual pleasure.

Some of these behaviors are quite traditional and socially acceptable by almost everyone: having sexual intercourse with one's spouse, for example. Some, such as incest, are clearly prohibited and go directly against the norms of society. Many are controversial, accepted by some segments of society and not by others, for instance, homosexuality. Others are in a socially ambiguous state and may be accepted by one's spouse and friends but not by society as a whole: mate swapping and swinging are examples.

It is important first that we understand the distinction between the terms *normative* and *deviant,* between *traditional* and *nontraditional,* or *alternative,* between *normal* and *abnormal.* All of these terms are used to describe different types of sexual behavior and they can lead to confusion. The terms cannot always be used interchangeably with any degree of accuracy. Moreover, people preferring certain types of sexual behavior may resent, quite rightfully, being judged as abnormal, in the sense of pathological or sick, when they see themselves simply as practicing a nontraditional, or an alternative, lifestyle, which serves their needs quite well.

Although these terms are often interrelated, for clarity, we will use the terms *normative* and *deviant* within the context of the sociological perspective, *normal* and *abnormal* within the context of the psychological perspective, and *traditional* and *nontraditional,* or *alternative,* as objective descriptors of what is generally widely practiced and what is not.

## The Psychological Perspective: What Is Normal?

A question people often ask is, Am I normal? Is what I enjoy doing sexually healthy or not? This can be a troubling question for two reasons. First, the individual's entire system of self-esteem, one's feelings about oneself, may be importantly influenced by his or her sexual activity. Second, there may be no one to speak to about it, someone with whom to compare notes. Even a traditional practice such as masturbation may be viewed as abnormal by some people, because no one they know personally has ever mentioned doing it!

In defining the parameters of normal versus abnormal, in the psychological sense of healthy versus unhealthy, the first question that arises is, How well is the person's sexual life integrated with his or her total interpersonal functioning? One of the chief criteria of healthy sexual functioning is that it be integrated with a person's emotional life (Freid 1975). We can consider the enjoyment of sex with a person we love and loving the person with whom we have sex as psychologically healthy signs. We do not mean to suggest that we shouldn't necessarily be able to enjoy sex with a range of people but merely that in our society love and sex should be able to support and fuel each other in the healthy personality.

Emotional integration

Psychiatrists and psychologists, the public arbiters of mental health, have disagreed, often vehemently over the years, about what specifically constitutes the normal and the abnormal. The public debate about homosexuality is the most obvious case in point, but alternative practices such as group sex, voyeurism, promiscuity, and extramarital relationships have all been subjects of heated contention.

Normal vs. abnormal

These debates still linger, but in general it is agreed that almost any of the nontraditional sexual activities can be viewed as ''normal'' if they are in the context of sexual foreplay between two consenting adults. The criterion of healthy sexual functioning, according to most psychologists, is that it lead ultimately to satisfying sexual relations. The same nontraditional activities become unhealthy, pathological, that is, abnormal, if they constitute the sole source of sexual pleasure. In other words, the psychologist looks at the activity in the context of the individual's total lifestyle and integrated sexual functioning. A specific sexual practice can be healthy or unhealthy, depending upon its integration in the person's emotional life and relationships with others.

## Gregory and Selma

Gregory enjoys looking at pornographic magazines and masturbating in bed. He also enjoys having sexual relations with Selma, his wife. One of the things they love to do as foreplay is for Selma to watch from behind the bed, out of Gregory's view, while he masturbates. He imagines that he is being watched by his mother, and then Selma steps out and gets into bed with him. This fantasy game makes them both passionate, and they have a very lively sex life.

Total functioning

A psychologist would probably say that this nontraditional practice is healthy, at least in the sense that it contributes to Gregory and Selma's marital functioning. From the psychological perspective then, the key elements of sexual normality are not solely what a society says is normal, but rather how well integrated the sexual practices are in the person's total functioning, how well related sex is with emotion, and how capable the person is of enjoying sex with the person he or she loves.

When we contrast the situation we just described with that of Tommy and Kate, we will see how the psychological perspective differentiates between the healthy and the unhealthy.

## Tommy and Kate

Tommy and Kate are married but don't have much interest in sex with each other. Tommy buys pornographic magazines and masturbates but does it out of view of Kate, who thinks it's sick and disgusting. It turns her off to see her husband doing this, and Tommy knows it. But he prefers to masturbate rather than make love to his wife, whom he considers boring. He often has to go into the bathroom to masturbate and feels guilty afterward.

Here the same behavior would certainly be viewed as unhealthy because it is not integrated with the interpersonal relationship and because the individual prefers masturbation to sexual relations with another, specifically, his wife. Thus, most psychologists would not regard this situation as an example of healthy psychological functioning.

## The Sociological Perspective: Normative vs. Deviant

The sociological perspective is somewhat different in emphasis, but basically consistent. Sociologists look more at the varieties of sexual experience in terms of norms and of deviations from the accepted norms, of what a society says is acceptable and what is not, and of why the society condones some practices and not others. Thus, like the psychological perspective, the sociological position is a relativistic one. For the former, the standard of comparison is the person's general emotional and interpersonal functioning, while for the latter, social definitions are the keys. Gagnon and Simon (1967, pp. 1–2), for example, point out,

Social definitions

> The major criteria of what is deviant are not to be found in the behavior as such, but rather in its definition as norm-violating behavior. There is no form of behavior, sexual or nonsexual, that is intrinsically deviant or deviant because of the behavior that it involves. In the area of sexual deviance (as well as in other forms of deviance) there is wide variation between cultures in which specific behaviors are defined as deviant. With the possible exception of incest . . . there are no age preferences or gender choices or styles of sexual behavior that are universally prohibited . . . *a form of behavior becomes deviant when it is defined as violating the norms of some collectivity.* Usually, the collectivities that are relevant are those formally empowered to sanction deviant behavior in general, though for certain forms of sexual behavior only informal and covert sanctions are applied by selected collectives (italics ours).

Normative vs. deviant

In examining deviant sexual behavior from the sociological perspective, we should keep in mind that a person who is practicing nonnormative behavior is automatically labeled a social deviant and many of the general principles relevant to the sociology of deviance apply,

## Normatively Accepted Sexual Practices

The range of nonmarital sexual behaviors can be divided into normative and nonnormative. Normative sexual behaviors are those that are widely practiced and socially acceptable within the culture.

Masturbation    *Masturbation* can be defined as sexual self-stimulation. Although many young people are troubled about masturbation, sometimes plagued by feelings of guilt and confusion, it is generally agreed by people who have studied adolescent behavior that masturbation is a normal part of the adolescent sexual experience (Dranoff, 1974). It is therefore considered a normatively accepted sexual behavior, even though talking about it may cause a person anxiety. According to most studies, approximately 95 percent of adolescent boys and 50 to 80 percent of adolescent girls practice masturbation. Despite this high rate, masturbation may cause the adolescent, and particularly the early adolescent, to experience guilt, self-disgust, and remorse. We know, for example, that attitudes toward masturbation change dramatically with age, and that "on the whole, males judge masturbation more permissively than females" (Schoof-Tams et al., 1976).

Whether or not masturbation is a helpful or harmful part of adolescent sexuality is open to debate. Masturbation is least problematic when it is accompanied by the appropriate attitudes; namely, if the adolescent realizes the normality of his or her masturbatory experimentation (Dranoff 1974). One particularly constructive use of masturbation is to learn to experience heightened sexual pleasure without guilt (Ford 1966). At this period of life, it is often through autoerotic activity that the healthy boy or girl learns to appreciate sexual response. The appreciation takes two forms: fantasy and bodily stimulation (Ford 1966). Through fantasy, the young person is able to appreciate the diversity and creativity of the sexual experience. Through bodily stimulation, he or she learns about areas of the body that are most sensitive to stimulation and stroking. It is through these two activities that the adolescent forms his or her feelings about sex. Through fantasy, for example, he or she may bring into sexual consciousness those others who will ultimately become sexual partners. Ironically, the adolescent may learn that sex, which is really a two-person activity, is beautiful through the stimulation of his or her own body.

*Fantasy or bodily stimulation*

*A learning experience*

Petting    The earliest type of overt sexual activity occurring between young people of the opposite sex is usually petting. Broadly speaking, *petting* is sexual activity that leads in the direction of and may or may not culminate in sexual intercourse. It includes kissing, touching parts of the body, oral stimulation of the erogenous zones, and mutual masturbation. Petting is a normal part of the adolescent experience and the prelude to satisfying adult sexual relationships. For many adolescents, petting can serve as a learning experience and a testing ground in which new styles of intimate behavior may be explored.

Petting and early sexual experimentation establish a sense of intimacy with the opposite sex. Through sexual experimentation sanctioned by the peer group, boys and girls learn to relate to each other in new, personally satisfying and socially fulfilling ways. Thus, sexual experimentation, in this respect, may be a means to an end. As Mitchell (1972, p. 449) suggests,

> Sexual behavior . . . can foster an openness which facilitates intimacy at levels other than the sexual. This is especially true among adolescents despite the commonly held maxim that psychological intimacy should precede sexual involvement. For adolescents with minimal meaningful involvement elsewhere, sexual behavior is a basic avenue for creating bonds of psychological intimacy.

In other words, it may serve important social and psychological purposes in the development of paired relationships.

Petting may also be the subject of much moral confusion. How far should I go? Is what I am doing wrong? What will others think of me? Mitchell (1974) points out that the adolescent's moral dilemmas transcend sexual activity and relate to such basic social questions as conformity, independence, and acceptance by others. In another paper, Mitchell (1975) specifies five major changes in the adolescent "moral structure" that can help us better understand how the adolescent deals with his or her moral dilemmas:

**Moral confusion**

1. Moral *outlook* becomes more abstract and less concrete.
2. Moral *convictions* become more concerned with what is right and less concerned with what is wrong; justice emerges as a dominant moral force in the adolescent's life.
3. Moral *judgment* becomes increasingly cognitive; therefore the adolescent is inclined toward analyzing social and personal codes more vigorously than during childhood and thus to make up his or her own mind on moral issues.
4. The adolescent's moral *judgment* becomes less egocentric.
5. Moral *judgment* becomes psychologically expensive to the adolescent because it may create emotional tension

**Conflict of values**

Religious values, held since childhood, may conflict directly with desires and behaviors. Values instilled by the parents and respected by the adolescent may also conflict with influences of the peer group or the media. This conflict may appear even more frequently in the adolescent girl, who may still be judged by herself and by others according to the double standard (Scales 1977).

Contraception    The sexually active person has to make an important personal decision about *contraception.* Whereas in the marriage relationship this is typically a mutual decision of the partners, for the nonmarried person it may be made independently, without a single sexual
partner in mind. In an ongoing, sexually active relationship, however, the
decision would probably be made much as it would be in the marital relationship (see chapter 9), with some slight differences.

Nonmarried vs.
married

   Two important differences between contraception decisions for nonmarried versus married women should be mentioned. First, if the unmarried girl is still living with her parents a dilemma may arise about
whether or not to inform her parents that she is using contraception. In
Philip Roth's novel *Goodbye, Columbus,* a college girl's mother discovers
a diaphragm hidden in her bureau drawer, setting off a major family conflict. The living-at-home single person usually has to take certain realities
into account, such as the parents' reactions or the influence on and reaction of younger siblings. While the same may hold true for the unmarried
boy, parents are more likely to accept sexual realities about their sons
than about their daughters.

   Second, the girl who is not presently involved with a boyfriend in a
sexually active relationship may still have to decide about whether or not
to use birth control pills, which cannot be used at the spur of the moment. This type of decision requires a conscious recognition that she is
planning, either in the long run or in the short run, to find a sexual
partner.

Information

   For both sexes, the decision about contraception may, to a large
extent, be influenced by overt or covert social policy; namely, how much
information the young person is provided, how the information is presented, and how readily available the contraceptive means are. After all,
an adolescent can only make a decision to the degree that information is
made available. In some areas, appropriate contraceptive information is
not supplied at all, and the decision is severely limited by the lack of available information (Reichelt and Werley 1975). For instance, Finkel and
Finkel (1975) found that even in districts where schools were teaching
about contraception, it was often several years *after* the students had begun having sex! Only 32 percent of sexually active young men interviewed knew that if a male withdraws his penis before ejaculation his
partner can still become pregnant. In part, there may be some social pressure against making information about contraception available because of
the belief that the availability of contraception encourages sexual promiscuity, especially for girls. This premise has been examined carefully and
found to be unsupported by Garris, Steckler, and McIntire (1976), who
found no differences in rates of promiscuity between informed and uninformed adolescents.

Nonmarital Pregnancy   Pregnancy that occurs outside a socially recognized marriage relationship, that is, *nonmarital pregnancy,* cannot be clearly categorized as either normatively accepted or deviant behavior. It is, in our heterogeneous American society, somewhere in between. Many factors affect how the unmarried pregnant woman is viewed by her family, her friends, and by others. The woman's age is important, as is her social status. A 14-year-old girl may be viewed as a "mixed-up kid," while a 25-year-old single working woman who makes a reasoned choice to become a single parent may be perceived by her friends as liberated and willing to take chances in life. Class differences play an important part too, as do religious orientations. For example, out-of-wedlock pregnancy is more accepted by the black lower class than by the black middle class. In the former case, it could be considered a normatively accepted behavior, while in the latter it would not be. Over half the black children born in this country today are born outside a marriage relationship, with this incidence considerably higher when we look at the black lower class. (U.S. Census Bureau 1978.)

Societal perceptions

The incidence of nonmarital pregnancy in general is rising, especially among adolescent girls. In 1962, there were approximately 100,000 out-of-wedlock births to women under 20. Six years later, there were about 166,000, an increase of 66 percent, despite the fact that the overall birth rate had been decreasing (Braen and Forbush 1975). In 1977, there were an estimated 1 million teenage pregnancies, 60 percent of which (600,000) resulted in the birth of a child (Cherlin 1978). The others were aborted or miscarried (involuntarily aborted). In 1980, it is estimated that over 1 million children will be born out of wedlock, most of these to mothers under 20 years of age.

Rising rates

There are several reasons why women may opt for pregnancy outside of marriage. One position stresses that young girls who have babies during their adolescent years have serious emotional problems, and that out-of-wedlock pregnancy, therefore, can be viewed as a sign of some psychological or family disturbance. This position is supported by a great deal of evidence; namely, many of these girls come from broken homes; there is a high incidence of parental alcohol abuse; there are often serious family conflicts and signs of violence in the home; there is a high frequency of sexually seductive fathers; these girls generally lack interest in socially acceptable activities or hobbies (Curtis 1974; Abernathy 1976; Hertz 1977).

A number of social factors have been identified as contributing to the increase in nonmarital pregnancies, for instance, the more liberalized sexual attitudes held by women. From this position, nonmarital pregnancy is

Contributing factors

viewed as an accidental consequence of sexual intercourse. The increasing teen-age population as a percentage of the total population also contributes to the increase in nonmarital pregnancies since teenagers make up the bulk of the total number of out-of-wedlock pregnancies. It has also been suggested that the new role of women allows them to raise children on their own, even while working, and that this has the effect of encouraging single women who want children to go ahead and have them without getting married.

## Betty Lou

Betty Lou just received the result of her pregnancy test and it is, as she suspected, positive. She'll tell Wade tonight at dinner, and she already knows his reaction. ''I can't get married now,'' he'll tell her, thinking that's what she wants. But she doesn't want to get married either, at least not now. She had decided a long time ago, ''If I get pregnant by Wade, I'll keep the baby and raise it on my own.'' After all, she reasons, ''I make good money at my job, and I can continue to work, at least part time, after I have the baby.'' Her older sister, who has a five year old, will probably babysit while Betty Lou works at the real estate office.

We will discuss the implications of single parenthood, both for the children and the parents, in chapters 9 and 10.

## Nonnormative Sexual Practices

Nonnormative sexual behaviors are those that are not practiced by any significantly large group in society, or those which a culture views as undesirable, and therefore tries to restrain. There are many kinds of nonnormative sexual preferences and practices, which psychologists may view as unhealthy and which sociologists may view as deviant. We now look at four types, which while only a fraction of what is practiced, are probably the most common to our experiences.

Voyeurism    *Voyeurism* is the practice of becoming sexually aroused by watching either ''live'' or through some medium, such as film, books, or videotape, another person or persons, partially or completely nude and involved in some form of sexual activity. Part of the excitement is that the person the voyeur is watching does not know that he or she is being observed. Most of us are, to some extent, voyeuristic; that is, we become aroused by erotically explicit stimuli (Steele and Walker 1974; see table 5.6). A healthy and normative version of this is to become excited as we watch our partner undress in front of us.

But voyeurism becomes socially unacceptable and psychologically unhealthy when we spy on people without their knowing it. The "peeping Tom" who secretly wanders through backyards looking through windows is considered unhealthy and deviant. There is a middle ground too.

**Pornography**

The person who enjoys attending sexually explicit films may or may not be considered deviant, depending on the social standard that predominates in his or her environment. Psychologically, whether this is healthy or not would depend on how this excitation is integrated into other activities. Is the person only capable of becoming aroused by pornography?

Although it has generally been assumed that men respond more to voyeuristic stimulation than do women—after all, we don't have any "peeping Janes"—, some recent research seems to indicate that the differences are smaller than have been suggested and that in general "the pattern and intensity of reactions to explicit sexual stimuli are in general the same for men and women" (Schmidt 1975, p. 355).

It may be that the woman has been socialized to not recognize and report the stimulation she feels, since her sexual excitement can generally be recorded biologically before it is reported by her.

## Exhibitionism

A person gets excited by being looked at, rather than by looking is called an exhibitionist. Although both men and women may get pleasure in this way, almost all recorded deviant cases involve men exhibiting themselves to women. The deviant exhibitionist becomes sexually aroused by exhibiting a part of himself, usually his genitals, especially to a shocked and unwilling onlooker. Generally healthy and socially acceptable exhibitionistic tendencies are expressed in the way we dress, in the way we conduct ourselves in public, and in the ways we seek attention in our interactions with others. As a pathological behavior, however, exhibitionism usually involves frightening a person with an inappropriate display of the genitals. An exhibitionist becomes aroused by the shocked reaction of the woman. McCary (1967 p. 276) describes a typical exhibitionist:

> Typically, the exhibitionist is a quiet, timid, submissive person who is beset with feelings of inadequacy and insecurity. He is usually described as being "nice" but immature. He was characteristically reared in a cultural atmosphere of overstrict and puritanical attitudes toward sex, and his formative years were

Table 5.6

**How Sexually Stimulating Men and Women Find Certain Types of Slides**

| Subject of Slide | Degree of Reported Sexual Stimulation | |
| --- | --- | --- |
| | Male | Female |
| Romantic | 7.4 | 11.3 |
| Sadomasochism, female on male | 2.5 | 1.7 |
| Sadomasochism, male on female | 3.0 | 1.7 |
| Triad | 10.9 | 2.7 |
| Homosexual anal coitus | 1.7 | 1.6 |
| Homosexual fellatio | 1.9 | 2.5 |
| Heterosexual coitus, male on top | 28.5 | 14.2 |
| Heterosexual coitus, female on top | 21.3 | 11.8 |
| Homosexual cunnilingus | 4.8 | 1.9 |
| Nude female, breasts exposed | 29.6 | 2.7 |
| Romantic petting | 21.2 | 19.8 |
| Heterosexual petting, partly clad | 3.9 | 4.5 |
| Heterosexual petting, nude | 20.9 | 9.7 |
| Heterosexual fellatio | 14.0 | 4.1 |
| Heterosexual cunnilingus | 11.2 | 8.2 |
| Masturbation, female | 10.4 | 2.8 |
| Masturbation, male | 2.2 | 3.0 |

Are men more voyeuristic than woman? Steel and Walker (1974) exposed men and women to a series of slides and examined their relative rates of sexual stimulation. Above we see some similarities and differences between the sexes.
Source: Adapted from Steele and Walker (1974).

dominated by a powerful, engulfing mother. Despite the fact that most of these men are married, the sexual relationship with their wives is a poor one. All these influences work to create in exhibitionists pervading doubts and fears concerning their masculinity.

Women have exhibitionistic tendencies too, but our society finds them more acceptable, and it is not usually considered a deviant behavior. Again, we should emphasize that exhibitionism can be an enjoyable part of a healthy sexual relationship. If our partner enjoys watching us and we enjoy watching our partner, this can be an exciting part of foreplay.

## Transvestism

*Transvestism* is the practice of dressing in the clothing of the opposite sex in order to attain sexual pleasure. The transvestite is not necessarily a homosexual. This confused idea persists because people assume that when a man dresses as a woman or a woman as a man, that person is necessarily homosexual. This assumption is simply not valid.

The transvestite, colloquially, the "TV," typically gets sexual pleasure out of public displays of his or her appearance in the chosen garb. The man enjoys passing as a woman, and some men have even carried on dating relationships with men, without the other man suspecting that he was dating a transvestite.

Women heterosexual transvestites are less common and are often taken for *dikes*—masculine lesbians. The *diesel dike* is a lesbian, usually of large proportions, whose dress as a man is accompanied by exaggerated "masculine" behaviors.

In some cultures, children are routinely dressed in the garb of the opposite sex. For example, young German boys in the early years of this century were garbed in dresses. But since this does not involve getting sexual pleasure out of the act, it is not technically considered transvestism. Transvestism then is almost always considered a deviant behavior.

## Fetishism

*Fetishism* is the process of attaching a sexual value to an inanimate object or to a part of the body, as opposed to the whole person. If a person is unusually attracted to brassieres, boots and leather objects, or lace, then this person has a fetish for inanimate objects. Sometimes, however, a person may be unusually attracted to one part of the body at the expense of the others: to breasts or to hair, for example. Such a person may relate only to part of the person and not be able to relate to the person as a whole. This is a different type of fetish.

Typically, the objects chosen for fetishistic value are those that society directly or indirectly associates with sex or with gender. People develop fetishes to things that are traditionally feminine or traditionally masculine; that is to things that are specifically identified with one sex or the other. Moreover, certain fetishes are reinforced by the media, where such things as a woman's breasts are glorified as erotic elements even in nonsexual contexts. In other words, we are taught to "worship" them and to find them stimulating. Advertising capitalizes on this worship by catering to our fetishistic fantasies.

*Not necessarily homosexual*

*Cultural and psychological components*

*Almost everyone feels some fetishistic interest. Healthy people make the transition between the fetishistic object and the whole person.*

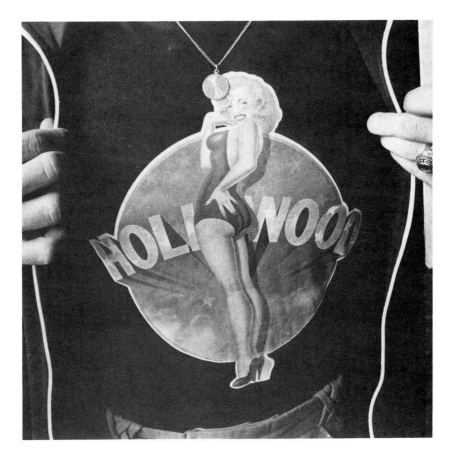

Fetishism may vary greatly in degree. On the one hand, every person exhibits some fetishistic interest; that is, there are certain parts of the body or items of clothes that we invest with more sexual interest than others. However, the healthy person, according to most psychiatrists, is able to make the appropriate transition between the fetishistic object and the whole person. That is, the fetish, in a healthy sense, serves as a prelude to the paired sexual relationship.

As a deviant behavior, fetishism either excludes the whole person or other individuals altogether from sexual activity or involves some antisocial behavior. The man who runs around stealing women's underwear from clotheslines is clearly exhibiting fetishistic deviant behavior. Generally, fetishism occurs in conjunction with some other forms of sexual perversion, such as exhibitionism, assault, or compulsive masturbation.

## Summary

1. During the adolescent years important cross-gender socialization occurs in the contexts of dating and sexual experimentation. Evidence seems to indicate that while there are major changes in premarital sexual standards there is not a sexual revolution, at least in the sense of massive social upheaval.

2. Many factors influence sexual standards and behaviors: the values of the peer group, the mass media of communication, and especially primary socialization in the nuclear family of orientation.

3. Decisions regarding abstinence and permissiveness are influenced by religious, social, and biological factors. Ira Reiss suggested in the 1960s that sexual abstinence was a declining practice, and it still seems to be declining today. Permissiveness is generally characterized by affectionate love, rather than by promiscuity.

4. A double standard of sexual behavior, in which men and women are judged differently, still exists, although its rigidity is changing with the times. Women's premarital sexual experiences are becoming more frequent.

5. The terms normative, deviant, traditional, nontraditional, or alternative, and normal and abnormal differ with the perspective being used. Normative and deviant can be used to denote what is and what is not socially accepted as seen from a sociological perspective. Normal and abnormal define what is mentally healthy or unhealthy from a psychological perspective, and traditional and nontraditional are objective descriptors of what is traditionally practiced and what is not.

6. There is a general consistency between the sociological and psychological perspectives of normal and normative of abnormal and nonnormative, or deviant.

7. Masturbation, petting, and contraception are some normatively accepted sexual behaviors. Nonmarital (out-of-wedlock) pregnancy may be considered normative or deviant, depending upon the subculture, but in either case it is an increasingly common occurrence in our contemporary American society. This increase is partially explained by the changing role of women, both with respect to premarital sexual standards and economic independence.

8. Voyeurism, exhibitionism, transvestism, and fetishism are four of the more common nonnormative sexual preferences and practices.

## Key Terms

These terms have been introduced and defined in this chapter. Definitions also appear in the glossary.

| | |
|---|---|
| abnormal | normal |
| abstinence | normative |
| alternative | normative sexual behavior |
| contraceptive | permissiveness |
| deviant | petting |
| double standard | promiscuity |
| fetishism | puberty |
| masturbation | secondary sex characteristics |
| menarche | sexual potency |
| nonmarital pregnancy | traditional |
| nonmarital sexual preference | transvestism |
| nontraditional | voyeurism |

## Discussion Questions

1. How do you remember your adolescent years in terms of your sexual awakening? Specifically, would you say this period was one of smooth development or a rocky bridge to adulthood? What social and psychological factors contributed to its smoothness or roughness? Did you form romantic attachments during your adolescent years that are still a part of your life? What, to you, were the most serious and difficult challenges of that period?

2. In what ways have you personally been affected by the double standard of sexual behavior. How would you describe it in terms of your values and your behaviors? What do you foresee as the possibilities of this double standard becoming a single, equalitarian standard in the next decade. Since no explanation of its source is universally ac-

cepted, how would you explain the origins and social purpose of the double standard as it now exists?

3. Look at some of the attitudes reflected in tables 5.1–5.5 (Kaats and Davis; Sorenson). How do they agree or differ from your attitudes and from those of your peers? Do you think these attitudes are in the process of change today? In what direction?

4. From your reading of this chapter and from the tables provided, list five of the chief characteristics of premarital sexual attitudes, standards, and behaviors in the United States today.

5. How do we determine if a sexual behavior is normative or non-normative? What is the relationship between the psychological and cultural determinations of what is normal?

## Suggested Readings

1. John H. Gagnon and William Simon. *Sexual Conduct: The Social Sources of Human Sexuality.* Chicago: Aldine, 1973.

An excellent, thorough-going social learning theory approach to the social bases of human sexual behavior by two extremely knowledgeable investigators in this field.

2. Morton Hunt. *Sexual Behavior in the 1970's.* Chicago, Playboy, 1974.

An extremely useful report on an empirical survey of contemporary American sexual behavior.

3. Alfred C. Kinsey et al. *Sexual Behavior in the Human Male.* Philadelphia: Saunders, 1948.

The ground-breaking classic work of one of the pioneers in the systematic survey of human sexual behavior. Despite the flurry of conceptual and methodological criticism, this volume (and its companion one on women) has stood the test of time and changed the nature of discussion and research into human sexual behavior.

4. Alfred C. Kinsey et al. *Sexual Behavior in the Human Female.* Philadelphia: Saunders, 1953.

This is the follow-up of the original Kinsey volume on men and perhaps was even more influential because of the general taboo on discussions about sexuality of women.

5. William H. Masters and Virginia Johnson. *Human Sexual Response.* Boston: Little, Brown, 1966.

A superb, detailed, and technical book on the results of laboratory studies of human sexual behavior. It is a useful companion to the Kinsey surveys of reported behavior.

6.  Ira L. Reiss. *Premarital Sexual Standards in America.* New York: Free Press of Glencoe, 1960.

An important analysis of the standards for premarital sexual behavior which lead to the development of a typology of premarital standards that have served as the bases of many studies to this day.

7.  Ira L. Reiss. *The Social Context of Premarital Permissiveness.* New York: Holt, 1967.

A report of what is probably the first sociological analysis of a nationwide probability sample of premarital sexual attitudes and behavior of adolescents and adults in the U.S., including the social constraints on such activities.

# Chapter 6

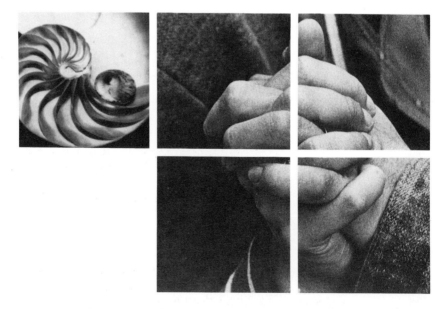

# Mate Selection

## Chapter Aims

1. To survey in detail the process of mate selection, considering the gamut of social-psychological factors that help define our choice of a marital partner.

2. To outline the social and interpersonal contexts of pairing.

3. To identify the social and interpersonal factors that serve to include or exclude other people from our "field of eligibles."

4. To look at some theories of why we choose to marry whom we do.

## Overview

At what point two people become a couple is influenced by other people's perceptions, the couple's mutual agreements about their relationship, their form of communicating with each other, and ultimately some sign that is visible, such as telling people of their plans together.

Why people become a couple is influenced by a range of social and psychological factors that are always interacting. Society limits our choice by sanctioning marriage only outside of close family and only within certain other groups, such as one's socioeconomic, racial, or age group. In choosing a mate from the group that society sanctions, your personality and other interpersonal, or social psychological, factors play an important role. These factors may include your needs and your self-image.

## How Free Are We?

Pairing is an integral part of our socialization. In the course of growing up, maturing, and experiencing life, we invariably explore relationships with many different people, enjoying some more than others, learning from some and not learning a great deal from others, profiting from some and finding others painful and empty. At some point in our growth most of us begin to look for, to feel the need for, a more serious and long-lasting attachment with another person. This need for a serious, long-lasting attachment is an acquired need. In our culture it is also an important mark first of adolescent and then of adult status.

Learned behavior

As we noted in chapter 1, in many societies throughout history, the selection of a mate was not left to chance or to the flights of romantic fancy. It was done by capture, purchase, or arrangement. But in our contemporary society, the idea of finding the ''right'' person for each of us is an important idea, one that deeply influences whom we choose to marry.

The ''right'' person

It is this contemporary belief that compels us to search. Sometimes, the search for the right person may require many years of effort in meeting new people and in forming new relationships. Eventually, we find someone special and establish a socially recognized and personally fulfilling relationship. We become paired with that person, and we are perceived, by those around us and by ourselves, as part of a *couple,* that is, of a socially recognized pair. The age at which this happens and the qualities of this process vary not only from society to society and from subculture to subculture, but from individual to individual as well.

A variety of forces help shape our choice of a mate. There are social forces that affect every person in a society, but each person in a different way. The specific way these forces are perceived and responded to has a major impact on one's perception of one's role in the mate-selection process as well as the mate one finally chooses. These forces are imposed from without, but processed within, thus the social and the psychological are combined. We each have our own personalities, our own unique psychologies, which are entwined with the social forces. These differ greatly from individual to individual.

For instance, consider the following situation, which illustrates the interaction of these forces:

### Sandra and Beth

Both Sandra and Beth were raised in the same Orthodox Jewish community in Boston. As they reached their late adolescent years, both their families put subtle pressures on them to find husbands and start families. Both were also given a clear, and basically identical, message of what type of person the husband should be: he should be a practicing Jew who keeps the Sabbath, either a professional or someone studying Jewish law fulltime; he should come from a "good" family; preferrably he should want to stay in Boston so the daughter would not have to move to another city. These and many more parental and peer expectations were taught to the girls as part of their socialization.

But even though they received the same messages, they responded quite differently. Sandra, an obedient girl, found exactly the kind of man her parents wanted. Beth, on the other hand, who is just as religious but also a bit rebellious, refused to look for a husband. She said she wanted to pursue a teaching career first and would find a husband later. When her parents objected strongly—"first things first," they said—she developed a relationship with Martin, who was not very religious and not a professional. Her parents are still trying to discourage her from marrying Martin, although they would not go as far as to prohibit it.

We see here how the two girls' individual personalities affected their choice of mates, even though both had been exposed to the same general social orientation.

While we like to believe we are completely free to make our own choices, there are a variety of identifiable social and interpersonal forces: from the environment around us, from our peers, from our family, and from the obvious and subtle cues provided by the culture. These help shape and influence our decisions.

# What Is Pairing?

At what point do two individuals become a couple? Is it when they recognize themselves as such? Is it when they act, or think, or feel in such a way that most people around them, such as friends, family, and colleagues, say they are a couple. Or, is it when some institution designates them a couple and indicates by certain signs and symbols that these two people have formed a partnership? We can say that for society to recognize two people as voluntarily paired, there must be a mutual exchange of affection in which each demonstrates his or her fondness and interdependence with the other. The psychological development of the person and the social customs that influence all of us provide some valuable clues about how this happens.

**Mothering one**

At the beginning of life the infant is paired to another person, to someone who is primarily responsible for his or her care and survival. Harry Stack Sullivan calls this person the *mothering one.* She or he is deemed by society to perform a certain role, to express certain attitudes about and behaviors toward the child. This mothering one has the responsibility for seeing that the infant is taken care of, that its physical and emotional needs are satisfied. At the same time, the mothering one is the primary agent in socializing the infant; that is, in teaching the infant the appropriate social attitudes, skills, and behaviors. The infant, sensing the care and concern, develops warm, loving feelings for the mothering one.

**Attachment**

This feeling is called *attachment,* and it becomes the prototype for later situations in which one becomes paired with another person.

The first prerequisite for pairing then is the feeling of attachment. Socially, however, it is not enough for one person to feel attached to another in order for pairing to take place. Rather, there has to be mutual attachment. When one person loves another and the other does not reciprocate,

**Unrequited love**

this is called *unrequited love.* A recurrent theme in many of the sad songs we hear, this is a most painful experience.

The mutual attachment that constitutes pairing develops within the relationship. It may first be observed by either or both of the individuals or by their friends. It is not uncommon to find that your friends know you are becoming seriously involved with someone even before you know it.

## Betty and Jarred

Betty and Jarred began to date casually in early May. They liked each other immediately, but they had both decided and made it clear to each other that they wanted to be free during the summer, when they planned to have active social lives and date many different people. Both of their sets of friends saw that they were "right" for each other from the beginning; and by the beginning of June when one was invited to a party, the other was invited also. By mid-June the two individuals, Betty and Jarred, had become a couple, recognized as such and treated as such by their contemporaries.

This is a good example of how, after a period of time, the people around two individuals may begin to designate them as a couple even before they are ready to acknowledge it themselves. We find the same situation true with respect to parents and their perceptions of their children's choices. If Betty's parents like Jarred, or if Jarred's like Betty, the parents may treat them as a pair in conversation and in practice, even before Betty and Jarred are ready to make the commitment themselves. The families may practice such accepted social conventions as inviting Jarred to Betty's family's Thanksgiving dinner or Jarred's cousin Louise inviting Betty to her wedding as Jarred's date.

## Implicit Behavioral Contracting

There are several signs inside the relationship to indicate that pairing is taking place. While the world outside is making its own assessment, the two people involved are also deciding whether or not they are to be partners. The *intrarelationship process of pairing* involves setting up an implicit, unwritten, sometimes ambiguous, and often flexible behavioral contract. This is worked out slowly, as the relationship evolves. This contract says in effect, "We can function as a couple under the following conditions." Several areas of agreement are then worked out. When these are adhered to, their "couplehood" is unchallenged. But, when parts of the contract are broken, the stability of the couple as a unit comes under attack and they either have to work out new clauses and stipulations or dissolve the partnership.

First and foremost is usually the issue of *exclusivity*. Whenever two people choose to date *only* each other, they invariably become perceived as a couple by themselves as well as by others. This perception is clear and simple, agreed to by the society and the individuals. However, some couples may choose to date outside their relationship, but only under certain conditions. Our society does not generally favor such an arrangement. Other people are reluctant to grant the status of "couplehood" to two love-struck individuals who request it but who do not agree to abide by the laws of exclusivity.

Intrarelationship process pairing

Exclusivity

## Ted and Julia

When Ted and Julia first decided they were right for each other, they both realized that their relationship would probably lead to marriage. But neither felt ready at that point, and they decided to date each other exclusively for at least two years before becoming officially engaged. But the following year, when Ted went away to graduate school in another state, he and Julia agreed that each should have the opportunity to socialize with others, as long as they remained sexually exclusive. Their revised contract now defined this status as "faithful," or exclusive. This new provision was communicated to their friends, and each told any dates they might have that it was only some companionship they were looking for. Nevertheless, people refused to believe them. It was generally felt that if their relationship was still going strong they would not be dating other people under any circumstances. The society now discouraged the designation of couplehood for Ted and Julia, even though both of them desired it.

## Couple Communication

As a relationship blossoms, the couple begins to develop intimacies of communication, which may be verbal or nonverbal (Goodman and Ofshe 1968). On the verbal level, these include shortcut expressions, key words, nicknames for themselves and for others, and other pet terms they enjoy. The two people get pleasure out of using these terms because it reassures them they are part of a small, exclusive group. Moreover, as these nonstandard uses of language are revealed in public, other people recognize the two individuals as a couple. Just as two speakers of the same foreign language would be recognized as a group, these two, speaking their own foreign language, are perceived as a group of two.

Verbal cues

In addition to verbal communication, there are important changes in nonverbal communication and body language that reveal a message to the outside world: "We are a pair." In one study, it was found that independent observers watching subject couples considered the time they gazed at each other most important in giving their relationship a positive rating (Kleinke, Meeker, and La Fong 1974). Other studies have also shown that our body language changes as we become more intimate with another (see chapter 4). This intimacy reveals to the world that the two people are functioning as a couple.

Nonverbal cues

## Social Symbols

Finally, there may be recognized *social symbols,* such as a piece of jewelry, to indicate the binding of one person to another. These may include a formal or informal engagement ceremony or announcement or simply a casual talk about marriage in the near or distant future. Two people beginning to plan their lives together, acknowledging a common future, is the clearest sign that they have now become a pair.

In our culture, in which relatively free marital choice is the norm, this symbolic gesture reflects the couple's voluntary consent to be perceived in terms of and to function as a pair. It is a social affirmation of their freedom to choose and a recognition that society will go along with their choice. They are, in effect, by their overt actions, telling others around them, particularly friends and family, "We are now attached to each other in a special way; one presumably and traditionally leading to a permanent relationship." This type of gesture is a recognized form of social communication, one that informs others that the expectations of the two individuals have been changed and that new perceptions of the two individuals are to be expected. Such a message is required only where free choice in marriage selection prevails, and historically this has not always

Free choice

*People have clear, non-verbal ways of communicating to the rest of the world that they are a couple.*

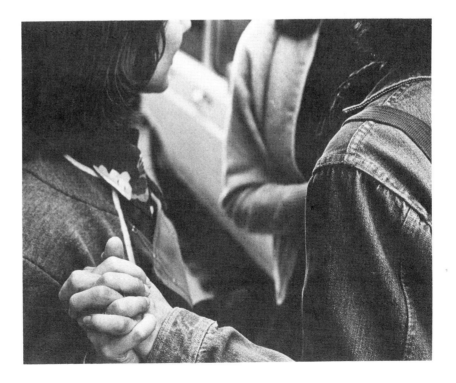

been the case. In fact, throughout the course of history, in most societies the choice of a mate was not made voluntarily by the couple, but was dictated by parents or other individuals with a vested social interest in the young people's marriage choice. In such situations, social guidelines were used to determine who was to marry whom, as well as to warn others to stay away.

## The Effects of Choice on Pairing

Complexities of choosing

Whenever a society does afford its members a relative amount of free choice in the selection of a mate, the complexities of choosing come into question. We should keep in mind that while we are free to some extent, there are many factors that limit and shape our choice. While having the freedom to select a mate of our own choosing is certainly good, it also presents us with many problems we would not have if our mate were selected for us, as in the case of marriage by arrangement. How, for example, do we go about making this choice? What factors influence us? How do we know whether we've made the correct choice or not? "Although basing a marriage on love creates instability because of the irrational nature of emotion," Cox (1974) points out, "certainly few can deny that individual freedom has been increased by it. With individual freedom there is greater opportunity to maximize potentials" (p. 22).

Even as we begin to understand how the couple forms the paired relationship, we still do not see why one person chooses another as a mate. We will divide the factors that influence this choice into two categories: the social factors and the interpersonal, or social-psychological. We should keep in mind, however, that these groups always interact.

## Social Factors in Pairing

No society leaves mate selection to chance. Marriage and the creation of a family are such critical social acts and have such potentially important and far-reaching consequences that society cannot afford the choice of a mate to be left unregulated.

Field of eligibles

As we select our mate, we are not selecting from all the people in the world, but rather from a limited range of individuals, who constitute the available population. This discriminate group is called the *field of eligibles*. This field of eligibles is not of our own making; it is determined by an interaction of social pressures that make themselves felt. Individual feelings of romance that may blossom early in a relationship soon give way to the realization that certain people are right for us and others are

## Figure 6.1
### Operation of Exogamy and Endogamy in the Field of Eligible Partners

The field of eligibles is defined as the area between the circles and the arrows.

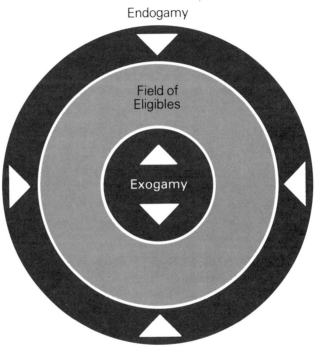

not (Falk 1975). The field of eligibles becomes clear to us through social approval and disapproval.

Across the world there are two key regulations that help shape our field of eligibles. These are exogamy and endogamy. As shown in figure 6.1, they operate jointly to define the socially sanctioned pool of potential marriage partners that sociologists call the *field of eligibles*.

**Social approval and disapproval**

## Exogamy

*Exogamy,* requiring marriage outside a specified group of people, is probably the more fundamental regulatory principle of mate choice. It defines those categories of individuals with whom one should not mate (for example, members of one's own sex). It is probably more fundamental than endogamy, marriage inside a particular group, in the sense that the loca-

**Outside the field of eligibles**

tion of those who clearly are to be excluded from the "field of eligibles" is generally more important than how large the pool is to be. The two major exogamous principles involve sex and kinship. Kinship exogamy is better known as the incest taboo and deserves further elaboration.

Incest taboo

The incest taboo, the prohibition against sexual or marital relations among family members, is the best-known application of the rule of exogamy. All societies have an incest taboo that puts members of one's immediate family outside of the sexual and marital pale. There are only a handful of exceptions to this generalization, in ancient Egypt and with the Incas to name two. But these exceptions always involved members of the royal family and not the general populace, which, even in the societies showing these exceptions, was subject to the incest taboo. However, there is no cross-cultural universality as to who else is included.

Consequences of exogamy

One important consequence of the operation of the rule of exogamy is that it creates alliances by forcing people to marry outside of a relatively narrow kinship circle. Such social pressure serves not only to enlarge the number of groups within society, but it keeps the individual free from being wholly contained within a single social group, such as one's family, total commitment to which could threaten allegiance to the society as a whole.

## Endogamy

At the same time as we are influenced by exogamy, we are influenced by a counter force, *endogamy*. Every society has an outside boundary to the field of eligibles. The delineation of this outer limit on socially acceptable marital partners is called endogamy. Marriage is not only a personal act; in fact, in most societies around the world its personal component is its least important feature. It is, above all, a social act, and the rule of endogamy is often seen as protecting the composition and internal social structure of the society. It unites different families and social groups; it creates or cements alliances; it provides for the inheritance of scarce resources; money, property, goods, and magic rituals, for example. Most importantly, the application of the principle of endogamy plays an important part in maintaining the solidarity of the society or, in large, complex, and differentiated societies, the appropriate social subgroup.

Inside the field of eligibles

The boundary set by endogamy is almost always the same as the boundary defining the group itself. That is to say, the endogamous principle is coextensive: it covers the group's domain. Thereby it serves to reduce, if not to eliminate, intergroup marriage whether the group is defined in terms of clan, religion, race, ethnic background, social class, community of origin, or any other important sociological characteristic.

To understand these principles better and how they interact, let us

*The influence of social norms on mate selection is revealed in the conventional height differences between men and women in paired relationships.*

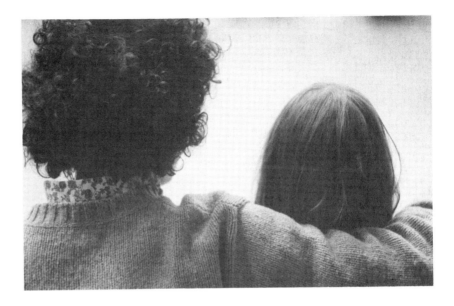

*The influence of social norms on mate selection is revealed in the conventional height differences between men and women in paired relationships.*

look at some specific variables that are affected by endogamous pressures.

### Socioeconomic Level

Throughout most of recorded history, wherever a society has been characterized by different social classes, there has always been a powerful social bias that people should marry within their own social and economic class. A *social class* can be defined ''as any group of people who occupy similar positions on a scale of prestige which is determined by educational, occupational, and economic achievements'' (Hughes 1971, p. 131). Individuals have traditionally selected their mates in response to the endogamous social pressure to marry within one's class. A novel such as Theodore Dreiser's *American Tragedy* illustrates how even in the presumably egalitarian United States there is immense pressure to maintain socioeconomic class endogamy. Clyde Griffiths, the protagonist, is compelled to murder when the lower-class working girl he had been dating becomes pregnant, ruining his chances to marry into a higher class with the new girl he has found. Dreiser is perceptive of people's reactions and sensitive to the social sanctions against boys of a lower class marrying girls of a higher class. In the classic New Haven study of youth, Hollingshead (1950) found that when class lines were crossed in mate selection, it was most often the man who married a woman from a lower class. There was a much lower incidence of a higher-class woman marrying a man from a lower class. Historically, the choice of a marriage partner has even caused nations to have major

Social class

internal crises. Henry VIII's choice of a new wife, which required that he get divorced, contributed in part to his country breaking away from the Church of Rome. In this century, the marriage of the Duke of Windsor to Wallis Simpson, an American divorcée and a commoner, forced him to give up the throne and made him persona non grata in his own country.

*Social mobility,* the tendency of people to move from one social class to another, has certainly had a profound impact on mating patterns in the United States. It is no longer totally unacceptable, or even shocking, for a person of the lower class to marry a person of the upper class, and marriage between lower and middle is quite common. Yet, it is not as common as marriage between people of the same class. A number of reasons have been suggested for this phenomenon. The most important of these is *propinquity,* the nearness and accessibility of a person.

People tend to live with their own kind. Out of choice or out of necessity, a large segment of society lives in neighborhoods with others sharing many of the same social characteristics. For the prosperous this may be more a result of choice; for the poor it is necessity. Some families select a neighborhood because it has appropriate places of worship for them or good schools for their children. In New York City, hundreds of young artistic couples with children have settled in a former factory district, called Soho, which is now considered a very "arty" place to be raised.

In growing up and socializing, therefore, we have more opportunities to meet people of our own socioeconomic level. The people at the country club where we socialize, on the streetcorner where we hang around, or in school or on the job are all probably from the same socioeconomic group as we are. Obviously, if we go to college, we are more likely to meet a college-educated person than if we are not exposed to people at college.

Second, there is a tendency for members of the same socioeconomic class to share a relatively common set of experiences. Because common interests and shared values, which come with shared experiences, are an important part of intimacy, they make it more likely that people of the same social class will find each other more suitable partners for marriage. The person who was raised in a welfare home will understand the pains and difficulties of growing up poor better than a person who has grown up in a wealthy home. The person from the middle-class family may not be able to understand how important it is for the rich person to travel to Europe every summer.

**Sharon and John**

Sharon and John met at a party given by a mutual acquaintance. As they began dating they enjoyed each other's company because of the attraction they felt for each other and be-

*Social mobility*

*Propinquity*

cause of the excitement in finding someone new. But as the relationship became more serious the deficits of it became apparent to both of them. Sharon's father was a bank president and Sharon simply ''had to'' spend her summers on Shelter Island. The city, she said, was unbearable. John was used to working in the unbearable city during the summer and could hardly afford a weekend off and certainly not the whole summer. Sharon knew good restaurants and enjoyed good food; John didn't know frogs' legs from pâté de foie gras. Sharon loved theatre, while John couldn't see wasting fifteen dollars on a ticket for a show when he could see a movie for four bucks. Sharon was an avid reader; John preferred TV. Sharon loved tennis; John played baseball. When they broke up after about five months of dating most people felt that Sharon was the spoiled rich girl who couldn't ''lower'' herself. But the truth was that because of their class differences, their upbringings, and their values, Sharon and John had real trouble understanding each other and sharing the same pleasures in life.

Compatability of Beliefs and Experiences   There is evidence that we choose to pair not only with people from the same socioeconomic class as our own, but within that class with people who have beliefs and attitudes similar to ours. We know that within any socioeconomic class there is great variation, *intraclass variation,* and there is a tendency in choosing a mate toward similarity: toward finding people whose beliefs, education, religion, and world view are similar to our own.

This may involve mutual interests as illustrated above or even deeper beliefs. In selecting a mate, especially during the earlier stages of pairing, one tries to find out how many shared beliefs there are between the other person and oneself. Since the likelihood is that some, or many, of our friends share our belief systems, there is the distinct possibility that if we choose someone whose beliefs are very different from our own, we are risking the loss of some of these friends and people we consider important.

This risk has been especially true of religious beliefs. There has always been a strong tendency for the organized religions to teach the child from the earliest years that one should marry someone from the same religious group, and there have been all kinds of punishments against individuals who marry outside the group. For example, in some religious communities if you marry outside your religion, you are virtually banned from the community. Yet, there is an increasing, and some religious

*Intraclass variation*

people say "alarming," tendency for young people today to marry outside the religious group. This is explained in part by a slackening of religious fervor and dogmatism and in part by the mobility of young people
and the opportunities this affords to meet people of different religious
backgrounds.

## Age, Educational Attainment, and Other Social Fac-
tors   We have become accustomed to certain rules governing the selection of a mate. The man is typically somewhat older than the woman, but
not more than two or three years older. There may be social pressures
exerted against very large age differences. These pressures are different if
the older party is a man from those exerted if the woman is older.

*Age sanctions*

### Beth and Paul, Lawrence and
### Elizabeth

In a small community, two unusual marriages recently took
place. Beth, aged 22, married Paul who had been her college
professor and was in his late 50s. Although there were many
comments about this seemingly incongruous pairing, the
people of the town were basically willing to accept it, since no
marriage had been broken up because of it and since it appeared that Beth was not marrying Paul for money, a question
that had been raised by the townspeople earlier. However,
when Lawrence, in his midtwenties married a widow, Elizabeth
Peal, who was 20 years his senior, eyebrows were raised and
censure became the order of the day. "He must be overly attached to his mother," neighbors speculated. "I think it's disgusting that a woman her age is marrying a man so much
younger," others said. There seemed to be much more anger
at the older woman with the younger man than at the older
man with the younger woman. In both of these cases, you notice, motives other than love were looked for, since the age difference is viewed as an abnormality until proven otherwise.

In the New Haven study cited earlier, it was found that "the age-
sanctions that impinge on a woman with reference to the age of a potential husband narrow her marital opportunities to men her age, or to
slightly older men" (Hollingshead 1950).

This limitation as to age of male and female partners also extends to
educational differences. Generally, the social pressure is for a person to
marry someone of his or her educational level. The male college graduate

**Sex-role biases**

will most likely not be chastised for marrying the female high school graduate, but the female college graduate is expected to marry a man who has at least completed college. There is also a great deal of pressure against the career woman who chooses to marry a nonprofessional, a blue collar worker. Yet, the professional man can easily get away with marrying a "housewife," as long as she is able to function within his social circle. Again, as we have seen in many instances throughout this book, these examples reflect a sex-role bias against women.

**The strongest endogamous pressure**

**Race**  Probably the pressure to marry within one's own race is the strongest of all the endogamous social pressures. Hollingshead (1950) found that "racial mores place the strongest, most explicit, and most precise limits on an individual as to whom he may or may not marry (p. 619). So strong is this taboo traditionally that in many states such marriages were prohibited by law. Of course this has changed drastically over the past three decades, but interracial marriage is still frowned on by many who would more easily tolerate marriage between partners of different religious affiliations or social or economic classes. This reluctance is socially significant according to Porterfield (1978), who has written a book on the subject, because the public's attitude toward black-white marriages is "one of the most accurate indices for measuring the extent to which a group is achieving social, economic and political equality. If complete acceptance comes to pass, it is likely that discrimination in the United States, based on race or skin color, will cease to exist" (p. 14).

Petroni (1973) has studied interracial dating patterns in more recent years. In addition to the pressures against whites who wish to date blacks, he finds that there is a tremendous pressure against black girls from their parents and friends if they wish to date a white boy. Petroni (p. 144) also points out that,

> Those who date interracially pay a price. In the game of imputing motives, few are convinced that the daters merely like one another. Rarely is the couple not accused of promiscuity.

**Interracial marriage**

Stuart and Abt (1973) have edited an excellent volume on the literature of interracial marriage, pointing out many of the adjustment problems interracial couples face and the pressures that are brought to bear upon them. In a detailed research study, in which the available literature and a large amount of statistical information was analyzed, Monahan (1976) found that all socioeconomic groups participated about equally in interracial marriages without any clear pattern of marrying "up" or marrying "down." But "when there was a difference between blacks and whites, whites more often married blacks of lower status" (p. 175).

*Although interracial marriage has become more common, the pressure to marry within one's race is still the strongest endogamous social pressure.*

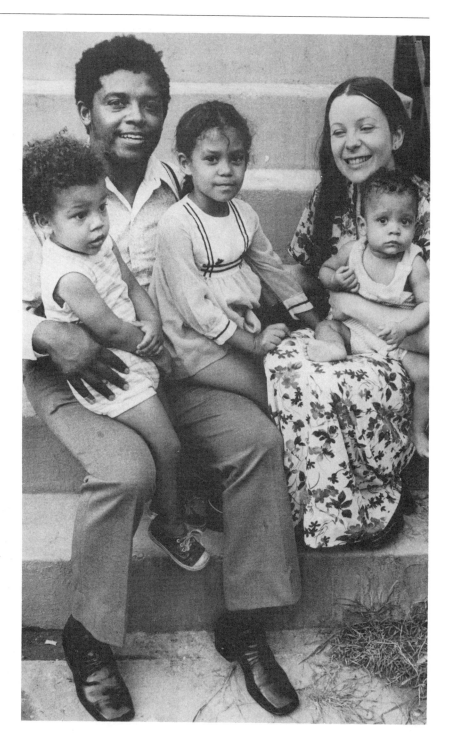

## Interpersonal Factors

After reading the preceding section, you may be under the impression that our choice of a mate is governed almost entirely by social factors. This is far from correct. While social factors play an important part in defining the field of eligibles from which we choose, there are powerful interpersonal, or social psychological, factors that influence one's choice of a specific partner within the socially constructed arena of values and attitudes enumerated above. As Levinger (1977) points out, there are actually four units embedded in the intimate pairing relationship: (1) the individual partner, (2) the pair unit, (3) the social group, and (4) the larger society. Each of these units requires some attention, some perspective. One's personality and interpersonal functioning combine with social factors to shape the individual's choice of a specific mate, within the context of those four units.

Four units in intimate pairing

As we attempt to examine the interpersonal, or social psychological, factors that influence our choice of a mate, we will see how the different types of personalities, with different configurations of needs, play a role in making an individual prefer one person over another. We will see how each of us has needs that must be met and how we try to find people who meet these needs, either in a healthy or an unhealthy way. Then, we will see how one's personality structure influences the choice of love object and how the person one chooses becomes integrated into one's own personality.

## Self-Image

Each of us has an image of self, a sense of who and what we are and how we fit into the world around us. This sense of self has a profound personal value, called self-esteem. Some of us think very positively about ourselves: we feel deserving, wanted by others, able to accomplish things; in general, we have a sense of mastery over our environment and a feeling that life is important. Others of us may have a considerably less positive sense of self: we may feel worthless, have little self-esteem, and feel essentially incapable of mastering our circumstances. In most cases, we fluctuate between these extremes.

The way we feel about ourselves largely influences our choice of mates (Satir 1967). We choose mates to a considerable extent who reflect our self-images. This can happen in several ways. The other person may act toward us as we feel about ourselves. For example, psychoanalysts believe that if we feel worthless we may choose someone who treats us poorly, that is, who makes us feel worthless. Or, the choice of a mate may be a way of compensating for our deficit feelings. If we feel

worthless deep inside, we may choose someone who treats us well because that treatment makes us feel better about ourselves. To more
clearly understand the relationship among self-image, needs, and mate
selection, let us look at some theories that have attempted to explain this
relationship.

## Individual Needs

Each of us has many needs that cry out to be met. Human needs are essential to our understanding of the individual's behavior, including the
choice of a mate. A number of systems have been suggested to help us
better understand our matrix of needs: to classify and organize them in
some way that we can make sense of them and understand their relationship to each other. Two of the most widely accepted systems of need
theory are those of Abraham H. Maslow and Henry A. Murray.

Maslow's hierarchy

Maslow classified human needs in a hierarchical arrangement: from
the most basic needs for food and air to the most profound needs for social esteem and the respect of others to the ultimate needs for self-actualization and growth (see figure 4.1). As the person is able to satisfy one
level of needs, Maslow argues, he or she is then able to concentrate on
the higher-levels needs. The person remains primarily on a certain level of
need until that level is achieved. Thus, an important part of human motivation and growth is going from level to level while adequately satisfying
the needs at each level.

Murray also offers a theory that considers the relationship between
the individual's needs and his or her motivation as a factor in satisfying
these needs. He breaks all the human needs down into 12 physiological
and 28 psychological needs. Physiological needs include the need for
water, sleep, and elimination of waste products; psychological needs include the need for status, autonomy, abasement, that is, criticism and
submission. A person's behavior can be explained in terms of how he or
she satisfies these inner needs against the demands of the realities of the
outside world, which Murray refers to as *press.* Corsini (1977, p. 408)
points out,

Press

> Murray's theory can be seen as a theory of motivation: The inner
> person and the outer world interact to lead to differential behav-
> ior. This means we must consider what is in the brain of the
> individual in terms of what gets there from inside (needs) and
> what gets there from outside (press), which combine, fuse, inter-
> act, and lead to differentiated action.

Theories of mate selection inevitably take human needs into account.

Since we are constantly in the process of trying to satisfy our needs and since selecting a mate is an important part of this process, a full understanding of the integral relationship between satisfying needs and choosing a mate is essential.

## Homogamy and Heterogamy

There is a popular saying that opposites attract: that the quiet and reserved guy will be drawn to the outgoing girl; that the friendly, gregarious young man will find himself attracted to a more withdrawn and diffident girlfriend. One reason this saying is so interesting is that it contradicts another widely held belief; namely, that people of similar personalities, beliefs, likes, and dislikes are attracted to each other, that "birds of a feather flock together." When a couple are obviously not "birds of a feather," the convenient saying of "opposites attract" helps explain why the two people are attracted to each other.

### Bert and Denise

The students in the dorm are at first puzzled by the seemingly incongruous pairing of Bert and Denise. Bert is one of the most popular guys at school: the captain of the basketball team, a smooth speaker in public, and an all-around charming and friendly person, always eager to lend a hand to someone who needs help. Denise, on the other hand, tends to be sarcastic and somewhat curt; she is not the type to be warm and intimate with others. She prefers to keep to herself, reading and painting in her room, and has no close friends to speak of. It is true that Denise and Bert are both taller and more physically attractive than the average person, but this similarity seems to be all they have in common. When commenting on their relationship, most people say, "You know how it is. Opposites tend to attract."

What in fact does the research show? Do opposites or likes tend to become attracted to each other?

Homogamy = alike

The term *homogamy* is used to describe the marriage of people who are alike. Its opposite is *heterogamy* the marriage of opposites. Throughout much of the research in mate selection, social researchers have attempted to see if the principle of homogamy adequately explains how we choose our mates. Also considered in this research is the possibility that

Heterogamy = opposites

people become more alike through the proximity and exposure of being married to each other. This process is called *association.*

In a classic paper, Burgess and Wallin (1953) reviewed and evaluated all the research literature available at that time. First, it was found that in studies reporting statistically significant results, couples tend to be more similar than different. Neither or only one of the pair may have any strong feelings about music; but if one likes classical music very much and the other does have a strong musical preference, it is likely that it will be toward classical music. Although in some cases there is little apparent similarity between the attitudes and beliefs of the two people; when we break down their complex of traits including attitudes and physical traits, we still find more like traits than different traits. This similarity is found more in areas such as religious beliefs than it is in physical characteristics and more in attitudes about marriage than in abstract opinions.

Complex of traits

Despite the many studies that tend to support the principle of homogamy, theories built solely on the concepts of either homogamy or heterogamy are basically oversimplifications. In reality, the matter of marital choice is never so simple that it can be broken down into such clear-cut categories. In any given relationship, people are alike in some ways and different in other ways. A good theory has to account for these different dimensions. Also, as we pointed out earlier, the related social pressures of exogamy and endogamy interact here with the psychological tendencies.

From the 1950s onward several more sophisticated, complex, and empirically verifiable theories have been developed. These theories tend to take into account three things: first, that once we are constricted to the field of eligibles, different personality factors and psychological factors play a role in our specific choice; second, that the satisfaction of our needs is a central part of our choice of a marital partner; and third, that any theory must account for the full complexity of human choice. We will look at the two most widely discussed theories: the complementary needs theory of Robert F. Winch and the Stimulus-Value-Role theory of Bernard I. Murstein.

## Theory of Complementary Needs

Robert F. Winch has introduced a theory that clearly goes beyond the principles of homogamy and heterogamy. It is an important theory that, although lacking solid empirical support, still finds many adherents.

Winch's position in brief states that ''in mate-selection, each individual seeks within his or her field of eligibles that person who gives the greatest promise of providing him or her with maximum need gratification'' (Winch 1967). Winch's concept of needs is based directly on the work of Henry A. Murray, from which he has selected twelve basic needs and three general traits to measure. Rather than limiting himself to same or different needs, Winch uses the concept of complementarity to account for the relationship. His theory is called appropriately the *theory of complementary* needs.

Winch defines two types of *complementarity. Type I complementarity* occurs when "A's need *X* is gratifying to B's need *Y* and B's behavior in acting out B's need *Y* is gratifying to A's need *X*" (Winch 1958). *Type II complementarity* involves two different needs. For instance, if one person is high on the need to be nurtured, to be taken care of, the other person will be high on the need called *succorance,* meaning nurturing or helping behavior. Using Murray's categories of needs, Winch, Ktsanes, and Ktsanes (1954, p. 243) offer examples of Type I and Type II complementariness:

**Complementarity**

> An example of Type I is found in the case of a person desirous of attention and recognition (need recognition) who finds gratification in a relationship with a person who tends to bestow admiration on the former (need deference). Type II is illustrated in the interaction between a person who wants others to do his bidding (high need dominance) and one lacking the ability to handle his environment who is looking for someone to tell him what to do (low need dominance). It will be recognized that this definition of complementariness embraces two forms of heterogamy.

*Marriage is not only a personal act but also a social act which maintains the solidarity of society.*

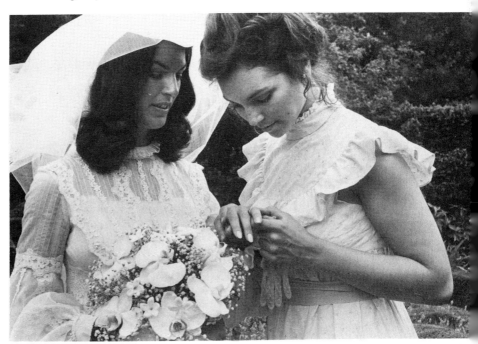

The existence of both of these types of complementary needs have been tested in a series of studies, but at the present there is generally insufficient support for this theory (Wagner 1975). Winch has modified his theory in recent years to include the effects of social roles enacted by the spouses as an integral part of the stability of the relationship (Winch 1974), but this phase of it still remains untested.

## Stimulus-Value-Role Theory

Bernard I. Murstein has developed a theory that has replaced Winch's as the most widely accepted today. Murstein's recent publications, including *Who Will Marry Whom?* (1976), have thoroughly investigated and evaluated the available literature. What makes Murstein's theory especially valuable, besides it's substantial empirical documentation, is that it recognizes that mate selection is a fluid and dynamic process, one that may involve different factors and different stages along the way to final selection. Moreover, Murstein takes into account the importance of social role in this process as we see below when we look at *R*. The *S*, the *V*, and the *R* of his theory reflect the different stages of the mate selection process.

SVR theory

*Stimulus-Value-Role Theory,* which is commonly abbreviated S-V-R, states that ''(1) marital choice involves a series of sequential stages . . . that are labeled stimulus, value, and role, and that (2) at any given point of the relationship, its viability can be determined as a function of the equality of exchange subjectively experienced by its participants'' (Murstein 1973, pp. 23–24). What this means simply is that at the beginning of a relationship what is most important is the stimulus value of the other person. If Michael turns Harriet on and her friends think he is a good date, these constitute sufficient reasons to begin dating him. As the relationship progresses, however, personal values held by each partner become important. As Harriet begins to recognize Michael's commitment to social change and personal sacrifice for the common good, she realizes this directly conflicts with her wish to marry a man who will make a lot of money—for them! Later on, considerations of role become paramount.

S = stimulus value

We may be initially interested in people because they are physically attractive to us, because of their *stimulus value.* They enjoy a high prestige position in social situations and this serves to stimulate our interest. This is called the stimulus stage because we are not responding to something about the inner person, but to initial impressions, to perceptions that are stimulated inside us by external factors.

## Bob

Bob has decided that he will ask Marlene to the party. He made this decision after considering a number of alternative possibilities. She is very attractive, the most popular at school, and would, for him, have the highest prestige value. Thus, his choice is based on her stimulus value as an individual; not on anything that could be considered a relationship.

The relationship develops further and gets more serious during the next stage, the "V" stage, that of *value comparison*. "The primary focus of the value comparison stage," Murstein points out, "is information gathering by verbal interaction with the other" (Murstein 1976, p. 123). He goes on to illustrate (p. 124) what happens in this stage:

V = value comparison

> The value comparison stage occurs when the couple has not as yet developed sufficient intimacy to learn and confess the innermost precepts, fears, aspirations, and concerns that each has. Nevertheless, there is much public and private information that each learns about the other in this period. Information is gleaned about religious orientation, political beliefs, attitudes toward people, parents, friends, interests in sports, the arts, dancing, and the like.

During the value comparison stage, "the importance of the stimulus variables has waned somewhat" (124), and therefore the values expressed by each partner becomes important in understanding and relating to the other partner. Murstein (1973, pp. 24–25) explains how this works:

Shared values

> Should the couple find that they hold similar value orientations in important areas, they are apt to develop much stronger positive feelings for each other than they experienced in the stimulus stage. One reason for this is that when an individual encounters another who holds similar values, he gains support for the conclusion that his own values are correct; his views are given social validation. Providing we have a reasonably positive self-image, we tend to be attracted to those persons whom we perceive as validating it. Also, perceived similarity of values may lead to the assumption that the other likes us, and there is empirical evidence that we like those individuals who we think like us.

During this stage, the two people discuss their views and find that they have a lot in common. As they discover their shared values they come to like each other more; they each feel better able to understand the other.

Finally, we come to the *role stage*. During this stage, each partner tests the other's ability to function within a given role. It is during this stage that the individual realizes he or she is heading toward marriage, and "faced with this awareness, he is apt to reappraise the qualities of his possible spouse" (Murstein 1976, p. 125). A part of this reappraisal is measuring the stimulus qualities and value comparison qualities against the more permanent quality of the other playing the role of spouse.

R = role stage

## Bob and Marlene

Now that they have been dating for almost a year, Bob and Marlene are beginning to look at each other and at themselves as part of a couple differently. They have stopped dating others and are considering the possibility of getting engaged or of living together or even of eloping. As these ideas go through their minds, each thinks about how the other will be as a partner. What will my parents think? How will my friends react? What kind of parent will he or she make if we decide to have children? These are some of the role questions that are asked during this stage.

According to Murstein, the relative values of S, V, and R in the relationship vary at different points in the courtship.

The strength of a relationship, its viability, at a given point depends on how equally the two partners are giving to each other as well as receiving from each other. Murstein calls this the principle of *equity*. Murstein goes on to add other complex dimensions to this theory, dimensions involving the perceptual and behavioral expression during the three stages. He also applies to mate selection an increasingly useful social psychological perspective, *exchange theory;* namely, that each partner offers to the other an amount roughly equal to what he or she gains from the relationship. According to this principle, each partner attempts to *profit* from the relationship, "profit being defined as the rewards he gains from the interaction minus the costs he must pay" (Murstein, 1973, p. 26).

Exchange theory

## Summary

1. There are personal and social symbols that tell others that two people have consented to function as a pair. These include bodily gestures, intimacy of communication, explicit and implicit contracting, and such standard symbols as the engagement ring. As others recognize that this pairing is taking place, they confer the role of couple on the two people.

2. Social factors play an extremely important role in mate selection. Society establishes a field of eligibles from which a person should select a mate. This group is determined by the principles of exogamy, choice outside of a group, and endogamy, choice inside other groups. Endogamy governs such social factors of choosing a mate as finding one within the same socioeconomic, religious, age, racial, and educational group.

3. Interpersonal, or social psychological, factors influence mate selection from within the field already determined by social factors. What causes people to choose certain mates from the field of those eligible? Self-image and the needs of the individual are at the foundation of choice and especially of marital choice. Two popular theories of mate selection are Winch's theory of complementary needs and Murstein's Stimulus-Value-Role Theory. Winch proposes that within the field of eligibles we find mates whose needs complement our own or who are able to gratify our needs by their behaviors. Murstein's theory of mate selection states that marital choice typically involves a sequence of stages, from reliance on the stimulus value of the other to a more intense relationship involving values and role considerations. The available evidence seems to favor Murstein's position.

## Key Terms

The following terms have been introduced and defined in this chapter. Definitions also appear in the glossary.

| | |
|---|---|
| association | press |
| attachment | profit |
| couple | propinquity |
| endogamy | role stage |
| equity | social class |
| exchange theory | social mobility |
| exclusivity | social symbol |
| exogamy | stimulus value |
| field of eligibles | Stimulus-Value-Role Theory |
| heterogamy | theory of complementary needs |
| homogamy | Type I complementarity |
| intraclass variation | Type II complementarity |
| intrarelationship process of pairing | unrequited love |
| mothering one | value comparison |
| pairing | |

## Discussion Questions

1. Observing the people around you, what specific social symbols are most frequently used to indicate to others that a person is attached? How effective are these symbols in communicating this information?

2. Looking at all the factors we suggested play some part in the selection of a mate, which would you say that you have personally found most relevant in your own marital or close relationship choice? Specifically, how would you characterize your field of eligibles in terms of how it differs from the general population? Would your field of eligibles be substantially different if you were from a different social class? A different racial or ethnic group? If you lived in a different type of geographic area, such as city vs. rural? If you were from a different religious group?

3. Using as an example the most intimate romantic relationship in which you are or have been involved, test out the theory of complementary needs and the S-V-R theory to see which better explains your reason

for choosing the person you did. Would you say that one theory is consistently a better explanation than the other or are there varying factors that determine which is a better theory?

4. What would attract two very different people to each other? Why might they find it easier to get along than two people who are very similar?

5. From your reading of this chapter, what would you cite as the main factors limiting mate selection? As you construct your answer, use in context as many of the terms from the preceding questions as you can.

## Suggested Readings

1. Ernest W. Burgess and Leonard S. Cottrell, Jr. *Predicting Success or Failure in Marriage.* Englewood Cliffs, N.J.: Prentice-Hall, 1939.

A landmark study of the sociological factors that lead to successful marriage and their incorporation into a scale to predict marital success.

2. William R. Catton, Jr., and R.L. Smircich. "A Comparison of Mathematical Models for the Effect of Residential Propinquity on Mate Selection," *American Sociological Review,* No. 29 (August 1964), pp. 522–529.

A technical analysis of the importance of residential proximity as a factor in mate selection.

3. Alvin M. Katz and Reuben Hill. "Residential Propinquity and Marital Selection," *Marriage and Family Living,* No. 20 (February 1958), pp. 27–35.

A thoughtful attempt to understand the reasons why residential propinquity plays an important role in mate selection. The authors develop what they call a "norm interaction" hypothesis that stresses the role of available opportunities for interaction, the attendant rewards and costs of such an interaction and possible alternative opportunities.

4. Bernard I. Murstein. *Who Will Marry Whom? Theories and Research in Marital Choice.* New York: Springer, 1976.

A detailed analysis of theories of mate choice and the development of a view that recognizes mate selection as a dynamic process. Murstein's S-V-R (stimulus-value-role) theory has become the major sociological alternative to the earlier dominant psychoanalytically based Theory of Complementary Needs of Robert F. Winch.

5. Robert F. Winch. *Mate Selection.* New York: Harper, 1958.

Until recently this book (and several articles) by Winch formed the basis for the most influential general theory of mate selection. It has at its base the psychoanalytic view of the importance of the attraction of opposites. More recent research (e.g., Murstein's work among others) have suggested a more restrictive role for Winch's theory in this area.

# Part THREE

## Contemporary Patterns of Bonding

**7. Challenges and Roles in Marriage**
**8. Alternative Styles: The "Outsiders"**

In the preceding part of the book, we focused on the social psychological processes through which two individuals join to create a paired relationship characterized by intimacy, mutual affection, and sexual activity. We considered some of the key issues: why we are attracted to another person; why we chose *that* person over another from the field of eligibles; what the social recognition and psychological implications of a paired relation are. We also looked at different kinds of sexual attitudes and behaviors outside of or peripheral to the marital relationship.

In this part, we will direct attention to the social structures and intrarelationship processes of paired relationships, including traditional heterosexual marriage, homosexual partnerships, nonmarital cohabitation, singlehood, and communal living.

In Chapter 7, "Challenges and Roles in Marriage," we will examine a range of issues related to marital roles and patterns of communication between marriage partners. We will also concern ourselves with these key questions:

- What kinds of expectations do people have when they enter marriage? Are these expectations realistic?
- How do men and women find mutually effective roles in marriage?
- Are there ways that husbands and wives can communicate more effectively with each other?
- How do the differences between men and women with regard to

their sexual perceptions and sexual arousals affect the development of marital sex roles? Is there really a battle of the sexes?

- In modern marriages is the husband or wife generally the more powerful and authoritative? Or is there a new equalitarianism in marriages?
- Do most men feel comfortable with a mate as intelligent or more intelligent than they are? Do most men want to marry a woman who will pursue an occupation?

In Chapter 8, ''Alternative Styles: The 'Outsiders,' '' we will look at some contemporary models of bonding outside the traditional monogamous marriage relationship. Without attaching value judgments, we will attempt to examine objectively the strengths and weaknesses of:

- communal living
- nonmarital cohabitation
- singlehood
- paired homosexual relationships

We will examine how these forms work and how they are viewed by people engaging in more traditional lifestyles.

## Chapter 7

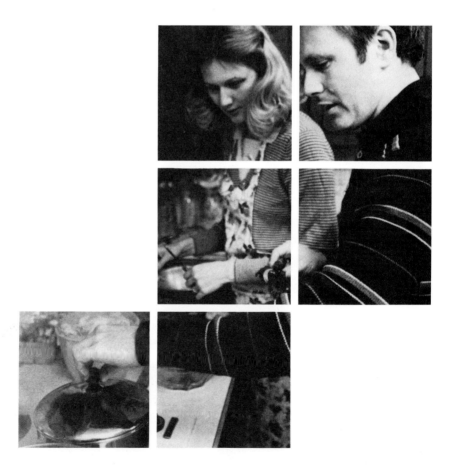

# Challenges and Roles in Marriage

## Chapter Aims

1. To view marriage in terms of the development of mutually satisfying marital roles and to examine the challenges implicit in learning and maintaining these roles over a period of years.

2. To consider the criteria of effective interspousal communication and to see how this can improve role performance and marital satisfaction.

3. To look at the allocation of power and responsibility in the marriage relationship.

## Overview

What do you expect from marriage? The roles in marriage are determined culturally, but many details are left to the couple. Men and women often bring to marriage different sets of expectations about what roles they are to perform and about how they are supposed to behave sexually. Which roles and the number of resources a partner has may influence the amount of power he or she will have in the marriage.

Back and forth communication between the partners makes it possible for both to find roles in the marriage that are acceptable to both. Acting defensively is a major obstacle to this communication.

## The Partner of Your Choice

Marriages, we all know, are not made in heaven. In fact, as we have noted throughout this book, it is a cultural rarity that such romantic notions as love, attraction, mutual interests, and being right for each other emotionally even play a part in the choice of the person we marry. The cultural norm is less romantic, less personal.

Expectations

We might expect marriage to be a relatively easy, natural, satisfying state for people lucky enough to select their own mates. After all, isn't it much easier to get along with someone you have selected as right for you, as opposed to someone you were involuntarily paired with because that person's family happened to own land next to your family's farm?

The answer is yes and no. In some ways it is easier, but it can also be more difficult because of our initial expectations, especially if these expectations are unrealistic. The partners in a contemporary marriage face many tests as they seek a happy, fulfilling relationship. What makes a marriage successful and how realistic are the expectations people have of marital satisfaction?

## Initial Expectations of Marriage

Most couples, when they enter into a marriage, have implicit and explicit expectations of what marriage will be like. Some of these expectations are realistic and others are probably unrealistic. Some are based on the rela-

Implicit and explicit expectations

tionship with the intended spouse; others develop from earlier socialization. For instance, the way marriage has been depicted on TV and in the movies shapes a part of our expectations, as does what we have seen in the home situation between our parents.

One of the most commented upon of the initial expectations with which couples enter marriage is the illusion of romantic love. Since this powerful, pleasurable feeling has permeated their relationship during the courtship period, they tend to expect it will maintain its full force, or some semblance of it, over the many years of marriage. Of course, it does not.

"There are two main forces that create [these] unrealistic, romantic expectations," Krich and Blum (1974, p. 58) point out.

The first is social: We as a society retain a concept of romantic love that has no place in marriage, and in fact cannot exist in marriage. . . . One certainly can love one's husband or wife, but to remain madly, jealously, selfishly, worshipingly in love would be to perpetuate a temporary state of lunacy. . . . The second force is personal. Each of us comes into marriage with unresolved problems. The degree to which we believe in romantic tradition combined with the severity of our neurotic needs determines how well or how poorly we react to the disappointments inherent in marriage.

If the persistence of romantic love is an unrealistic expectation, our next question is, What is a realistic expectation with which to enter the marriage relationship? There is no single answer to this question, but we can make some progress in answering it if we understand that marriage is an evolving relationship, one that changes over time, as the individual partners change, as their family and financial circumstances change, and as the society itself changes. The central concept of marital role, which we will explore in this chapter, will help us understand how these factors interact to affect individual marriages.

**An evolving relationship**

## Finding Mutually Acceptable Roles in Marriage

**Marital role**

*Marital role* can be defined as the set of attitudes and behaviors a spouse is expected to demonstrate in the context of the marriage relationship. A marital role comprises cultural expectations, associated with the husband or with the wife. A husband, for instance, may be expected to be the provider and head of the family and the wife a homemaker and companion. Or, the wife may be expected to be the strong one, upon whom the husband can rely. There are infinite possibilities or at least as many possibilities as there are marriages; but by far most of the accepted marital roles are culturally determined, with only the fine details left to be worked out by the partners.

There are many different kinds of marital roles. Nye et al. (1976) identified these eight as the chief roles: *providing, housekeeping, child care, child socialization, sexual, recreational, therapeutic,* and *kinship.* Table 7.1 shows briefly what these roles are. "Traditionally," Nye et al. (1976 p. 13) points out, "housekeeper, child care, and sexual roles have been assigned by the norms to the wife, with provider assigned to the husband, and kinship and child socialization roles to both. However, there has been a tendency in recent years for wives to share enactment of the provider and husbands the housekeeper and child care roles." With these new possibilities of changes in roles, it is necessary that there be some clarification, usually explicit, so that the partners understand their respective marital roles. Without such a clarification, there is always the possibility of confusion, especially by retreating to the traditional

Table 7.1
**Delineation of Marital Roles**

| | |
|---|---|
| PROVIDER | Assumes responsibility for the financial support of the family. With this is usually the responsibility for providing safety and security. |
| HOUSEKEEPER | Involves obtaining, preparing, and cooking the food, maintaining a habitable house, caring for clothing and household furnishings. |
| CHILD CARE | Provides basic physical and psychological conditions to assure the normal development of a healthy organism. |
| CHILD SOCIALIZATION | Includes the basic child-care role but goes much further. Involves all integrated efforts to produce a socialized, competent individual. This role combines a mixture of intellectual, social, and emotional goals in child-rearing. |
| SEXUAL | Functions as a satisfying sexual partner, within the context of a mutually enjoyable, and usually exclusive, sexual relationship, includes initiating and responding to the partner's sexual advances. |
| RECREATIONAL | Is responsible for organizing and carrying out family recreational activities. |
| THERAPEUTIC | Assists the spouse in coping with and resolving problems of a psychological nature, is supportive and emotionally facilitative. |
| KINSHIP | Assumes the obligation to maintain contact and good relationships with kin. |

Adapted from: Nye, F. I. et al. *Role structure and analysis of the family.* Beverly Hills, CA: Sage Publications, 1976.

husband-wife roles that have been an integral, although possibly subtle, part of the socialization for marriage.

## Peter and Niki

Peter and Niki view themselves as a modern couple. Both work as teachers and earn about the same amount of money. But Peter still feels that it is Niki's responsibility to clean the house and do the laundry. ''I take care of the car,'' he answers, when she chides him for not helping out in the house. ''I also painted the whole place,'' he adds. In fact, he just doesn't feel comfortable participating in the housekeeper role, even though his wife participates equally in the role of provider.

*Traditional husband-wife roles have been an integral part of our socialization. Departing from them may require clarification between the partners.*

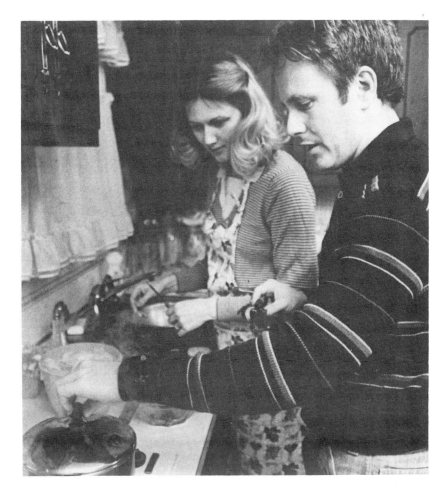

Typically, a young couple entering marriage does not explicitly state what their respective roles will be, although this may be understood implicitly. As the relationship changes over time, the implicit role expectations may come to the fore. Of course, today, there are such profound changes in what is expected of men and women that there is no longer a defined husband role and wife role. Options are now available, and they are being explored. "Many couples are searching for a different formula. A few are experimenting, tearing down the old barriers, reversing roles, living separate social lives. Getting away from the stifling, conventional idea of togetherness is of crucial importance" (Russell 1973).

**Communication**

What enables a modern marriage relationship to endure and to remain stable in the midst of these rapid social changes in husband-wife role designation is good *communication* about marital roles: when one partner can openly and uninhibitedly tell the other what is expected of him or her and the other partner can respond. When there is a sharing of ideas through communication, roles can evolve with more flexibility. Communication allows a couple to make explicit to each other the role expectations that may have been implicit. It also allows for the development of mutually acceptable marital roles.

We can state then as our general principle that the specific challenges of marriage usually revolve around the task of finding mutually acceptable marital roles and communicating one's expectations effectively to one's partner.

## What Is Effective Communication?

The core of a stable continuing relationship is the ability of the pair to be able to change with situations: to adapt their marital roles as their partners' needs change and as they grow and their needs change. It is essential, therefore, that they be able to communicate effectively with each other. Effective communication between partners provides a solidifying bond, a stabilizer, in the marital relationship.

In recent years, as research in this area has intensified, a number of specific factors have been identified as important in facilitating enriched marital communication. Miller, Corrales, and Wackman (1975) point out, for example, the following concepts that have frequently been cited in the literature: awareness, rules, disclosure and receptivity, skills, and esteem building. Let us look at each of these briefly to understand some of the foundations of effective communication in marriage.

**Awareness**   *Awareness* means accurately sensing and perceiving the people and things around you, and understanding your relationship to these people and things. The term *awareness* is used in its general meaning but is also broken down into component parts, which Miller, Corrales, and Wackman call topical awareness, self-awareness, awareness of partner, and relationship awareness.

*Topical awareness* means that we are aware of things outside of the immediate environment, things that are going on in the world. Topical awareness means we are not living in a shell limited by our own experiences. *Self-awareness* refers to our ability to understand our emotions, sensations, and thoughts. The clarity with which one can understand him- or herself often affects how well one deals with others.

*Awareness about one's partner* ''involves knowing accurately what it is your partner is experiencing in terms of his own self-awareness'' (p. 145). It is the ability to be sensitive to your partner, to experience empathy and see the world and the relationship as it is experienced by your partner. It is much like the condition of empathy we discussed in the development of intimacy.

Finally, there is *awareness of the relationship,* which focuses on the interaction of the couple rather than the behavior of each alone. This type of awareness helps each spouse clearly see the relationship in its full perspective. It helps both of them understand how they express their feelings to each other, what the balance of their rights and responsibilities are, and how symmetrical, or equal, their footing in the relationship is. In short, it touches the inner pattern of the relationship and helps reveal the structural rules by which the relationship is governed.

Rules     Every marriage relationship has certain *marital rules.* These can be expressed in terms of ''who can do what, where, when, and how, for what length of time'' (p. 147). Marital rules may be complex, changing from situation to situation. But because they are rules, they can always be understood in their complexity by both partners, who are able to make adjustments to the rules or to change them by mutual agreement. It is through these rules, moreover, that roles evolve and change.

Marital rules

Disclosure and Receptivity     A partner conceivably can be aware of much that is happening in the relationship but unwilling to express it. *Levels of disclosure and receptivity* refer to the ability and willingness of a partner to disclose his or her feelings to the spouse and the ability and willingness of the spouse to be receptive to those feelings. This ability is integral to ''helping a couple look at their typical patterns of interaction, sometimes for the purpose of creating change in the way they relate'' (p. 148).

*The better two people know each other, the more efficient their communication becomes.*

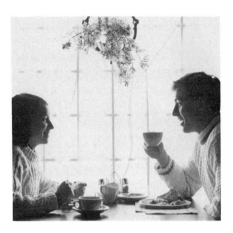

## Relationship Communication Skills
*Relationship communication skills* are specific behaviors and skills that facilitate communication in a relationship. These include such general communication skills as "speaking for self and owning one's own statements (usually done by using personal pronouns which refer to oneself), giving specific examples (documenting interpretations with specific sensory data), making feeling statements (verbally expressing what it is one is feeling at that moment), and so forth" (p. 148). These communication skills will be explored in greater detail below, when we look at feedback.

## Esteem Building
Interpersonal communication generally functions on two levels: one, a *level of content* and the other a *level of intent.* Intent, which can be viewed as the underlying feeling or intention behind a message, is emotionally more important than the content of what is said. Also, if there is a discrepancy between content and intent, it leads to incongruity, to a double message, which produces confusion in the relationship and may lead to discord.

Level of content

Level of intent

*Esteem building* is often a part of the intent level of messages couples routinely send to each other. "Messages," Miller, Corralee, and Workman (p. 149) point out, "tend to either value or devalue self and partner." The intentions behind many of our messages can be explicitly stated only if we are aware and receptive, and then we can see if it is esteem building or degrading for our partner.

### Laura and Van

When Laura and Van were visiting their friends, Van was just delighted as Laura related step-by-step how Van had put a new roof on the house. ''C'mon, you're boring them,'' he protested feebly, but inside he felt really great hearing Laura tell about it. The emotional message she was communicating was how proud she was of Van, how he had pleased her, and what a successful job he had done. This helped build his self-esteem in front of others.

These communication factors—awareness, rules, disclosure and receptivity, skills, and building of esteem—serve as the beginning in our efforts to understand how partners communicate marital roles to each other. To the degree that they are successful in these areas, there is a greater likelihood of their being able to establish mutually agreeable and satisfying marital roles. One concept that can probably help us understand this in even more depth is the idea of feedback.

## Feedback

Feedback is a key concept in understanding all human communication but especially between partners in intimate relationships. *Feedback* can be defined as a response to an individual's behavior that is reflected back to the individual by specific others or by the environment. We say an obscene word and the person to whom we are speaking winces, feeding back to us the effect of what we have said. Or, when one whispers a sweet endearment to one's spouse and watches how his or her face lights up, this response feeds back that one has said the right thing.

Feedback is always a reciprocal process. First, we act; that is, we say something or do something to communicate with those around us. We give a message. Our action initiates a response in the other person. This response is then fed back to us. This process allows us to infer what effect our action has had on those around us. Sometimes, of course, our inferences are wrong; but the more common the situation and the better we know someone, the more likely we are to interpret their responses correctly (Goodman and Ofshe 1968; Weinstein et al. 1972.)

A reciprocal process

Effective communication depends, to a large extent, on one person's ability to assume for the moment the role of the other; to interpret information within the context that the other person is offering it. The better two people know each other, the more efficient the communication is between them because ''the more two people are able to take accurately each other's role (to 'tune in' to one another), the fewer communicative units are required to transmit information or meaning between them'' (Weinstein et al. 1972, p. 248). When two people begin to date, they usually have to work out a communication pattern so that each understands what the other is saying. As they become more intimate, there is less ambiguity in the communication between them, and it is more efficient. When they have lived together for a period of time, they understand each other so well that their feedback is far more efficient and accurate an indicator than it was at the beginning. They have learned to "read" each other.

Feedback may be positive or negative, verbal or nonverbal. If a woman gives her spouse a gift and his eyes light up with appreciation and love, even if he says nothing, this is an example of feedback. If a man spends all day preparing a meal and as soon as his wife takes her first bite, she makes a horrid face, this would be an example of nonverbal, negative feedback. In these cases, something we have done, some behavior we have engaged in, some communication we have with others, or some involvement we have had with our environment, produces a response that tells us the effect of our action.

*Positive or negative*

*Verbal or nonverbal*

## Feedback Loop

In understanding how most continuing communication, as that in a marital relationship, actually works, the concept of the *feedback loop* becomes important. A feedback loop is a model of how feedback is used by individuals communicating with each other.

Whenever two people interact, and the first conveys some kind of message to the second, and the second in turn effects a change of condition, which then requires the first to communicate new information to the second, we have an example of the feedback loop. It is called a loop because it is a continuous process in which the conveyance of information is constantly changed along with the position of the communicator, in order to adjust to the response being fed back by the other person.

*A continuous process*

This may sound complicated but is easily demonstrated by typical family situations, which illustrate how the feedback loop works. We will use a simple diagrammatic format to represent the transaction. If A and B are communicating with each other, we can represent it as:

$$A_{msg.} ------> B_{comp.} \quad (1)$$
$$B_{msg.} \quad \quad > A_{comp.} \quad (2)$$
$$A_{msg.} ======> B_{bhv.} \quad (3)$$

where *msg.* stands for the content of a message and *comp.* stands for the comprehension of a message, and *bhv.* stands for the behavioral change (or change of condition) resulting from the comprehension of the message. In this scheme, A's message is understood by B [1]; B in turn offers a message which is understood by A [2]; and the response message by A causes a change in B's behavior [3].

### Dan and Norma

When Dan (D) comes home from work ten o'clock at night, he knows he has a lot of explaining to do to Norma (N) his wife. As he walks through the door, she gives him an angry look ($N_{msg.}$-------->$D_{comp.}$). He smiles, as if to erase her look ($D_{comp.}$------->$D_{bhv.}$), and stumbles for an explanation. "Sweetheart," he begins gently, but sees at once by her expression that this is the wrong approach ($D_{msg.}$--------->$N_{comp.}$ ------>$N_{bhv.}$). He makes a serious face. "I got tied up at the office and I'm exhausted" ($D_{msg.}$------->$N_{comp.}$). She gives him a disbelieving look ($N_{comp.}$------->$N_{bhv.}$). Perhaps she called the office? "I left at seven, but then my tire went flat on the freeway." She looks like she believes him now ($D_{msg.}$------->$N_{comp.}$). "I was driving and all of a sudden the car swerved. . . . God, honey, I thought I was gonna smash into a pole." Her expression turns sympathetic and he continues this fine narrative ($D_{msg.}$------->$N_{comp.}$------->$N_{bhv.}$).

We see in this situation how oral communication and visual feedback from the wife, who did not utter a single word, were used in the form of a feedback loop through which the husband constructed his story.

## Convergent and Divergent Feedback

Whenever we are fed back information, it may be convergent or divergent. *Convergent feedback* is that which is consistent with our expectations, while *divergent feedback* is inconsistent.

Convergent feedback, therefore, brings a predictable result, consistent with our expectations, while divergent feedback brings an unexpected and often undesired result. In the example above, when Dan first walks in the door, his presence elicits an angry look from his wife. He smiles but she feeds back more angry looks, indicating to him that this is not the right approach. He sees that his use of the endearing "sweetheart" is also a mistake. It is only after he appeals to her sympathy that he gets the convergent feedback that tells him he is on the right track.

There are many different factors that contribute to convergent, predictable feedback. Successful and effective communication in marriage can be defined as a convergent feedback loop, with the marriage partners accepting the same symbols and able to understand each other and respond to each other. If A and B are communicating, the conditions for good communication are:

$$A_{msg.} \quad \text{-----} \!\!> B_{comp.}$$
$$B_{msg.} \quad \text{-----} \!\!> A_{comp.}$$
$$A^{mng.} < \!\!===== \!\!> B^{mng.}$$

where *mng.* stands for the meaning of the message. In this scheme, A's message is understood by B; B's message is understood by A; and the meaning attributed to the message is the same for A and for B. On the other hand, an example of poor communication is,

$$A_{msg} \text{:} \not{-}\not{-}\not{-}\!\!> B,$$

where A's message is not acknowledged at all by B, or,

$$A^{mng.} \text{:} \not{=}\not{=}\not{=}\!\!> B^{mng.},$$

where A's meaning about a communication is different from B's meaning.

There are factors that contribute to successful communication and those that work against it. One of the most important of these, defensiveness, works against communication.

## Defensiveness

Defensive behavior is often responsible for a divergent feedback loop. As a general rule, the less defensive the partners are, the more efficient the feedback between them and the more effective the communication in the relationship. Psychoanalysis offers an informative explanation of how *defensiveness* contributes to divergent feedback. Whenever a person acts defensively, this position suggests, he or she distorts, blocks, or changes the reality. The *defense mechanisms* are used to describe this type of behavior. Defense mechanisms are psychological strategies for handling anxiety, strategies that do not lead to healthy adaptation.

Defense mechanisms

In many ways the defenses are the opposite of empathic communication. They prevent us from accurately understanding what is happening because they don't allow us to see the situation from the other person's role. These psychological strategies, derived from psychoanalysis, are insightful descriptions of many types of social behavior and are compatible with role theory.

Parapraxis

Repression    *Repression* is the most common defense mechanism. In its most basic form, repression simply means forgetting. We repress feelings and situations, thoughts and occasions, often because by repression we get rid of anxiety or reduce some other emotional tension. A common manifestation of repression is the so-called *Freudian slip,* technically called a *parapraxis.* A Freudian slip is when we say one thing when we intended to say something else. This type of behavior, according to Freud, is an attempt of the repressed material to break free, to come to the sur-

*Defensive behavior prevents us from understanding what is happening because we can't see the situation from the other person's role.*

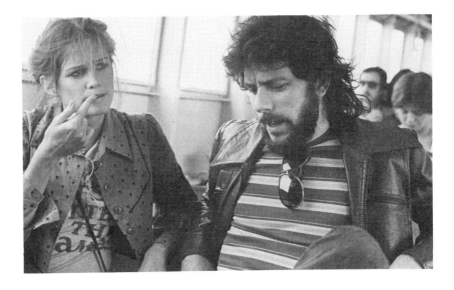

face and be revealed. In other words, when we make a Freudian slip we do so because on one level we want the other person to be aware of some of our deeper feelings.

### Janet

Janet is horrified when in the midst of petting she calls her present boyfriend by her former boyfriend's name. It is only later, when she goes home and reflects on this, that she realizes that she was thinking of how her former boyfriend was more romantic with her and that she really wanted to be with him! She then realizes the reason she may have made the slip.

One other reason repression is important is that since many of our impulses are socially unacceptable, it is necessary to "bury" them in order to conform to social expectations.

Refusing to accept

Denial   The mechanism of denial is sometimes confused with repression, but it is different. *Denial* occurs when we consciously refuse to accept that something is happening. For instance, there is the saying that often holds true that the husband or wife is always the last to know when the partner is cheating. It could be that the knowledge is so painful that he or she denies it is happening. Best friends and family may be aware of what is going on and ask, "How can Lance be so blind to what is happening?'' The answer is that Lance is using the prerequisite mechanism of denial.

Reaction Formation   The common defense of *reaction formation* involves acting in a way that is completely opposite to the way a person really feels. While a person is acting in this way, however, he or she is unaware of the deeper level of feelings and, therefore, unable to recognize ths mechanism at work. In this way it protects the mind from harmful thoughts, feelings, and impulses.

**Actions vs. feelings**

### Ray and Vivienne

Ray is shocked when Vivienne tells him she wants to break up with him. Sure they've had their troubles during the two years they have been living together, but during the past few months Vivienne has been nicer than ever. Almost a new person, Ray says! At last, she had been paying more attention to Ray, showing an interest in his schooling, talking to him about things of mutual interest. Recently she even bought him a very expensive watch, and she had never before been a present giver. What Ray didn't realize is that Vivienne had been reacting to her deep feelings of wanting to break up with Ray: she was acting in the very opposite way than the way she really felt, without realizing she was doing so.

One way to tell if an individual is using the mechanism of reaction formation is to note if a behavior is a sudden change from past patterns, from the expected, or if it is very extreme, dogmatic behavior. Because reaction formation is an attempt to block out a deeper feeling it is often a fanatical behavior, stronger than we would normally expect.

Rationalization   Rationalization is a mechanism in which a person develops a false explanation for actions, attitudes, or consequences. For instance, Paul says he spent money for a vacation in Europe in order to please his wife, even though she would have actually preferred to save the money for a down payment on a house. When she complains, he says, ''Well, we would have squandered it anyway—you know how we are. At least this way, we enjoyed ourselves.''

   There are three types of rationalization. In the first type, a person attributes a more favorable motive to his or her behavior, as we saw in the example above where Paul claimed he spent the money to please his wife. A second type is commonly referred to as *sour grapes,* after the famous Aesop fable of a fox who tried repeatedly, without success to get a bunch of grapes. Failing time and again, the fox finally gave up his attempts, rationalizing that the grapes looked sour anyway.

The third type is sometimes called *sweet lemons.* Something unpleasant happens, but the person rationalizes and says this is all for the best anyway, like trying to smile while sucking a lemon. For example after Vivienne told Ray about her plans to move out, he thought to himself, "Well it's better it happened now than after we got married. This way I found out what kind of person she is before getting tied in the marital knot."

Projection    *Projection* is the process of attributing to another person or to an object feelings that emanate from within oneself. A person who feels that no one likes him, for example, may be projecting his own internal feelings of hostility on to all of the people around him.

Jealousy is one form of projection that can cause severe marital problems. When people constantly feel, without justification, that their partners are cheating, it may be that they really want to cheat themselves, that they are projecting their own sexual wishes.

### Carol and Bob

Carol is somewhat amused, but also somewhat troubled, by her husband Bob's suspicions that she is carrying on with some man at the office. After all, there is no real reason to be suspicious, since she believes in loyalty. What she doesn't realize is that her husband's own sexual feelings, stirred up at his job, make him uncomfortable. Rather than thinking about these feelings, he thinks about the possibility of his wife having an affair at her office.

There is another interesting dimension to projection. We sometimes imagine that others are attracted to someone we are really attracted to.

### Bill's father

Bill's father fixed him up with a girl from his office, raving for weeks about how Bill would be crazy about her, how beautiful she was, and how interesting she was to talk to. When the big night came, Bill couldn't stand her. He found her unattractive, grandiose, and boring. It seems that Bill's father—*not Bill!*—had these wonderful feelings about her. But because Bill's father was married and an older man, he couldn't acknowledge that he was attracted to her; so he projected these feelings, assuming that his son would have these reactions.

Another case of this type occurs when a woman or man imagines that the partner is attracted to someone whom the partner actually finds totally neutral.

### Sid and Jeanette

After a party, as they are getting ready for bed at home, Sid mentions casually that he noticed Jeanette looking at that muscular guy in the T-shirt, "trying to be Nick Nolte." In fact, Jeanette was very interested in the little Al Pacino type and hadn't even noticed Mr. Muscles. Sid had been projecting his feelings, because on one level he was attracted to the muscle man and didn't feel comfortable with those feelings.

*[handwritten margin note: Edward (leaving home)?]*

Regression    Finally, we have the mechanism of *regression,* which means returning to a more childish type of behavior. Typically, when a person feels overpowered by feelings that he or she can no longer handle, one way of dealing with the situation is to return to a more primitive level

*[margin note: Primitive level of behavior]*

of behavior. For instance, Carla has been having lots of problems with Chuck lately. But instead of dealing with these problems, instead of facing up to the conflict, she eats, eats, and eats. This is a more childish way of dealing with frustration, one indicative of an earlier point in life.

Effects of Defensiveness    We see then that defensive behavior can be an inhibitor of effective communication between people. In terms of the development of mutually agreeable marital roles, a prerequisite for a fulfilling marriage, defensiveness does two things. First, it limits the

*[margin note: Defensive behavior = inefficient communication]*

realistic negotiation of roles by preventing one or both partners from realistically assessing (1) what is expected of him or her, (2) what he or she expects from the spouse, and (3) how he or she and the spouse feel about these expectations. Second, overdefensiveness makes effective convergent feedback impossible and leads to arguments and discord, which could result in severe marital strain.

## Marital Sex Roles

New expectations

Along with the wide-scale social changes in premarital and adolescent sexual behavior discussed in chapter 5 have come new expectations of marital sex roles. The traditional set of role expectations, in which the man was the sexually aggressive partner and the woman the compliant, childbearing, less impulsive one—an expectation with which many men and women entered marriage—is slowly giving way to a more flexible and idividually adaptable range of roles. These new roles have greater potential to offer both partners in terms of increased levels of sexual and emotional satisfaction, because they recognize the unique needs of both partners.

Basic differences between men and women

Despite these changes, a large majority of existing marriages still contain many elements of traditional sex-role practices. For example, as we noted earlier, men and women are socialized to be different sexually, and this difference does have to be taken into account. They tend to approach sex with different styles, experience sexual feelings in different ways, are aroused by different kinds of fantasies, and perceive sexually related situations from different vantage points. These basic differences, which extend from the superficial levels of observation to the profound levels of inner experiencing, are responsible, directly or indirectly, for the perennial battle of the sexes we hear about. These basic differences also have profound implications in the development of marital sex roles.

## Differences in Sexual Perception

Socialization in our culture leads to important differences in the ways that men and women perceive sex, and many of these differences have the potential to lead to incompatibilities. Our language reflects this bias. To the man, sex often involves ''taking''; to the woman, it involves ''giving.'' Socially, when the boy engages in sex, he has ''gained'' something; when the girl engages in sex, she has ''lost'' or ''sacrificed'' something.

Biases reflected by language

Looking at the words used to describe sexual activity, it becomes clear that this discrepancy between men and women infuses much of our sexual perception. When a boy sleeps with a girl, he is likely to say, ''She put out,'' ''She gave in,'' ''She's a free girl,'' ''I took her,'' ''I had her (or, she was had by me),'' ''She let me.'' Men are more likely than women to ''get some action.'' These kinds of expressions are used by many young boys, particularly when they first start dating girls. While the expressions are not used as the person matures, the stigma lingers on that the girl who has sex is *giving* something and that the boy who has sex with her is *taking* something.

Young girls also often reflect this bias in their language. The girl perceives herself as "giving" something when she "submits" to the boy. Her friends may exclaim, "You let him do it," thereby agreeing that it was done *to* her. The girl "puts out" for the boy. While the boy does it *to* her, she does it *for* him.

**Incorrect perceptions**

This foundation perception, reflected in the language that we use, leads to other biases in perception. The man's idea of "scoring" with women indicates that each new girl he sleeps with increases the score, or that the "more" he "gets"—lips, breasts, genitals—increases his score. The girl "goes" further as the boy "gets" further."

The relationship between taking and giving reveals a lot about the differences between the sexes, differences that should be taken into account when looking at marital sex roles. After all, we usually have to like a person before we give that person something, and it is easier to take from someone from whom we feel little or at whom we are angry. Thus, a husband may not have to feel as much to take from his wife, while the wife would probably have to feel some strong affectionate feelings in order to give to her husband.

## Corrinne and Danny

Corrinne can't understand why Danny would even want to make love to her after they've had a fight. She's so angry at him that she feels she can't bring herself to make love. But Danny seems to see lovemaking as a way of making up: "If you do this for me, baby, then everything will be all right." But Corrinne's attitude is, "If you want to make love to me, honey, then do something to deserve it."

Likewise, if the wife finds out that her husband "took" from another woman, it is often not considered quite as serious an offense as if the husband found out that his wife "gave" to another man. The essence—although not the basis—of the double standard in marriage is found in the language that is used to express sexuality.

## Differences in Sexual Arousal

Are there measurable differences in sexual arousal levels between men and women? How does this affect the development of marital sex roles? We now have some ways of answering this first question, since studies have revealed a number of subtle differences in sexual attraction and arousal between the sexes. For example, Waters (1974), using a test known as the *Sensation Seeking Scale,* found that men were generally less inhibited than women, more likely to seek thrills, and basically more adventure seeking. Other differences, which we will discuss below, have been found in men and women's ability to realize when they are "turned on," and to respond to erotic stimuli.

### David and Marion

David and Marion have been married for ten years. As they describe their relationship, it would appear that they have a generally good, stable marriage, that they share mutual interests, particularly in bringing up their two children, and that generally they communicate well with each other. The one problem they have, as they see it, is that "things aren't working out sexually." They feel a sense of loss in their marriage.

As we get to know them, a pattern of their home life begins to emerge. David, who is a sales manager for a textile firm, comes home about seven, "gobbles down" his dinner, and puts away a couple of drinks. As soon as he is done with dinner, he lies down on the couch and sips wine while he watches TV or reads the evening newspaper. Marion finishes the dishes and sits with him while he reads or watches TV. About eleven they go up to their bedroom and watch the Eleven O'Clock News. When the news is over, David shuts off the television, and either goes to sleep or on many nights tries to make love to Marion.

David gets angry as he discusses his wife's rejection of him. "She makes me feel inadequate, like she doesn't find me attractive any more. Why, all day I have women flirting with me at the office, and when I come home what do I get? Nothing!" Marion is apologetic in relating her half of the picture. She feels at fault: "I know David wants to make love, but I'm so tired after taking care of the house and the kids all day that by eleven I don't have any strength left. But I really do still find him a very sexy man."

In truth, Marion is bothered by David's nightly advances; she finds them obnoxious and suspects she is being made to feel guilty because she can't respond with passion. David, on the other hand, feels that Marion should be flattered by his sexual attention. "After all," he reasons, "it's not every husband who's so turned on to his wife that he wants to make love to her all the time." He can't understand why she is not flattered nor can he comprehend why she doesn't feel like making love to him if she really finds him as attractive as she says she does.

This marital difficulty is a case of two people perceiving themselves and their partners incorrectly. Things become clearer when we look at the situation from their respective points of view, taking into account the differences in sexual arousal between men and women, and how this affects their marital roles. David is out of the house all day, exposed to attractive women who flirt with him. This situation triggers his fantasies, and he begins to improvise, building up a sexual pressure inside him. By the time he gets home, he is internally aroused and need only unwind for a couple of hours before he is "raring to go."

Marion, on the other hand, is home all day, deprived of the kind of attention and stimulation that would arouse her. She needs the stimulation of a man she cares about making her feel important and wanted. When David comes home, he fails to provide the kind of attention and interest she needs to become aroused. He takes it for granted that she can become excited as he does, which of course she cannot.

Perhaps if he brought her flowers, took her out to dinner, asked her about her day, showed some interest in her as a person, she would begin to become as aroused as he is. But why should he? After all, they're married, aren't they? David fails to realize that his wife's requirements for sexual arousal are different from his; that she needs some romantic attention from the person with whom she is emotionally involved—that is, from her husband. His sexual perception does not help him understand his wife's frame of reference.

The different mechanisms involved in men's and women's sexual arousal can be explained in terms of a social psychological concept described with *cues*. An *internal cue* is any stimulus inside you. Feeling hunger in your stomach is an internal cue. Having a sexual fantasy that arouses you is an internal cue. Feeling tired after a hard day's work is an internal cue. An *external cue* is something outside yourself that triggers the same kind of response an internal cue would. Seeing an advertisement for a juicy steak an hour or two after dinner could trigger hunger, even though internally you are not hungry. You are then responding to an external cue. Being sexually aroused by looking at a sexy movie is another example of external cueing. Feeling tired and going to bed because it's eleven o'clock and that is your bedtime is a response to the external cue of time.

Each of us responds more strongly to either internal or external cues

Internal cue

External cue

in different areas of behavior. Much psychological research has been conducted in an attempt to understand how this process works.

Cueing seems to have an important influence on our sexual arousal. Men tend to be externally cued more easily than do women. Of course, this is not the case for all men or for all women: individual differences are greater than gender differences.

**Gender differences in sexual arousal**

Some gender differences were explained in a study of men's and women's sexual arousal conducted by Dr. Julia Heiman (1975) at the State University of New York at Stony Brook. Male and female college students were hooked up to a sensitive recording device that detects even mild levels of sexual arousal by measuring the blood volume in the penis or clitoris. The subjects were shown neutral and erotic films and asked to tell when they felt sexually aroused. Their self-reports of arousal were then compared with the results of the physical measurement, in order to see if they were aware of when they felt aroused.

In general, it was found that on a physiological level men and women experienced about the same levels of arousal for the same kinds of film matters. But what turned out to be most interesting was this: while all of the men readily acknowledged their arousal, even when it was very slight, more than half the women who were sexually aroused, even at a high level, as indicated by the measuring device, did not acknowledge it! In other words, even though the women's bodies responded to the stimulus, they did not actually report feeling aroused.

**Socialization for sexual roles**

The results of this study show that the differences in sexual arousal between men and women are the result of socialization, not of biology alone. Men are apparently better able than women to define the symptoms of sexual arousal and to integrate them into their thought processes regarding sexual activity. Men often fail to understand this aspect of women. Perhaps some training in this direction would be helpful. Part of the husband's sexual role in marriage should be to provide the external cues, the romantic environment, that can help his wife acknowledge her sexual arousal.

And yet, it should also be pointed out that there is some research that indicates more similarities than differences when the sexes respond to erotica as opposed to responding within a relationship. For example, Fisher and Byrne (1978) conducted an experiment where two groups watched an erotic film, portraying petting. One group was told that the couple petting was in love, while the second group was told the woman was a prostitute and the man a "John." They found that generally "men and women were more sexually aroused by the casual sex theme than by those involving love or lust. Apparently," they go on to conclude, "romantic or affectional emphasis is not a precondition for female arousal by erotica." (p. 117)

## Differences in Orientation

There is another point regarding how men and women are socialized for their sexual roles in marriage. The woman's sexual role, according to Chilman, is a "dual" role, oriented not only toward the mate relationship but also toward reproduction and motherhood. Moreover, because "most females have been socialized to accept dependency and the importance of interpersonal relations they may be more open to the complex emotional aspects of the mate relationship and readier to combine sex with love, commitment, and dependency" (Chilman 1974, p. 130). She goes on to point out,

> Cultural norms generally support the value that a female finds
> her identity primarily through a close relationship with a male
> and as a mother to their children, but that a male wins his right to
> such a relationship and to fatherhood through establishing his
> identity in the outer world. Thus, in mating, he feels counter-
> pulls to escape from its entanglements and barriers to achieve-
> ment and independence.

**Inherent conflicts**

Thus, there may be inherent conflicts in the different patterns of socialization. Because of the many differences in marital sex roles, it is especially important that open communication between husband and wife be vigilantly maintained.

## Power and Responsibility

In addition to marital sex roles, there are many other important roles in the marriage relationship. We mentioned earlier some of the roles suggested by Nye et al. (1976): care and socialization of children, therapeutic, recreational, kinship, sexual, and the provider and housekeeper roles. The enactment of many of these roles contributes substantially to the balance of power and the division of responsibility in the family. In fact, we can almost view some of these roles as job descriptions for the husband and wife. The more complicated question, however, is which

**Designation of roles**

jobs are designated to the husband and which to the wife. And, we might ask, how do they become designated: Is it through mutual agreement, by necessity, under pressure, or what?

As we look at the social and interpersonal interaction embedded in these roles, we will note some of the subtle implications of role division in the family.

A landmark study in this area was Blood and Wolfe's *Husbands and Wives,* published in 1960. They studied several hundred families in the Detroit area by interviewing the wives about certain marital topics. Their sample was from the middle class but included 731 urban wives and 178 farm wives.

One of the questions Blood and Wolfe concerned themselves with was how power is divided between husbands and wives. Recognizing that the traditional rules of authority no longer held sway in most marriages, they wanted to find out if men and women had general patterns of power dominance and what factors specifically influenced it. To find out, they asked the wives a series of questions about decisionmaking in the family: questions such as "Who usually makes the final decision about where to go on vacation?" or "Who usually makes the final decision about what house or apartment to take?"

On the basis of their interviews, they were able to characterize three types of marriages: *husband-dominated, wife-dominated,* and *equalitarian,* which included two subtypes that are not important to our discussion.

Blood and Wolfe explain the differences in power allocation through a *resource theory,* which says in effect that power in the family accrues "to the partner who has the greatest resources at his [or her] disposal." These resources include financial ability, social status, educational attainment, competence, and so on. As the wife gains more resources—say, she gets a job or takes on new responsibilities—she gains more power in the family. This compares in many ways to the exchange theory of interpersonal attraction we discussed in chapter 6. That theory, you recall, says we maintain a relationship with another when we are able to gain more than we have to give up.

The Blood and Wolfe research has been greatly criticized for relying solely on the wives' perceptions, for the kinds of questions about decisionmaking asked, and for other reasons. It does, however, provide some tentative insight on the power balance in the family.

*Three types of marriages*

*Resource theory*

## Division of Responsibilities

In every marriage there are concrete responsibilities that have to be attended to. There is keeping the house clean, providing an income, taking care of the children, bringing the car in for a tune-up. There is calling Mom and Dad on Christmas, paying the phone bill, sending a wedding gift to the Joneses. The division of these concrete responsibilities has traditionally been taken care of by assigned marital roles. But nowadays, as we pointed out earlier, more options are available and couples are making their own decisions about how to divide the labors of marriage. Take the example of the Koturs, who handle two houses, two children, and two jobs (adapted from Russell 1973, p. 49, 106).

*In every marriage there are concrete responsibilities, such as cleaning the house. Assigned marital roles traditionally took care of these.*

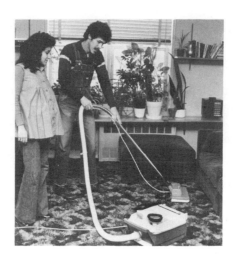

## Bob and Sheila

"Before we married, Sheila said, 'I do want a family but I also want to work at my career,' and I said, 'Fine, if that's what makes you happy; I'm sure you could do both, so do it.' I was born and raised in a small town in Ohio and I've seen what happens when a fellow goes out to work and a wife stays at home and gets a bit bored with life. I'd rather have a stimulated woman than a subservient one." Reflecting now is Robert Kotur, a dynamic, handsome, market research expert who married his English wife Sheila Camera, a fashion artist, seven years ago and is sharing the task of bringing up their two daughters, Fiona, six, and Alexandra, three.

"I really think I'm not cut out to take care of children and be very domesticated full time," adds Sheila. "I need to be stimulated. It wasn't easy to carry on work after I had children. The pressure is sometimes very wearing, especially as I work from home as a free lance. But Bob's very liberated, although I really don't think he realizes it. I've noticed whenever he's telling Fiona history stories at bedtime he always selects as many tales about famous women as men, so as not to be too one-sided."

The success of the Koturs's life has been very much built on Bob's understanding attitude toward the running of their households: they also have a weekend country house 100 miles away from their city apartment. "They have to run and you can only run them if you treat it like a job and make plans," he insists. "Otherwise confusion in the city is compounded by confusion at the other end, in the country." His responsibilities include the hiring and firing of live-in nursemaids who look after their children, organizing all the people involved in renovating the country house, and other things like arranging for carpets to be sent away and cleaned.

Decorating, choosing, and buying furniture have always been Sheila's jobs. Everything to do with food, shopping, cooking and entertaining concerns her too. She always takes both children to the doctor or dentist when necessary because, as Sheila says, "I like to know what's going on."

Bob happily shares the supervision of the children on weekends, when their nursemaid takes time off, if Sheila has a rush art job to complete; and he always takes Fiona to school in the morning. "It's a good chance for her and me to have a little chat. I feel a mother and father should get to know their children. That's part of enjoying life, enjoying the family."

Nowadays, many couples, with and without children, young and old, newly married or married for years, are developing and testing their own marital roles that allow for mutual satisfaction. As we noted in our discussion of the marriage contract in chapter 1, some couples are even taking the opportunity to put into writing at the beginning of marriage what their role expectations are. For those who do not take the opportunity at the beginning, it is never too late. After years of marriage some couples sit down and try to get into writing their mutual obligations. Best-selling author Alix Kates Shulman and her husband Martin, a successful textile manufacturer, worked out a written agreement of their marriage roles and responsibilities on a "50–50 basis" after being married seven years (Shulman 1972).

## Social Factors in Role Assignment

Just as the traditional marital roles were largely the product of overt and covert cultural forces, even in so-called *modern* marriages, the development and assignment of marital roles is influenced by a variety of social factors, including social class, sex-role stereotyping, educational level, and so on.

Mirra Komarovsky has shed light on some of these social influences in the development of marital roles. Her book, *Blue-Collar Marriages,* provides us with a comparative picture of the similarities and differences between working-class and upper middle-class marital role assignments and expectations. Unlike the Blood and Wolfe study, moreover, in her work both husbands and wives were interviewed, thus providing a presumably more balanced perspective.

What are some of her observations? First, we know that in middle-class marriages part of the therapeutic role is being able to share one's problems with one's spouse. Middle-class husbands and wives expect to be able to talk freely to their partners about how they feel. They expect to have a *companionate relationship,* in which the husband and wife are friends. Is this equally true in blue-collar families?

**Companionate relationship**

Komarovsky found that although there was no uniformity in their answers, the therapeutic marital role was noticeably hindered in the blue-collar families by a number of factors. There was, for instance, the working man's tendency of viewing the masculine role as characterized by an emotional reserve. This view prevented him from sharing freely with his wife. The idea of talking openly and expressively with another about personal feelings was viewed as a feminine trait. Moreover, she found, "even when a couple was exposed to the ideal of the companionate marrige, this lack of interpersonal competence occasionally hindered its realization. Indeed, the intellectual acceptance of such an ideal aroused in some couples feelings of inadequacy. *They knew that husbands and wives should talk to one another, but they found nothing to say.*" (1964, p. 337, italics ours).

We should point out, however, that there is some conflicting data on this, perhaps due to the twenty-odd years that have intervened. Nye et al. (1976) point out that "present data suggest that sharing one's problems with one's spouse or the reaction of the spouse to the problem is not, to any extent class-related" (p. 127). Perhaps the blue-collar marriage today is in the same process of liberation we have noted in other areas.

## Changing Sex-Role Norms
In a later study, Komarovsky (1973) examined the effects that some of the recent social changes in normative sex-role behaviors have been having on men. She found that about a third of the college men interviewed felt somewhat insecure in

**Intellectual equality**

relationships in which the woman was their intellectual equal. The majority of men were willing to accept the idea of their female partner as an intellectual equal, at least in theory. The men were then asked about their attitudes toward their future wives' occupational roles. Twenty-four per-

---

Table 7.2

**Readiness of Women to Play Down Intellectual Abilities (%)**

|  | Wallin 1950 | Sociology Class 1970 | Advanced Sociology Class 1971 |
|---|---|---|---|
| When on dates how often have you pretended to be intellectually inferior to the man? | | | |
|     Very often, often, or several times | 32% | 21% | 15% |
|        Once or twice | 26% | 36% | 30% |
|        Never | 42% | 43% | 55% |
| In general, do you have any hesitation about revealing your equality or superiority to men in intellectual competence? | | | |
|     Have considerable or some hesitation | 35% | 21% | 13% |
|        Very little hesitation | 39% | 33% | 32% |
|        None at all | 26% | 46% | 55% |

SOURCE: Komarovsky, M. Cultural contradictions and sex-roles. *American Journal of Sociology*, 1973, 78 (4), pp. 873–84.

---

cent of the men wanted to marry women who would be happy to stay at home and take care of the house. They were called the "traditionalists." Sixteen percent approved theoretically of their wives working, but when it came to concrete details, they hedged or backed down. They were designated as "pseudofeminists." A small fraction (seven percent) of the men were willing to allow the woman full and equal occupational opportunities, even it if meant altering their own roles significantly.

Almost half the men (48 percent) took what Komarovsky calls a "modified traditionalist" position. They envisioned a sequential pattern for their wives: work at the beginning of the marriage, withdrawal from work for childrearing, and eventual return to work. "They varied as to the timing of these stages and as to the aid they were prepared to give their wives with domestic and childrearing functions. The majority saw no substitute for the mother during the child's preschool years. Even the mother of school-age children, were she to work, should preferably be at home

Table 7.3

**College Women's Attitudes toward
Work and Family Patterns (%)**

|  | Random Sample of Sophomore Class at Women's Liberal Arts College 1943 | Class in Introductory Sociology, Same College 1971 |
|---|---|---|
| Assume that you will marry and that your husband will make enough money so that you will not have to work unless you want to. Under these circumstances, would you prefer: | | |
| 1. Not to work at all, or stop after childbirth and decide later whether to go back. ... | 50% | 18% |
| 2. To quit working after the birth of a child but definitely to go back to work. | 30% | 62% |
| 3. To continue working with a minimum of interruption for childbearing. | 20% | 20% |

SOURCE: Komarovsky, M. Cultural contradictions and sex-roles. *American Journal of Sociology,* 1973, 78 (4), pp. 873–84.

when the children return from school'' (p. 87). The remaining 5% saw marriage as so remote that they had no opinions in this matter.

In the same study, Komarovsky looked at women's attitudes about their roles in a paired relationship. Using survey data from three studies, one in 1950 and two in the 1970s, she wanted to determine if women willingly played down their intellectual abilities in their interactions with men. As table 7.2 indicates, women are less likely now to play down their abilities than they were during the 1940s (as reflected in Wallin's 1950 survey), but still do so to some extent. Even more striking is the change in women's attitudes toward work and family, reflected in table 7.3. In 1943, half the women chose to not work at all or to stop after childbirth: by 1971 only 18% chose this option. In 1971, 62% of the women indicated they would quit work to have a child but would go back to work later. In 1943, only 30% of the women chose this option. Finally, we see one area where there has been no change over the past quarter century. Only one-fifth of the respondents in 1943 and 1971 indicated that they would not interrupt their working for childrearing.

What can we interpret from this? Although there is some notable change in the way men think of their future wives' occupational roles and changes in the way women think of themselves in relation to work, marriage, and childrearing responsibilities, there is still a clear-cut role division between men and women, with the man being viewed as the long-term provider and the woman responsible for raising the children.

## Summary

1. The initial expectations with which a couple enters marriage may affect how much satisfaction they are able to derive. One of the common unrealistic expectations is that romantic love will persist through many years of marriage.

2. Marital roles are the set of attitudes and behaviors a spouse is expected to demonstrate in the context of the marital relationship. They are culturally determined. The main marital roles are: housekeeping, providing, sexual partner, caring for and socializing the children, organizing family recreation, maintaining relations with kin, and functioning as a therapeutic friend and comforter for the spouse.

3. Effective communication allows the partners to define and readjust their marital roles as necessary. One model of marital communication divides it into awareness, rules, disclosure and receptivity, communication skills, and esteem building.

4. Feedback is used to explain the reciprocal nature of marital communication, in which each partner not only initiates communications but responds to them. The feedback loop is used as a model of how the information is used in the relationship.

5. Defensive behavior can inhibit communication effectiveness and role definition. Some common defense mechanisms are repression, denial, reaction formation, rationalization, projection, and regression.

6. Sex roles are defined in part by differences in sexual perception and differences in sexual arousal. They are also influenced by a number of cultural factors.

7. Women are socialized to view engaging in sex as ''giving'' something, where the man is socialized to see it as ''taking'' something. This language difference reveals some functional differences.

8. Studies have revealed differences in sexual arousal. Men are apparently better able than women to recognize and define the symptoms of sexual arousal and to integrate them into their thought processes regarding sexual activity.

9. There are different theories on how power and responsibility are divided in the family. Blood and Wolfe propose a ''resource'' theory that suggests power accrues to the partner with the greater resources.

10. The traditional division of responsibilities is changing, as more men and women decide for themselves how to appropriate the chores and tasks. There is greater overlap today than in the past.

11. There may be some differences between blue-collar and upper middle-class marriages in terms of expectations about companionate marriage. The blue-collar spouse appears to be less likely to seek friendship from the partner and is less able to speak freely about feelings.

12. Although there are some changes in men and women's attitudes, most men still expect that even if the wife works at the beginning of the marriage she will stop working in order to raise the children.

## Key Terms

The following terms were introduced and defined in this chapter. Definitions also appear in the glossary.

| | |
|---|---|
| awareness | communication |
| awareness about one's partner | companionate relationship |
| awareness of the relationship | child care |

child socialization
convergent feedback
cue
defense mechanisms
defensiveness
denial
divergent feedback
equalitarian marriage
esteem building
external cue
feedback
feedback loop
housekeeper
husband-dominated marriage
internal cue
kinship role
level of content
level of intent

levels of disclosure and receptivity
marital role
marital rules
parapraxis
projection
provider
rationalization
reaction formation
recreational role
regression
relationship communication skills
repression
resource theory
self-awareness
sexual role
therapeutic role
topical awareness
wife-dominated marriage

**Discussion Questions**

1. Describe in your own words, with examples, the eight chief marital roles delineated by Nye: provider, housekeeper, child care, child socialization, sexual, recreational, therapeutic, and kinship.

2. As an exercise, conduct an informal survey among married people you know, establishing the following information: how long they have been married; how many children they have and their ages; how they would rate their marriages on a scale of 1 to 10 with 5 as "just ok"; and in what three areas they find the most potential or actual sources of conflict. What conclusions can you draw from your data and how do these conclusions compare with the information presented in this chapter?

3. Using the factors important to effective communication outlined in this chapter, how would you rate yourself as a communicator in the various interpersonal family relationships in which you are involved: marital, parental, sibling, and others. Does your rating as an effective communicator change from one relationship to another; that is, are you more or less effective with some people than with others?

4. Define each of the defense mechanisms discussed in this chapter. For each one, present an example of how it can cause a communication problem in a marital relationship.

5. What qualities of your parents' marriage would you hope to be present in your marriage? Which would you want to avoid?

## Suggested Readings

1. Robert O. Blood and Donald M. Wolfe. *Husbands and Wives: The Dynamics of Married Living.* Glencoe, Ill.: Free Press, 1960.

An early, though important, empirical study of over 700 city and 175 farm families around Detroit in terms of family behavior, focusing particularly on decisionmaking and distribution of power. This study has been widely criticized for generalizing from a limited number of selected decisions of presumed equal importance and the use of wives' reports of family behavior to substitute for both husbands' and wives' of perceptions of family behavior.

2. John Cuber and Peggy Harroff. *Sex and the Significant Americans.* Baltimore: Penguin, 1965.

An examination of marital and sexual activity of over 200 upper-middle-class men and women which lead to the development of a typology of marital interaction that has continued to prove useful in studies of the family.

3. Gerald Handel (Ed.). *The Psychosocial Interior of the Family.* Chicago: Aldine, 1967.

A nice collection of separate papers from several social science disciplines that view the family in terms of its integration as a whole and focuses both on the family's internal dynamics and on its relations with external social entities.

4. Mary W. Hicks and Marilyn Platt. "Marital Happiness and Stability," *Journal of Marriage and the Family,* No. 32 (1970), pp. 553–574.

A useful review of the literature on marital happiness and stability.

5. Mirra Komarovsky. *Blue Collar Marriage.* New York: Vintage, 1967.

One of the few solid, empirical studies that focuses specifically on stable marriages among working-class men and women. Komarovsky uses the case study approach to provide both depth and richness to her analysis.

0. Peter C. Pineo. "Disenchantment in the Later Years of Marriage," *Marriage and Family Living,* No. 23 (February 1961), pp. 3–11.

An important paper reporting the results of a follow-up study after 18 to 20 years of marriage of 400 couples. The study suggests a systematic decline in marital adjustment and satisfaction over time. However, there are substantial flaws in the study that cast doubt over the validity of its general conclusions.

7.  Boyd C. Rollins and Kenneth L. Cannon. ''Marital Satisfaction over the Life Cycle: A Re-evaluation,'' *Journal of Marriage and the Family,* No. 36 (May 1974), pp. 271–282.

A cross-sectional analysis of over 1,500 individuals at various stages in marriage that, like the Pineo study, also shows a steady decline in marital satisfaction, with the sole exception of the period when the children have left the home. This study too has some serious methodological problems that weaken its general conclusion.

8.  Anthony Pietropinto and Jacqueline Simenauer. *Husbands and Wives: A Nationwide Survey of Marriage.* New York: Times Books, 1979.

This ambitious survey of married Americans presents findings on why people marry, how they select their mate, the quality of the marriage relationship, how children affect marriages, and other issues relating to marital stability and marital satisfaction. Interspersed with the research are quotes from survey respondents which reflect a diversity of views on marriage.

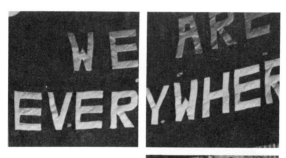
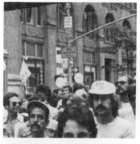
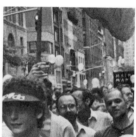
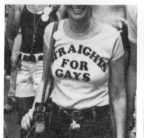
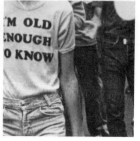

# Alternative Styles: The "Outsiders"

## Chapter Aims

1. To survey some of the alternative styles of pairing, bonding, and child-rearing.

2. To consider some of the ways in which communal living arrangements have existed historically and to point out how the commune is designed to replace the nuclear family.

3. To explore nonmarital cohabitation and singlehood, both of which may be viewed either as transitional stages to marriage or as end stages in themselves.

4. To understand better the paired and single homosexual lifestyle, differentiating the homosexual preference from the gay lifestyle.

## Overview

Although monogamous marriage and nuclear families are common in the United States, there are other paths that people follow: in a group, with one other person, or alone.

Individuals may live together in groups, sharing a common purpose and dividing responsibilities. An individual might choose to live with one other person of the opposite sex or to live alone. Each of these states is practiced as an alternative to or as a prelude to marriage. For people who prefer sexual activities with people of the same sex, there are options in terms of living with one other person or of living alone. Homosexuals sometimes turn to the gay community when they need support for their behavior, which is viewed as nonnormative by many people.

## An Approach to Alternative Family Forms

Status of monogamy

While monogamous marriage is still the preferred form in the United States, the special situations and opportunities of our society have challenged some of the foundation assumptions of heterosexual monogamy. During the past two decades the permanence of monogamous marriage as a social institution has come under scrutiny. While experimental family forms have clearly flourished and a new permissive sexuality has increased the opportunities for experimentation, the evidence at this time still overwhelmingly indicates that marriage as an institution is going to survive for a long time. However, "by learning new ways to communicate effectively, to find identity, and to socialize children through shared responsibility, experimental families may influence improvements in more traditional marriages" (Cogswell and Sussman 1972, p. 506).

In this chapter, we will survey some alternative styles of pairing, bonding, and childrearing. These are not presented as viable substitutes for traditional family forms, but rather as alternative styles that *do* exist and at times even flourish. Some may be transitional stages, on the way to marriage and parenthood; others may be substitutes for the traditional lifestyle and role expectations. "If one agrees with the proposition that traditional family forms, despite their historical contributions, no longer meet significant needs of a growing number of their members," Schulterbrandt and Nichols (1972 p. 429) suggest, "then maintaining an open mind toward emerging alternative family forms becomes essentially a spontaneous and nonthreatening response." It is with this attitude that we will approach our subject matter.

## Communal Living

During the mid to late 1960s and into the 1970s, there was a resurgence in the United States of what is actually a very old idea: the communal living movement. Many reasons have been cited for this revival. Among the most important are the "hippie" culture, partly a product of young peoples' protest against the Vietnam war (Baum 1973), the wider use of psychoactive drugs, including LSD and marijuana, which created in young people a sense of "tribal" identity outside their nuclear families (Speck and Speck 1975), and the rise of a coherent "countercultural social movement": one that was directed mainly "toward the creation of a sectarian society distinct from dominant society, which it considered irrelevant" (Westhues 1972, p. 87). All these forces combined to create a revived sense of communalism, which was fully covered and glamorized by the mass media of communication.

Of course, communal living was not limited to the young, non-married, drug-using, Vietnam protester. Older married couples, sometimes prompted by the media popularization of this adventurous style of living, began to form communes as well. Entertainer Orson Bean and his friends formed a small commune, in which several nuclear families lived together in a spirit of cooperation. In fashionable East Hampton, Long Island, temporary communes were formed on an experimental basis by successful lawyers, accountants, and advertising executives with their families.

The commune, as we will see, is not so much an alternative to nuclear family form as much as it is a structure that supersedes the family. The commune, in practice, can include families or weaken the family form. In answering the question, "Do communes themselves constitute

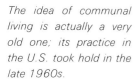

*The idea of communal living is actually a very old one; its practice in the U.S. took hold in the late 1960s.*

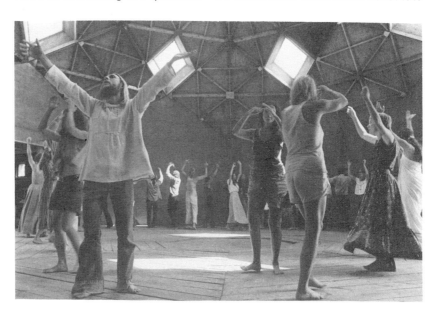

'families,' or do communes contain families in their midst?,'' Kanter (1973, p. 279) says,

> My answer is that communes are a larger, blanket social order that contain or potentially contain smaller family units, but in many cases smaller families have given up their autonomy and separation and have merged with the community. The commune takes over ''family functions.'' Stronger communes involve such elimination of the boundaries between families because this builds a more cohesive community.

In this section, we will look briefly at some aspects of communal living to see how well it fares as an alternative arrangement to traditional marriage and family forms.

## What Is a Commune?

A *commune* can be defined as a group of individuals living together, either in a single dwelling or within a prescribed area, sharing a common purpose and with assigned roles and responsibilities normally associated with the nuclear family. In some communes, there is a sharing of sexual relationships, in some there is monogamy, and in still others there is celibacy. In some there is equality of all role assignments, and in others there is a structured and fixed hierarchy of roles. Some are built on the principles of a socialist society, while others are built on the idea that the only way to a workable social order is through religion. Most believe firmly that they are encompassing the highest or best principles of social living.

Historically, there have been a surprisingly large number of social experiments in communal living. Some were founded on religious ideologies, and others were attempts to find a Utopia, or perfect society, in this world.

Of the latter, the most notable efforts were those of the nineteenth-century French social reformer Charles Fourier (1792–1837), who developed a complex economic theory of communal living based on *phalanxes,* socially and economically cooperative communities of 400 families that would be related around the world and would trade together. His ideas inspired several communes in the United States, but none remained viable for more than a few years.

Most of the communes have been based theoretically on religious ideologies but in practice on very strong leadership. The Oneida community in upstate New York was founded in the mid-nineteenth century by John Humphrey Noyes, a theologian who insisted that all people must strive for perfectionism, even at the cost of their individual personalities. A form of group marriage, called *complex marriage*, was practiced. In this

Phalanxes

Complex marriage

form there was a general attachment by all group members to each other, and they were, with certain limitations, free to engage in sexual relations with various members.

**The Amana community**

The Amana community of Iowa, which we now associate with refrigerators and ovens, was originally formed in 1843 as a religious commune, called the "Community of True Inspiration," by a group of German immigrants. They dissolved as a commune during the depression of the 1930s, but even today former members and families still produce electrical appliances. They also make famous grandfather clocks with the same traditional care as when the community was founded.

**The New Harmony communities**

The two New Harmony communities of Indiana flourished for a period in the early nineteenth century. Originally in Pennsylvania, the followers of "Father" George Rapp came to the banks of the Wabash river in 1814 and built a successful town they called Harmonie. Their official practice was celibacy, although observation of it was apparently not enforced. They developed several successful businesses, and their trademark, the "Rappite Rose," became associated with a guarantee of quality in the same way we now associate the Rolls Royce sign with the best in cars. But disagreements with neighboring communities forced the Rappites to sell their land and return to Pennsylvania in 1824.

The thriving town was bought by Robert Owen, a rich eccentric Englishman who believed in the possibility of a Utopian society not based on religion. He named the town New Harmony and invited "one and all" to join him at his expense until the town could become self-supporting. Unfortunately, he attracted mostly lazy people, who contributed nothing, and the town died out by 1828. Today, the site of these famous communal experiments is a national historical landmark, with many of the original buildings still intact.

**Twin Oaks**

Among the more notable of the contemporary communes is the Twin Oaks Community, an 80-member egalitarian community in Virginia founded in 1967 largely on the practical principles of behavioral psychology and social cooperation that B. F. Skinner developed and depicted in his book *Walden Two*. One of the founders of Twin Oaks was Kathleen Kinkade, who views the experiment as proof that a planned egalitarian society can exist (Kinkade 1974). Ms. Kinkade, along with her daughter and granddaughter is the subject of an extensive interview by Wenig and Coffman (1978), in which they show the life there.

**Hippie communes**

To a great extent, the "hippie" communes of the 1960s and early 1970s differed from the historical ones because they were not based on religious or on financial principles but were "small in size, anarchic in philosophy, and seeking family-style intimacy without much else in the way of a utopian platform" (Kanter 1972, p. 635). They were more rebellious against what was rather than visions of what could be.

## Sociological Considerations

Despite the many different types of communes we have noted and their widely disparate styles and purposes, there are some general features of communes that help us better understand them as social institutions. Most importantly, communes always attempt to replace the nuclear family to varying degrees and in different ways. This attempt is made either by new role assignments or by physical arrangements that make traditional nuclear family living impossible. Rosabeth Moss Kanter (1973) has studied contemporary communes extensively and has pointed out the four main characteristics of social organization of almost all communal arrangements:

Attempt to replace the nuclear family

1. Minimal differentiation of nuclear families within the community (regardless of the prevailing specific marital and parenting arrangements).
2. Performance of "family" functions by the entire collectivity.
3. Minimal differentiation between domestic and economic life.
4. A flexible division of labor.

She also explains in detail some of the ways the commune replaces or weakens the nuclear family as the primary social unit. Some communes eliminate the emotional and erotic bonds and authority rights that act as a basis of differentiation for the nuclear family. Power in areas of decision-making, such as having children and where to live, may be removed from nuclear family units and left to communal leaders, whose decisions consequently affect every area of functioning in the family, from family size to domestic policy. Finally, by controlling property and territory, the commune exerts a powerful influence over the mobility of the family and its social and organizational ties. In short, "In communal systems . . . nuclear families or couples may not be as differentiated from other families or from the whole community as they are outside the communes" (p. 294).

In recent years many of the communal living arrangements that have received the most attention in the public eye are the poorest examples of communal living as a viable social form: Jonestown, the Manson "Family," and domestic terrorist organizations, such as the Symbionese Liberation Army. Probably the best illustration of how communal living can work effectively is found in the Israeli kibbutz.

## The Kibbutz: A Special Arrangement

We mentioned the kibbutz briefly in chapter 2 as a possible exception to the universality of the nuclear family. But of even greater relevance, soci-

Differentiation of
nuclear families

First large-scale form

ologists have focused their attention on the kibbutz arrangement in Israel because it is the first large-scale social effort in Western culture to rear children collectively and accurate measurement of the psychological, intellectual, and social effects are readily available. It is, in short, the largest experimental "laboratory" on communal childrearing in our history.

A *kibbutz* is a social-economic collective, where many individual families work together to produce goods for the community. It is based on the political principles of democratic socialism, and women are afforded equal status with men. Schlesinger (1970, p. 256) lists the four main objectives of the kibbutz system:

1. To abolish parental authority, particularly the patriarchal authority of the father.
2. To free the female from the impediment of being assigned only a few special roles in society, such as homemaking and childrearing.
3. To perpetuate the value system of the communal society.
4. To provide the children with the most democratic education possible.

Emancipation of
women

One of the integral goals of this social structure was the emancipation of women, especially from the burdens of childrearing. "By instituting a system of communal socialization, it was believed it would be possible to achieve part of this goal . . . And if her children were reared by professional nurses, the woman would not only be free from that responsibility, she would be spared the chores of housekeeping as well, since she and her husband would require little room" (Schlesinger 1970).

Because having children is encouraged and yet women are required to participate in all the labor and in the administration of the kibbutz, a unique arrangement has been established for the raising of children. This arrangement is based on the use of comprehensive collective care facilities for the children; that is, the children are raised by the collective, as Devereux et al. (1974, p. 270) describe:

> The most distinctive feature of kibbutz upbringing lies in the fact that the children live, not with their own parents, but in special "children's houses" nearby, with a cohort of age-mates, under the care of a trained *metapelet* [caretaker]. Typically, the kibbutz has a whole colony of such houses, divided by age level from the infants' and toddlers' houses up to those for teenagers. This system was planned both to allow the mothers to participate fully in the extrafamilial work and citizenship duties of the kibbutz and to contribute to the goal of assigning equal responsibilities to both husband and wife for the home and family.

Within the communal context occur all the processes of socialization: formal education, learning of the language, peer interactions, learning of values and moral development, and participation in the work experience. The kibbutz becomes for the child a home with many siblings, and learning to function in this communal home is the integral goal of the entire educational experience.

**Socialization of children**

The *metapelet,* or caretaker, and teacher, functioning as substitute parent and educator, provide this integral experience. While the child does retain his or her identity as a family member, he or she has a simultaneous identity as a member of the collective.

**Metapelet**

For most of the day the child is away from the parents, although special provision is made for continuity of the family structure. This is the main argument used to refute the statement that the kibbutz is an exception to the universality of the nuclear family. Devereux et al. (1974, p. 271) point out that

> while a major part of the socialization process in the kibbutz has been extended to other agents—to the peer group, the teacher, and the *metapelet*—the plan also allows for close contact between parents and their own children. In the later afternoon, after the day's work is done, the children return to their parents' apartments for the customary "four o'clock meal" where they spend the time until supper together. Since the parents have little need to be engaged in household tasks and meal preparation at this time, they usually give the children their full time and attention during these hours.

**Research Findings**   Much research has focused on the effects of this type of upbringing. Two influential books have had an impact on our understanding of the fascinating socialization context. Neubauer (1965) edited an early volume that presented research findings of that time. A few years later, psychoanalyst Bruno Bettelheim wrote his classic work on the subject, *The Children of the Dream.* In recent years there have been hundreds of studies about the children of the kibbutz.

**Order of influence**

Bettelheim points out that in the kibbutz, the major influences on the child's development are the peer group, the collective itself, and the parents, in that order. He shows that socialization instigated and molded through the peer group and collective is generally no worse than the traditional socialization through the family. However, as the child reaches adolescence, according to Bettelheim, there are some definite deficiencies including less empathic understanding in relationships and less individual identity than children raised in the traditional nuclear family setting. These findings have been challenged in other studies (Jay and Birney 1973), and the results are not entirely clear, although certainly no major social or developmental problems of children raised on the kibbutz have been found.

What the kibbutz does show is that the alternative style of communal living does have viable possibilities and can be made to work, especially under conditions of larger societal support.

## Nonmarital Heterosexual Cohabitation

At one time, a couple living together without being married would not have received much social acceptance. In fact, the term "living in sin" was widely used to describe what sociologists call nonmarital cohabitation, and it was viewed as a deviant behavior. Nowadays, however, this attitude is changing. Nonmarital cohabitation has become a more acceptable and certainly more prevalent, alternative style of bonding. "Nonmarital cohabitation," Macklin (1978) points out in her thorough review of the literature and demographics, "is fast becoming a part of the dominant culture in this country and it seems likely that in time to come a majority of persons will experience this lifestyle at some point in their life cycle" (p. 2).

Definition of roles

*Nonmarital cohabitation* exists when a couple, often with "serious intentions," lives together with the overt or covert idea of ultimately joining in marriage or a permanent relationship. Roles in such a living arrangement are not always as clearly defined as in marriage, and there is usually a spoken or unspoken question about if and when the couple will marry at all. Also, parents, friends, neighbors, people at the job, and others may feel uncomfortable with certain aspects of the situation, because it is outside of a traditional marriage arrangement.

### John and Diane

"It was funny when John and I took our first apartment together. I was so uncomfortable every time I'd see the super, because I could tell he didn't know whether to call me Mrs. Collins or Miss Collins or Miss Lustgarten, John's name. Also, you could see with the neighbors that they weren't sure whether to say, 'Your husband' or 'Your roommate,' or 'Your friend.' It was . . . well, it was just uncomfortable."

Why do some individuals choose nonmarital cohabitation? There are many reasons, including the widespread but not yet proven, belief that a marriage will have a better chance of success if the partners live together first (Ridley, Peterman, and Avery 1978). It is sometimes assumed that people who choose nonmarital cohabitation are rebels, who are rejecting the social norm. Yet, this assumption does not hold up under scrutiny. Investigations of individuals involved in experimental cohabitation have revealed that in general they are neither less traditional nor more nonconforming than individuals involved in traditional relationships but are somewhat more likely to have been involved with more sexual partners than have noncohabitors (Markowski, Croake, and Keller 1978).

By and large, the data do not seem to support a strong conservative view of marriage as over and against cohabitation. Specifically, when we look at the statistically significant findings, we see that although both men and women who were married have had fewer group sex experiences and fewer sexual partners than those who were cohabitating, they are on the whole more satisfied with the majority of their intercourse experiences, and for the men also with their first intercourse experiences. The point we want to emphasize then is that this evidence does not suggest that the cohabitational life is one of more erotic satisfaction; rather it suggests the opposite.

Whatever the reasons for choosing this lifestyle, the couple has to make several types of adjustments. Since we are primarily socialized for marriage rather than for cohabitation, some of the accepted marital roles we have learned and that we take for granted may be more critically examined and questioned in a cohabitating situation (Trost 1978). Several questions couples must come to grips with are:

- How should we arrange the financial conditions of this relationship? Should the rent and expenses be shared equally, shared in proportion to our respective earnings, or handled in some other way?
- How will household responsibilities and decisionmaking be divided between us?
- Are we planning to maintain an exclusive sexual relationship? To what degree are outside relationships permissible? What about nonsexual friendships with people of the opposite sex?
- What will we do in case of unplanned pregnancy?
- Would we be willing to marry if we had a child?
- How will the assets acquired during our cohabitation be divided if we break up? What about sacrifices made during this period: What compensations will there be for these?
- In what ways will we respond to and interact with our nuclear families?

Table 8.1

**Summary of Responses to Some Sexual History Variables for Cohabiting and Married Individuals**

| | Satisfaction with First Intercourse | | | |
| | Unsatisfactory | Satisfactory | Very Satisfactory | $x^2$ |
|---|---|---|---|---|
| Male-Cohabiting | 16 | 29 | 5 | 8.54* |
| Male-Married | 7 | 28 | 15 | |
| Female-Cohabiting | 14 | 27 | 9 | |
| Female-Married | 11 | 27 | 12 | |

| | Number of Partners in Sexual Intercourse | | | | | | |
| | 1 | 2–5 | 6–10 | 11–20 | 25–50 | Do Not Remember | |
|---|---|---|---|---|---|---|---|
| Male-Cohabiting | 7 | 15 | 15 | 6 | 4 | 3 | 15.60** |
| Male-Married | 23 | 15 | 5 | 4 | 2 | 1 | |
| Female-Cohabiting | 13 | 16 | 9 | 7 | 2 | 3 | 32.78*** |
| Female-Married | 39 | 10 | 1 | 0 | 0 | 0 | |

| | Satisfaction with Majority of Intercourse Experiences | | | |
| | Unsatisfactory | Satisfactory | Very Satisfactory | |
|---|---|---|---|---|
| Male-Cohabiting | 2 | 33 | 13 | 7.89* |
| Male-Married | 1 | 21 | 27 | |
| Female-Cohabiting | 10 | 21 | 17 | 9.73** |
| Female-Married | 1 | 19 | 27 | |

| | Number of Group Sex Experiences | | |
| | None | One | >One | |
|---|---|---|---|---|
| Male-Cohabiting | 35 | 6 | 9 | 8.89* |
| Male-Married | 46 | 3 | 1 | |
| Female-Cohabiting | 44 | 4 | 2 | 6.38* |
| Female-Married | 50 | 0 | 0 | |

*$p<.05$
**$p<.01$
***$p<.001$

Adapted from Markowski, E. M., Croake, J. W. and Keller, J. F. Sexual history and present sexual behavior of cohabiting and married couples. *Journal of Sexual Research,* 1978, 14 (1), 27–39.

**Acceptance by nuclear families**

The answer to this last question especially depends largely on the degree of acceptance or nonacceptance by the nuclear families. Some parents happily accept their cohabiting offspring, while others go so far as to disown their son or daughter who is living in a nonmarital relationship. Many parents are somewhere in between, pressuring the child either into marriage or into dissolving the relationship.

**Legal definitions**

Until recently there was little legal definition of cohabiting couples. They did not have the rights nor the obligations of a legally married couple. Then, in 1976, in a landmark California Supreme Court decision *(Marvin* v. *Marvin,* C-23303), Michelle Triola Marvin won the right to sue for equal property rights the man she had cohabitated with for several years, actor Lee Marvin. Although the final disposition of that case made it clear that living together does not assure joint property rights as does marriage in California and although Michelle Marvin won only a small sum for what the judge called "rehabilitation" purposes, the case did illustrate that the law is recognizing the increased incidence and acceptance of nonmarital cohabitation. As *Newsweek* magazine (April 30, 1979, p. 68) reported,

> The significance of the case . . . is that she [Ms. Marvin] got inside the court at all. "The important decision was the [court] recognizing for the first time that unmarried couples can sue each other," says Columbia University law Prof. Ruth Bader Ginsburg. "It illustrates the further breakdown of the legal line between marriage and unmarried union."

Nonmarital cohabitation is in no way threatening the survival of traditional marriage. More times than not, in fact, it serves as a transitional step between dating and marriage, with the period of cohabitation viewed as a "part of the courtship phase" (Macklin 1978, p. 8). Among the college population, especially those who live away from home, there is a higher incidence of and preference for nonmarital cohabitation than among working-class people who remain at home until they marry. "It appears that although marriage is still the first preference for a post college living arrangement," Jacques and Chason (1978) conclude from their study, "for a substantial minority, cohabitation—not marriage—is the preferred arrangement. Further, if students have experienced a cohabiting relationship prior to graduation, they are even more likely to prefer cohabitation to marriage after college" (p. 147). In short, for college students much of their subsequent pairing will be influenced by the styles they developed during their college years

Figure 8.1
## U.S. Singles Under 35 as of 1976

More people under 35 are living alone—more are divorced—and more are staying single

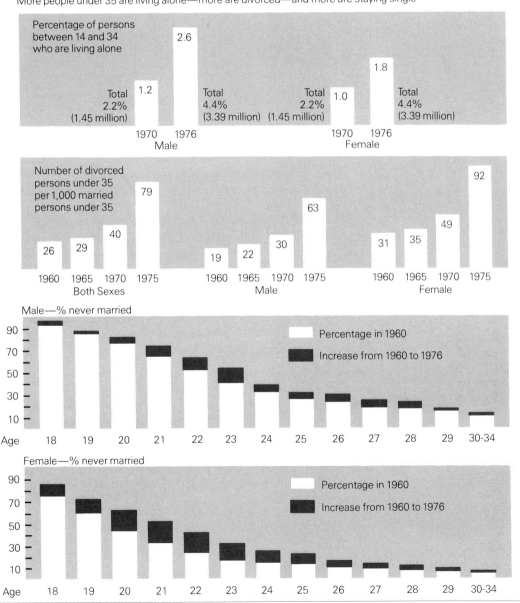

# Singlehood

*Singlehood* is a broad term used to describe an integrated social lifestyle based on the options an unmarried adult has. Being single is a social status. Rather than thinking of singlehood as the absence of marriage it is now viewed more as an individual's positive voluntary choice of a lifestyle appropriate for his or her needs. As figure 8.1 shows, a number of people under 35 are single today.

**Positive choice vs. absence of marriage**

Single people come from every age level, socioeconomic level, and ethnic group. There are significant functional differences, of course, between younger singles and older singles, between formerly married and never-marrieds, between childless singles and single parents, between heterosexual and homosexual singles. There is also a difference between what Stein (1978) calls the "voluntary temporary single" directed toward mating as a future goal, and the "involuntary stable single," who is not happy in that state. Table 8.2 shows a range of possibilities. But there are also common problems and common experiences shared by all individuals in singlehood.

The single person has different problems and responsibilities than the married person, the cohabiting person, or the person involved in communal living. The single is probably responsible for his or her own support; and since there is some truth to the adage that two can live as cheaply as one at least in terms of rent and owning a car, it may be difficult to support oneself as comfortably as one would like.

There are some stigmas attached to singlehood, and, despite a changing attitude, many have persisted over the years. The stereotypes vary especially according to age level. A few common ones are:

**Stigmas**

- Single people are basically selfish, immature, and unwilling to make a long-term commitment.
- Young, attractive single girls are promiscuous.
- Young, unattractive single girls don't get married because they can't find husbands.
- Single men over the age of 30 are probably gay.
- Singles tend to have swinging, freewheeling lifestyles, or, conversely, being single is always a lonely, depersonalizing experience.

**Increasing acceptability**

None of these stereotypes is essentially true. Of course there will be individuals who fit various categories, but they are not limited to single individuals. Fortunately, attitudes are changing and, "with decreasing emphasis on children, remaining single attains a modicum of respectability. Although the society still discriminates against the single person, remaining unmarried to devote oneself to career or to avoid the perceived difficulties of marriage is becoming more acceptable" (Cox 1974, p. 132),

The life of the single person depends a great deal on a myriad of circumstances. The single parent usually has the dual responsibility of finan-

Table 8.2
**Typology of Singlehood**

|  | Voluntary | Involuntary |
|---|---|---|
| Temporary | —younger never-marrieds postponing marriage for a few years<br>—recently divorced persons who are ''single again'' but seeking mates<br>—never-marrieds who were not interested in marriage for a number of years but are now actively seeking a mate<br>—cohabitators who now want to marry | —the divorced, widowed, and deserted seeking remarriage<br>—single parents seeking mates<br>—younger never-marrieds actively seeking mates |
| Stable | —men and women choosing to be single<br>—single parents not seeking spouses<br>—religionaries<br>—cohabitators not intending to marry<br>—formerly marrieds not seeking to remarry | —older widowed, divorced, and never-marrieds who wanted to marry or remarry, have not found a mate, and have accepted the idea of singlehood as a probable life state<br>—never-marrieds who are impaired physically or mentally in some way and not able to succeed in the marriage market |

SOURCE: Stein, P. J. The lifestyles and life chances of the never-married. *Marriage & Family Review*, 1978, 1 (4), 10–14.

cially supporting and raising a child or children while trying to maintain satisfying social relationships. These roles can conflict.

## Phyllis

"Men find me attractive and bright," Phyllis nonchalantly acknowledges, "but as soon as they find out I have a little boy at home, I can sense their reluctance to get involved. And there are practical problems. I can't just get up and go out on the spur of the moment. I have to arrange with a babysitter first. And then there's the problem of bringing men home. I have a policy: no sex in my apartment because it is kind of small and the baby could be disturbed. Well, my attitude is if the man likes me enough, he'll make the concessions necessary to date me. If not, forget it."

Single parents

The single parent also lacks much of the social support given to the couple who is raising a child. Single mothers or fathers may find that their children are perceived as "different" because of the parents' singlehood. And, when other parents get together, the single parent may not be invited because it is viewed as a threat to have a single person around socially.

Despite the increasing number of single-parent families, the mass media, religious institutions, and social organizations are still geared for the two-parent family. It is not unusual to encounter the embarrassment of a parent or child having to explain to a school or public official that there is no father or mother present at home. This situation can be remedied with the advent of new social attitudes: Chester (1977, p. 113) concludes in his study,

> What is needed is recognition of the facts that a plural society
> necessarily produces pluralistic forms of the family. . . . Coupled
> with changing thought about the situation of women and a con-
> temporary tendency towards the de-differentiation of conjugal
> roles, this would lead to the further recognition of how far the
> many problems associated with one-parent families are the prod-
> uct of institutional and cultural factors which could be modified.

In 1979, for the first time, a regular television comedy series about an unmarried mother and her child was aired, in a manner that gave the tooling that this lifestyle was becoming more natural, acceptable, and normative. Unfortunately this series, *On Your Own*, lasted but a few months.

Another type of single who becomes the victim of gross social misunderstanding is the older single, especially one who has never married.

There is greater stigma attached to the older single woman than to the older single man. Such terms as old maid and auntie describe the subtle contempt felt for the woman whose choice was to remain single. As

*Although attitudes are changing, our society still discriminates against single people and stereotypes them.*

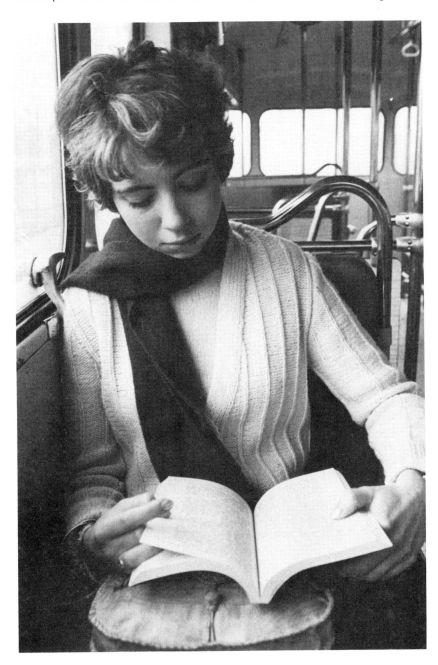

Older singles

people are living longer, however, there are increasingly more single people in the over-60 age group. One of the most denigrating attitudes toward this group is that it is disgusting, immoral, or inappropriate for older single people to be sexually active. The fact is often denied. While sex among young singles is viewed with a certain amount of romantic fascination, among the old it is viewed with skepticism and repugnance. Although we will discuss sex among the elderly in more detail in chapter 11, we should mention now that research has consistently demonstrated that an older person who is sexually active is far healthier than one who is not (Isaacs and Post 1978).

Permanent or temporary

One last point should be mentioned about singlehood as a lifestyle. As with marriage, it can never be known if it is permanent or temporary. So, that while the person develops his or her goals within the context of remaining single, the possibility and opportunity for marriage is everpresent. This means, in effect, that in the formation of friendships, in choosing a residence or a city to live in, in deciding between suburb or city, the possibility of future marriage and of dating opportunities—and for some, even the option of future marriage—may play a part in the single person's decision.

Now, we will look at the single and paired homosexual lifestyle, which differs in many ways from those we have been discussing so far in this chapter.

## Homosexual Lifestyles

The homosexual lifestyle is probably the most controversial of any we will cover in this book. For many years *homosexuality,* the preference for sexual activities with someone of the same sex, was considered a sign of psychological illness or deviant behavior, and the vast majority of homosexuals kept their sexual preference a secret. Many even married and raised families, living the straight—that is, heterosexual—life on the surface, while longing deep inside for a loving paired relationship they could relate to both sexually and emotionally.

Militant gay movement

Homosexuality only began to gain a modicum of social respectability in the late 1960s as the so-called *militant gay movement* became a potent, highly visible form of protest. With this "coming out of the closet" for the movement as a whole, many individual gay professionals, entertainers, business people, and others acknowledged their homosexuality as a fact. Often it had been suspected and whispered about by acquaintances anyway. In this section, while we will not be exploring in any depth the causes of homosexuality, we will look at its social implications and its practical consequences as a lifestyle. We will pay special attention to the social organizations that tie male and female homosexuals together and the changing attitudes about homosexuality.

## The Homosexual Preference

There are more theories about why people become homosexuals than there are theories about any other type of human behavior. There are probably so many theories because no one really knows the causes. At this point no one theory is supported by enough evidence to be considered more valid than the others. Therefore, we will only mention some of the more important ones and briefly summarize what they imply.

*Constitutional theory,* or *biological theory,* says that homosexuality is an inborn tendency, either neurological or glandular. Many proponents of this theory also believe it is genetic and transmitted from generation to generation.

*Classical psychoanalytic theory,* the most disputed, says that homosexuality is a consequence of a maternal deprivation or overprotection during the formative years of life. This position sees the homosexual, if not as ill, at least as lacking full psychosexual development.

*Social learning theory* argues that we learn homosexual behaviors either by modeling ourselves after same-sex figures in our lives or by being conditioned to respond sexually to people of our own sex and not to the opposite sex. Homosexuality, according to this theory, is a learned behavior that, under certain circumstances, can be unlearned.

*Sociological theory* suggests that homosexuality is an interaction of social, psychological and economic conditions that, from childhood to adulthood, result in a same-gender sexual preference. It states that a person's social situation provides the context in which his or her psychosexual needs are expressed (Ashworth and Walker 1972). Most likely, homosexual preference results from some combination of factors over a period of years, and the sociological theory seems to best take into account the mix among cultural and psychological factors, along with all other circumstances. It also allows us to better evaluate the influences of such variables as primary socialization, the mass media of communication, role learning, role confusion, and peer pressures. It is, in short, the most comprehensive way of understanding the homosexual lifestyle in a social context.

## Male and Female Homosexuals

Chafetz et al. (1974), among others (especially Simon, 1967), have pointed out important functional differences between male homosexuals and female homosexuals. Male homosexuals, for example, tend to be more promiscuous, less stable in relationships, and generally less committed to a single other person than do female homosexuals, who are called *lesbians*. Also, as a very general rule, lesbians tend to enter into sexual relationships only after establishing some kind of emotional in-

*There are numerous theories about why people become homosexuals, probably because no one knows the answer.*

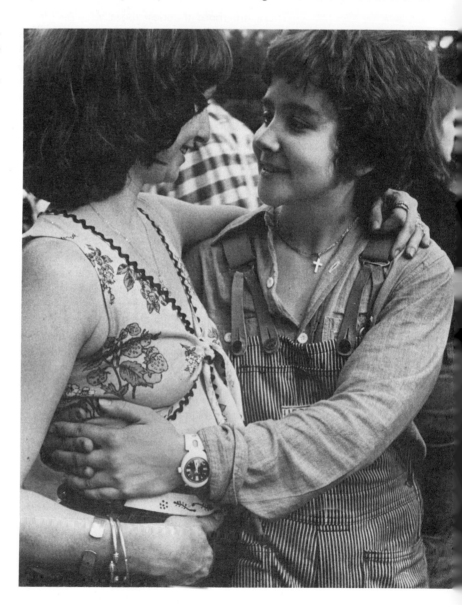

volvement with their partners, while men are more impulsive in their non-committal sexual behaviors (Gagnon and Simon 1967). Moreover, the male homosexual tends to have greater ties to the gay community than does the female homosexual, who is able to focus more on her relationship with another lesbian remaining relatively uninvolved with the gay lifestyle. Lesbians, however, may identify strongly with the feminist movement and the rights of women in general; gay and straight.

There is another important difference, the result of how male and female homosexuals are stereotyped. Gagnon and Simon (1967, p. 249) explain this in some depth:

> In a contrast between male and female homosexuals, it is probable that the former perhaps have a less complicated stereotype. For male homosexuality the severity of sanctions is sufficiently strong to organize and limit the content of the general social image. *The broader society is manifestly more concerned with repressing and sanctioning male homosexuality than with repressing and sanctioning female homosexuality.* It is possible that the level of anxiety in the general population evoked by male homosexuality is sufficiently high to place a constraint on the direct imputation of fantasy elements. The image of the female homosexual, however, is less likely to be organized by a single, strong theme; it may be more easily complicated by unmediated mixtures of anxiety and fantasy. *The lesbian, despite the general negative value attached to homosexual actors, remains a potentially erotic object to heterosexual males* in a way and to a degree that the male homosexual is unlikely to be defined (italics ours).

The point that heterosexual men still find homosexual women erotic objects has important practical implications. For example, a straight man may be extremely reluctant to hire a gay man for an office but would not hesitate to hire a lesbian, especially if he finds her sexually attractive. For female homosexuals it is not so much their homosexuality that stigmatizes them as it is looking too butch, too masculine. The feminine-looking lesbian in fact suffers far less social exclusion than the masculine-looking male homosexual does.

There is another aspect that should be mentioned. Because men are socialized to perceive other men as dominant and sexually aggressive, there is often the belief that a male homosexual will forcefully assert his homosexuality. The straight man may thus feel threatened by the gay man: he fears being coerced or seduced into homosexual submission. The straight man does not have this fear when dealing with the lesbian, however.

## Gay Lifestyles

It would be absurd to try to present a typical gay lifestyle, as if it were representative of even a fraction of a percent of the total homosexual population. For one thing, most homosexuals do not lead an overtly gay lifestyle. In reality, homosexuals are found in every occupation, in every socioeconomic level, as introverts and extroverts. They are as different and varied as are heterosexuals.

Yet, there is such a thing as a gay lifestyle, and as a subculture it does describe some of the role options open to and the behaviors exhibited by many homosexuals. Homosexuals do not segregate themselves from the heterosexual community; but when they seek reinforcement and support for their behaviors, they are more likely to turn to the gay community, where they can more readily find this support.

Fein and Nuehring (1975) have studied the organizational structures and functions of the *gender-integrated gay community,* where lesbians and male homosexuals interact with each other. They found that the two frequent places of social interaction are gay organizations and gay bars. The purposes of the gay organizations are to foster gay pride and self-awareness, to help gay people meet and establish a sense of social cooperation, and to improve gay-straight relationships with the broader society. In gender-integrated gay organizations, some women felt they were being subjugated to men in the same ways they would have been in straight society.

**Gender-integrated gay community**

The gay bars, Fein and Nuehring found, serve primarily as a social rather than a strictly sexual gathering place. It is a focal point of informal interaction among peers. Dancing is a popular activity, and men and women often mix in a friendly, natural style. Still, observation indicated that "within the context of even this ostensibly 'social' bar, differential patterns of sexual activity for males and females appear to be confirmed as has been noted in previous studies" (Fein and Nuehring, 1975, p. 154). Specifically, males tended, as we mentioned before, to be more promiscuous than did females.

**Gay bars**

In concluding their study, they point out some of the reasons for the existence of a gay community, in terms of what it offers the homosexual:

- The community offers social support, group identity, and validation of a positive self-image.
- The community provides opportunities for shared normative behaviors that enable members to overcome the ostracism they tend to experience from the straight society.
- The community provides informal social services, such as a place to stay overnight or a meal, not as readily available outside.
- The community serves as an informal, underground commu-

nications network, particularly concerning news about individual gays and the broader community.

- The community provides a secure setting in which to make sexual contacts.

Still, we should emphasize that for many homosexuals, even if they are ''out of the closet,'' their primary affiliation is not with the group that represents their sexual preference, but rather with some other group. A hard-working physician, for example, who happens to be a homosexual, rarely associates with other homosexuals aside from his lover because he is so absorbed in his work. He would much rather talk shop with other specialists in his professional field than go to a gay bar, where he would not feel that he had anything in common with the other gays.

## Single and Paired Homosexuals

There are many important differences between the homosexual lifestyles of a single person and the paired homosexual bond. Most of the same comments we made about singlehood in the preceding section would apply to the gay single. Likewise, many of the observations about marital roles and adjustment we will be developing in later chapters would apply to the paired homosexual relationship, especially if it is relatively permanent. There are some exceptions, however.

Need for support

Single heterosexuals have the support of the broader society, especially in seeking partners to date, in finding social contexts in which to interact, and in working out relationship conflicts. The gay person does not always find this support available. In fact, quite often at the very time the single homosexual needs this support it is not there.

### Bill

''When I first came to Dubuque,'' Bill, a handsome 30-year-old homosexual businessman says, ''I felt lonely and far removed from Akron, where I had been living most of my life and where I knew people. Everyone at the new office tried to fix me up with one woman or another—and even though I didn't hide my homosexuality in Akron, I didn't feel I could show it here. Not yet. In fact, I got the feeling that even though some of them knew about it, or suspected, they were secretly hoping that by fixing me up with the right woman, I would miraculously turn heterosexual overnight. I'll tell you, it didn't make things easy for me.''

**Adolescent homosexuals**

There is also an important difference that should be noted between the heterosexual and homosexual adolescent. At a period in life when acceptance by peers and conformity to images are of paramount importance, it is indeed difficult, if not impossible, for adolescent homosexuals to express themselves to their peers and to engage in the type of sexual activity and courtship that is available to their heterosexual counterparts. The main question that hangs threateningly over the heads of many homosexual adolescents is whether or not their feelings of homosexuality mean that they are "sick," even though much recent thinking is that homosexuality should be viewed as an alternative lifestyle rather than as an emotional illness (Jones 1974). This is also reflected by the American Psychiatric Association's decision to remove homosexuality from its list of psychological disturbances.

The homosexual adolescent may be exposed to ridicule and contempt by his or her peers. The class "fag" or "queer" often must bear the burden of repressed homosexual fears of some fellow students. Since the homosexual boy or girl is likely to experience more pressures than the heterosexual youth and, at the same time, to find less social reinforcement, it may be helpful if the student is exposed to some type of supportive counseling, when this is possible.

## Social Attitudes toward Homosexuality

**Homophobia**

When we look at the social attitudes toward homosexuality as a behavior and homosexuals as people, we are not only concerned about acceptance or rejection, but also about the powerful social phenomenon we call *homophobia,* sometimes called *homoerotophobia,* the irrational fear of homosexuality. People who are homoerotophobic virtually have such strong negative feelings about homosexuals that they dread even being near them (MacDonald 1976). This extends beyond the fear of direct homosexual behavior itself and reflects such individuals' stereotyped and rigid perception of the differentiation of male-female roles. Dunbar, Brown, and Vuorinen (1973, p. 174) point out that

> certain personality traits, interests, and professions are seen as being masculine or feminine. Those who exhibit behaviors which violate these sex-stereotypes are suspected of homosexuality. Thus a "feminine" male is thought to be homosexual by a highly homoerotophobic individual. Previous research has shown that those highly prejudiced against homosexuals also hold far more distinct concepts of masculinity and femininity than do less prejudiced subjects.

*Homophobia persists even though a majority of people feel that what consenting homosexual adults do in private is their business.*

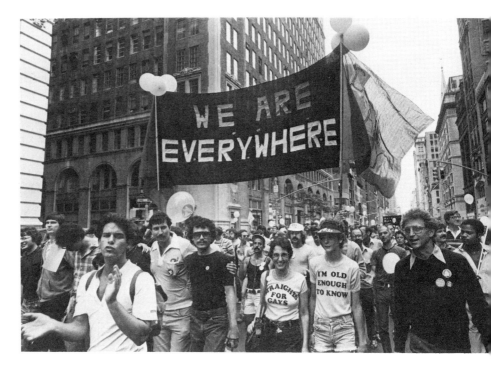

Although the overall attitude toward homosexuality is changing, especially now that very masculine figures, such as football stars have "come out of the closet," there is still homophobia and stigma is still attached, as shown in tables 8.3 and 8.4.

A 1970 survey found that judgments about homosexuality, as with heterosexuality, took into account the stipulation that affection be expressed as a concomitant, making it less "morally wrong" (Levitt and Klassen 1974). The results of this survey are shown in table 8.5. At that point in time and with that stipulation, 68 percent of the respondents agreed that "what consenting adult homosexuals do in private is no one else's business" (p. 43). This clearly shows that things are changing!

## Alternative Lifestyles and Deviance

With any of the alternative lifestyles we have discussed in this chapter, there is the distinct possibility that others may perceive the individual practicing it as a social deviant. Of the lifestyles considered, this possibility is most likely with homosexuality and least likely with singlehood. Communal living and cohabitation fall somewhere in the middle.

Deviant = outsider

The *deviant* is by definition an outsider, a person who differs from the accepted social standard. In his classic studies on the sociology of deviance, Howard S. Becker (1963) points out that although they differ in many respects, people that are labeled as deviant "share the label and the experience of being labeled as outsiders" (p. 10). The fact that they perceive themselves as deviant then assumes importance in their social interactions, especially with others who are exhibiting normative behaviors. As outsiders, they are relegated to view each social interaction differently than an insider would. Since, in the case of alternative lifestyles,

Table 8.3

**Opinions of Homosexuals as Dangerous, Homosexuality as Threatening, Offensive (Presented in Percentages)**

|  | Homosexuals are dangerous as teachers or youth leaders because they try to get sexually involved with children. | Homosexuals try to play sexually with children if they cannot get an adult partner. | Homosexuals are a high security risk for government jobs.* |
|---|---|---|---|
| Strongly agree | 44.7 | 35.1 | 43.1 |
| Somewhat agree | 28.8 | 36.0 | 15.8 |
| Somewhat disagree | 11.9 | 9.9 | 12.0 |
| Strongly disagree | 9.5 | 8.5 | 20.8 |
| Don't know | 3.9 | 9.8 | 7.2 |
| No Answer | 0.8 | 0.6 | 0.8 |
| Total percent | 99.6 | 99.9 | 99.7 |
| Total sample | 3018 | 3018 | 3018 |

*These three items provided responses concerning how many homosexuals are like this: "All or almost all?" "More than half?" "Less than half?" "Hardly any or none?" "Don't know," and a "No answer" category.
**This item provided five response categories: "Very much?" "Somewhat?" "Very little?" "Not at all?" and "No answer."

this status is primarily caused by their nonnormative sexual behavior, it means that this behavior, this part of their lives, infuses their entire social perspectives. In other words, their nonnormative behavior, which may be a relatively small part of their lives, becomes a major focal point. This understanding of their self-perceptions and the perceptions of others plays an important part in our understanding of how important lifestyle is to the individual's total functioning in the social order.

In the family context, for example, the deviant member may be ostracized, banished from the family, or singled out for special treatment. The

| Homosexuals tend to corrupt their fellow workers sexually.* | If homosexual men can't find men for partners, they try to force their attentions on women.* | Homosexuality is a social corruption that can cause the downfall of a civilization. | Homosexuality in itself is no problem, but what people make of it can be a serious problem. | To what extent do you think homosexuality is obscene and vulgar?** |
|---|---|---|---|---|
| 22.8 | 6.9 | 25.0 | 27.3 | 65.2 |
| 15.6 | 10.9 | 23.8 | 27.8 | 18.6 |
| | | | | |
| 19.0 | 22.2 | 18.8 | 16.9 | 7.4 |
| 35.0 | 45.4 | 24.6 | 23.0 | 7.5 |
| 7.0 | 13.7 | 7.2 | 3.8 | — |
| 0.6 | 0.6 | 0.7 | 0.8 | 1.0 |
| 100.0 | 99.7 | 100.1 | 99.6 | 99.7 |
| 3018 | 3018 | 3018 | 3018 | 3018 |

SOURCE: Levitt, E. P. & Klassen, A. D. Public attitudes toward homosexuality: Part of the 1970 national survey by the Institute for Sex Research. *Journal of Homosexuality,* 1974, 1 (1), 29–43.

Table 8.4

## Occupational Attitudes (Presented in Percentages)

Homosexual men should or should not be allowed to work in the following professions:

| | Court judge (7)* | School-teacher (8) | Minister (9) | Medical doctor (3) | Government official (5) | Beautician (2) | Artist (1) | Musician (6) | Florist (4) |
|---|---|---|---|---|---|---|---|---|---|
| Allowed | 22.8 | 23.1 | 23.4 | 32.3 | 32.6 | 71.7 | 84.5 | 85.2 | 86.8 |
| Not allowed | 77.2 | 76.9 | 76.6 | 67.7 | 67.4 | 28.3 | 15.5 | 14.8 | 13.2 |
| Total responding | 2957 | 2974 | 2970 | 2961 | 2954 | 2969 | 2960 | 2974 | 2972 |
| No answer | 61 | 44 | 48 | 57 | 64 | 49 | 58 | 44 | 46 |
| Total sample | 3018 | 3018 | 3018 | 3018 | 3018 | 3018 | 3018 | 3018 | 3018 |

*Parenthetic numbers in each column heading indicate the order in which inquiry was made in the interview.

SOURCE: Levitt, E. P. & Klassen, A. D. Public attitudes toward homosexuality: Part of the 1970 national survey by the Institute for Sex Research. Journal of Homosexuality, 1974, 1 (1), 29–43.

Table 8.5

## Moral Attitudes (Presented in Percentages)

| | What is your opinion of sex acts between two persons of the same sex when they: | | What is your opinion if a married person has sexual intercourse with someone other than the marriage partner? | If a teenager (boy/girl) 16–19 has sexual intercourse with a (girl/boy) without love? | If an unmarried adult (man/woman) has sexual intercourse with a (woman/man) when they love each other? |
| | have no special affection for each other? | love each other? | | | |
|---|---|---|---|---|---|
| Always wrong | 77.7 | 70.2 | 72.2 | 51.7 | 31.5 |
| Almost always wrong | 8.4 | 8.4 | 14.3 | 19.4 | 14.0 |
| Wrong only sometimes | 6.3 | 7.2 | 10.7 | 19.6 | 22.2 |
| Not wrong at all | 5.6 | 11.4 | 2.1 | 5.0 | 28.7 |
| Don't know | 1.6 | 2.2 | 0.4 | 4.0 | 3.5 |
| No answer | 0.1 | 0.3 | 0.1 | 0.1 | — |
| Total percent | 99.7 | 99.7 | 99.8 | 99.8 | 99.9 |
| Total sample | 3018 | 3018 | 3018 | 3018 | 3018 |

SOURCE: Levitt, E. P. & Klassen, A. D. Public attitudes toward homosexuality: Part of the 1970 national survey by the Institute for Sex Research. *Journal of Homosexuality,* 1974, 1 (1). 29–43.

Family reaction

family may try to be helpful to the person, but publicly disaffiliate itself from the deviant behavior. Pressure may even be brought to bear on the deviant family member to either conceal the deviance or move to a different place. The family may be unable to transcend its cultural limitations and understand the deviant member's choice of lifestyle for what it is and for what it means to that member. As Smrtic (1979, p. 9) suggests,

> We live in a middle-class oriented, contemporary American society. Within this society we have developed complex codes of conduct that constitute normal behavior in this specific cultural setting. We become so familiar with, and accustomed to, our way of life that often we have a tendency to view any behavior that does not fit in with the way in which people behave in our culture as being inferior, primitive, weird, threatening, or abnormal. We surround our eyes with cultural blinders that make us view behavior within very limited cultural guidelines.

Thus, to the degree that any of these alternative lifestyles are viewed as deviant and as long as the participant family member remains an outsider, there is the possibility of serious family conflict as a result. The implications of the individual's personal choice of lifestyle, then, can have an effect on all family members. For example, since the identity of the family is in part related to the identity of its individual members, the stigma of deviant would apply not only to the individual but to the family itself—at least to the extent that the family is seen partially responsible for the deviant behavior. Also, at a minimum, the family must spend some of its time, and possibly resources, to deal with the "deviance" and its consequences.

## Summary

1. A commune is a group of individuals living together, either in a single dwelling or within a prescribed area, sharing a common purpose and with assigned roles and responsibilities normally associated with the nuclear family. The commune is not so much an alternative to the nuclear family form as much as it is a structure that supersedes the family, at least functionally.

2. Despite the many different types of past and current communes, there are some general features of communes that help us better understand them as social institutions. To varying degrees and in different ways, communes always attempt to replace the nuclear family. This replacement is done either by new role assignments or by physical arrangements that make traditional nuclear family living impossible.

3. A kibbutz is a social-economic collective, where many individual families work together to produce goods for the community. It is based on the political principles of democratic socialism, and women are afforded equal status with men. It has enjoyed great success in Israel, where it has been studied extensively.

4. Some people choose nonmarital cohabiting situations instead of or as a prelude to marriage. Since we are primarily socialized for marriage, some roles we have learned and that we take for granted in marriage may be more critically examined and questioned in a cohabiting situation.

5. Singlehood is a broad term used to describe an integrated social lifestyle based on the options an unmarried adult has. It is now viewed more as an individual's positive voluntary choice of a lifestyle appropriate for his or her needs rather than as the absence of marriage.

6. The lifestyle of a single person depends on many circumstances. The single parent usually has the dual responsibility of financially supporting and raising a child or children while trying to maintain satisfying social relationships. These roles can conflict. The single parent may also lack the social support given to the married couple who is raising a child.

7. One type of single who becomes the victim of gross social misunderstanding is the older single, especially the single person who has never married.

8. For many years the homosexual lifestyle was considered a sign of psychological illness or deviant behavior, and the vast majority of homosexuals kept their sexual preference a secret. But homosexuality began to gain a modicum of social respectability in the late 1960s and the 1970s with the so-called *militant gay movement.*

9. There are more theories about why people become homosexuals than there are about any other types of alternative human behavior because there is not enough evidence to support any one theory alone.

10. The gay lifestyle as a subculture describes some of the role options open to and the behaviors exhibited by many homosexuals. Homosexuals do not segregate themselves from the heterosexual community; but when they seek reinforcement and support for their behaviors, they are likely to turn to the gay community, where this can be more readily found.

## Key Terms

The following terms were introduced and defined in this chapter. Definitions also appear in the glossary.

commune
complex marriage
constitutional theory of homosexuality
deviant
gender-integrated gay community
homophobia
homosexuality
kibbutz
lesbian
metapelet

nonmarital cohabitation
phalanx
psychoanalytic theory
    of homosexuality
singlehood
social learning theory
    of homosexuality
sociological theory
    of homosexuality

**Discussion Questions**

1. Briefly describe each of the following communal living arrangements: Oneida Community, Amana Community, the two communities at New Harmony, Twin Oaks, and the Israeli kibbutz.

2. Imagine yourself living in a communal arrangement. What philosophy would be most compatible with your views of what a satisfying and functional domestic arrangement should be like? What type of people would you want to live with? What type would you want to avoid? How would you feel about sharing all the responsibilities of the household? Do you think that living in intimacy with people that are in fact from different nuclear families of orientation can lead to much confusion, since their upbringings are so different?

3. How effectively or ineffectively do you think an urban kibbutz arrangement could work in the inner cities and ghettos of the United States? Particularly, do you think that large numbers of poor urban families, now on welfare or some other form of social assistance, could work together in manufacturing or providing services, using the same type of communal arrangement that has proven so successful in Israel?

4. Interview some single and married people whom you know or to whom you have access. Do the majority of the single people, as a general rule, indicate that they intend to marry at some time in the near or distant future, or do they feel that singlehood is a permanent way of life for them? Are most married peoples' conceptions of the single lifestyle borne out by the singles' experiences, or is there a tendency to glamorize and romanticize singlehood? Also, try to determine if singlehood for men and for women is a stigmatized status, if it is socially valued, or if it is neutral.

5. Try to determine the attitudes of your peers about homosexuality and toward homosexuals in general. Do you consider homosexuality a valid alternative lifestyle? A deviant behavior? Why?

6. From your reading of this chapter, what would you list as the three primary problems commonly facing the single heterosexual, the single homosexual, and the paired homosexual?

**Suggested Readings**

1. Bruno Bettelheim. *Children of the Dream.* New York: Macmillan, 1969.

A dynamic analysis of children raised on a kibbutz by one of the world's foremost psychiatrists that is both professionally responsible and humanistically perceptive.

2. Martin Hoffman. *The Gay World.* New York: Basic Books, 1968.

A well written, socially sensitive book by a psychiatrist who incorporates extensive case histories in writing about male homosexuality. Hoffman not only reviews the major current theories of homosexuality and the important literature, he also discusses the practices and problems of male homosexuals.

3. Rosabeth Moss Kanter. *Commitment and Community: Communes and Utopias in Sociological Perspective.* Cambridge, Mass.: Harvard University Press, 1972.

An important and useful analysis of the underlying bases of historical and contemporary utopian communities and of the psychosociological mechanisms—particularly commitment—in their formation and maintenance.

4. Roger W. Libby and Robert N. Whitehurst (Eds.). *Marriage and Alternatives: Exploring Intimate Relationships.* Glenview, Ill.: Scott, Foresman, 1977.

A collection of papers that are tied together by the view that contemporary marriage is too restricting for many and that alternative types of intimate relationships need to be discussed more widely and made more socially acceptable.

5. John Money and Anke A. Ehrhardt. *Man and Woman, Boy and Girl.* Baltimore: Johns Hopkins University Press, 1972.

A comprehensive analysis of the nature, development, and complexities of sex and gender identity.

6. Herbert A. Otto (Ed.). *The Family in Search of a Future.* New York: Appleton-Century-Crofts, 1970.

A collection of specially written papers, mainly by practitioners in one or more of the helping professions, about alternatives to contemporary marriage.

7. Melford Spiro. "Is the Family Universal?," *American Anthropologist,* No. 56 (1954), pp. 839–846.

A description of the "family" and "parenting" arrangements on an Israeli kibbutz as a possible exception to Murdock's view of the universality of the nuclear family.

8. Peter Stein, *Single.* Englewood Cliffs, N.J.: Prentice-Hall, 1976.

A report of a study of 165 men and women who chose singlehood as a life style. Stein uses both questionnaires and census data in his analysis and nicely summarizes the current state of knowledge and of ignorance in this important area of human activity.

9. Yonina Talmon. *Family and Community in the Kibbutz.* Cambridge, Mass.: Harvard University Press, 1972.

A careful and thoughtful examination of the nature of family and community within a kibbutz experience.

10. Clark Vincent. *Unmarried Mothers.* New York: Free Press, 1961.

Despite some methodological problems, this is a solid contribution to our understanding of an often taboo subject—the characteristics and experiences of unwed mothers. Because of their diversity in social background, personality, social circumstance, etc., Vincent found it difficult to make any simple generalizations about these women.

11. Leontyne Young. *Out-of-Wedlock: A Study of the Problems of the Unmarried Mother and New Child.* New York: McGraw-Hill, 1954.

A book written primarily for social workers and based on the author's direct experience in working with 350 unmarried mothers as well as drawing upon 1,000 other cases from case material and interviews with other social workers.

# Part FOUR

Parenthood: From Marriage to Family Life

The developmental passage from childhood through adolescence and into adulthood has as its social concomitant the transition from junior member of a nuclear family of orientation to one of the heads of a nuclear family of procreation. In the preceding two parts of the book, we examined many of the elements of this transition. We looked at how we develop intimate relationships, at the formation of romantic and sexual attachments, at the process of choosing a mate, and the establishment of normative and nonnormative paired relationships. In this part of the book we will look at an equally dramatic transition: the social psychological passage from early adulthood to old age. This journey in time will be explored in terms of its effects on marriage and family relationships. This will encompass the years from the early part of marriage to the existence of a mature family structure.

In Chapter 9, "The Creation of Families," we will look at the biological, psychological, and social aspects of reproductive behavior, including birth control and contraception, pregnancy, and childbirth. We will focus on several key issues:

- How do social and psychological factors affect one's choice of a contraceptive method? What are the relative merits and disadvantages of different birth control methods? How does a society overtly or covertly regulate the fertility and reproductive behavior of its members?

- To what degree is the experience of pregnancy, for the expectant mother and for the family, influenced by social and cultural factors? What psychological changes does a pregnant woman experience? What effect might these have on her husband? What changes is he experiencing also?
- How have attitudes toward labor and delivery changed in recent years? How do cultural values influence medical practice in terms of the attitude toward and treatment of the expectant mother and newborn infant?

We will then look at the years of childrearing in Chapter 10, "The Early Years of Family Life: Bringing Up Children." We will note how bringing up children is not necessarily something that comes naturally for everyone. Rather, childrearing is something that most people have to work at. In our complex, industrialized, urban society, which is rapidly changing, raising children is something we have to learn—not a totally natural thing. It is not a simple personal expression of the parents, but rather something more complicated, involving cultural guidelines and social restraints. Moreover, styles of childrearing have been associated with a number of factors, which we will look at in Chapter 10.

Finally, in Chapter 11, "The Mature Family," we will focus on the years from the time when the children have grown into late adolescence up through the period in which they have left the family home, leaving their parents in what has been termed the "empty nest." In these two chapters, we will attempt to answer the following questions:

- How do we learn the role of "parenting"? To what extent do we repeat our parents' parenting behaviors?
- What are some of the different "styles" of childrearing that have been identified, and how do they affect the child inside the family and outside?
- According to research findings, are children from single-parent families at a disadvantage either socially or psychologically? Does a mother working full-time affect her children's development and socialization? How do mothers and fathers contribute to the socialization of their children?
- What are some of the main discrepancies between social attitudes and stereotypes about older people and the realities of being old in America?
- What happens to the structure of the family and the strength of a marital relationship as the children of the family become adults and leave the home in which they were raised?

# Chapter 9

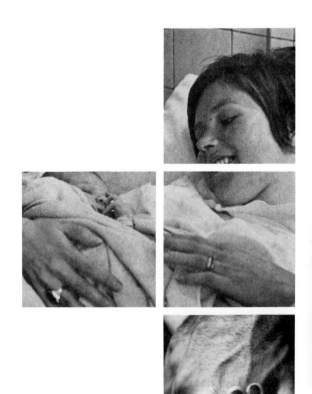

# The Creation of Families: Reproduction, Pregnancy, and Birth Control

## Chapter Aims

1. To examine the biological, psychological, and social aspects of reproductive behavior.

2. To consider the experiences of pregnancy and childbirth from the social as well as the psychological and biological viewpoints.

3. To survey the types of contraceptives available and to explore social and personal factors in deciding about contraceptive use and in regulating fertility control.

## Overview

Do you want children? How many do you want? And when? A couple plays a part in these decisions by choosing, or not choosing, from a vast array of methods: from those that you must think about each time you have intercourse to some that you never need think about after the initial decision is made. Biological, social, religious, and psychological factors influence the decision about which method to choose.

If there is nothing preventing it, the man and woman may each make a unique contribution to the process of human reproduction, which begins with the sperm and egg joining and ends with birth. During this period also, the man and woman have the opportunity to view themselves psychologically and in the social order no longer as just a pair, but as a family.

## A Pair vs. a Family

Rhoda and Fern grew up together, were the closest of friends virtually all their lives, came from very similar family backgrounds, and fondly referred to themselves as sisters, to let the world know how close they felt to each other. Even when they found boyfriends, they did it together. When Rhoda began dating Jeff, she asked him on the first date if he had a friend for Fern. The first two friends Jeff sent didn't work out well, but when Fern met Elliot it was—well, as she describes it, "instant lightning." Fern and Elliot, in fact, beat Rhoda and Jeff at becoming engaged, but only by a few weeks. During their engagements, the two couples decided to have a double wedding: an idea the girls' parents didn't like very much until it was pointed out that the brides and the grooms were willing to make some concessions about the elaborateness of the affair, saving them thousands of dollars.

They all honeymooned together in Mexico. When they returned to the States, they settled down not five miles from each other; Rhoda and Jeff in a small home they rented and Fern and Elliot in an apartment complex nearby.

It is now five years later. If you were to ask them, they would insist they still all love each other and feel as close as ever. The girls especially still feel like sisters. But as for the two couples functioning as friends—they don't double as much as they used to. Their similar interests have changed a bit, and there are a number of noticeable differences in their marital lifestyles. You could almost say that something has come between them, invisibly at first but most definitely a significant little force. Her name, in fact, is Amanda, and she is Fern and Elliot's first daughter.

Rhoda, that is, Aunt Rhoda, loves Amanda, ''her'' little Amanda, but doesn't plan to have children herself for ''many many'' years at least, ''if ever.''

''We value our freedom too much right now,'' Jeff explains, planning for their summer car tour of the country. ''And besides,'' Rhoda adds, ''we really can't afford to have me stop working.''

It's not that having children breaks up friendships, but it does change things dramatically.

*Marital lifestyles*  These two couples are learning that there are important practical differences between a married couple and a married couple with a child. The difference is that the latter is now a family, no longer just a pair.

One of the most important decisions a married couple has to make is whether or not to have children and, if so, how many children to have and when. This decision, like so many of the mate-choice, marital-related, and family-related decisions we have discussed in this book, is the result of a complex interaction among various social and psychological factors. To a large extent, the ways we are socialized affect our decision regarding family size. Many variables play a part, including class, socioeconomic level, working status, education, religion, and one's own family background (Coombs 1978).

## Human Reproduction: The Physical Process

*Perpetuation of the species*  The physical process of human reproduction, by all logical standards, is so impossible it just shouldn't work. It is characterized by a series of events, each so contingent upon many others and each fraught by nature with so many difficulties that it is absolutely amazing as we study it that we are in fact able to reproduce. And yet, nature has been clever and kind. For every danger of failure and every odd stacked against us, there is a biological loophole, one that allows, in the long run, for the consistent reproduction of people like us and the perpetuation of the species. And, reproduction serves as the biological foundation for the human family.

Together, the male and female reproductive systems are able to sponsor the biological merging of two reproductive cells. The female's system by itself is then able to support the prenatal development of a new social member.

Human reproduction involves three complex stages. In the first stage, as a consequence of sexual intercourse a sperm cell from the man meets an egg cell deep inside the woman. This results in *fertilization,* the biochemical process in which the two cells become one cell. This fertilized cell then begins to divide rapidly, as the reproductive growth process begins. During the second stage, which lasts approximately nine months, a baby is formed inside the woman's uterus. This process involves billions of divisions of cells. Cells reproduce other cells, while hidden genetic codes inside the cells direct the process down to the tiniest detail. Finally, the third stage, labor and birth, is characterized by this new human member of society being expelled from the security of the mother's body, down through the birth canal, and into the world.

Let's take a closer look.

## The Man's Contribution to Fertilization

The man's external genitals are much more obtrusive than the woman's. As figure 9.1 indicates, the prominent parts are: the pubis, the penis in-

Figure 9.1
**External Male Reproductive Anatomy**

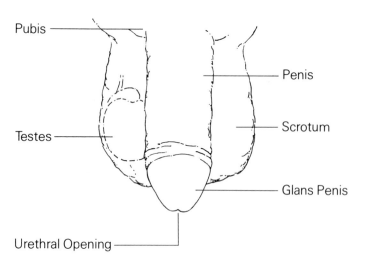

cluding the foreskin and glans penis, and the scrotum. The pubis is the sensitive area covered by pubic hair. The penis is an erectile organ that hangs loosely when it is not in a state of arousal. At the tip of the penis is the foreskin, a small flap of skin that for many boys was surgically removed in infancy by the process of circumcision. The scrotum is the sac that houses the testes which manufacture the hormone testosterone. Under the foreskin is a small hole, the urethral opening, from which the man's urine and semen are ejected.

The man's internal genital structure, shown in figure 9.2, is responsible for the basic reproductive functions. Inside the penis are three large masses of spongy tissue, which can become filled with blood. When they are filled, an erection occurs. The signal for blood to rush to these corpora cavernosa, as they are called, comes from the spinal cord. But the thought center of the brain also sends messages to the spinal cord, indicating that the erect penis is partly an involuntary physiological re-

Figure 9.2
**Internal Male Reproductive Anatomy**

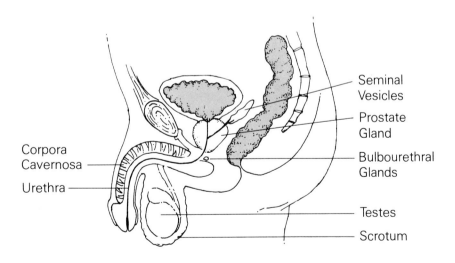

sponse and partly a result of thought. In fact, the penis can become erect under a wide variety of circumstances including sexual stimulation and erotic thoughts, of course; anxiety, although anxiety is more likely to cause impotence; a night's refreshing sleep after which ''morning erection'' can occur; feelings of affection and love.

Inside the scrotum are the two testes, the organs in which sperm cells, *spermatozoa*, and the hormone *testosterone*, are produced. Testosterone is responsible for the male secondary sex characteristics, such as facial hair and deepening of the voice. It is also necessary for the production of sperms. The sperms are produced through a process called *spermatogenesis*. Since viable sperm are produced at slightly less than body temperature, it is biologically necessary that the testes hang outside the body. The scrotum provides that environment. The production of sperm, interestingly enough, continues from puberty throughout life, as long as the male is healthy; and the average male produces about two hundred million sperm each day.

In order for the sperm to get out of the man's body and into the woman's, two things are necessary: first, a liquid in which they can be conveyed and, second, a process of conveying. The liquid is called *semen;* the process is *ejaculation.*

When the man ejaculates, the sperm are swimming in a seminal fluid, a translucent liquid substance, often thick and with a characteristic taste and odor. The purpose of this fluid is to keep the sperm healthy in their trip through the woman's vagina. This fluid is produced and stored through several processes involving the prostate gland, the seminal vesicles, and the bulbourethral glands, which together are responsible for getting the fluid out. When the man is ready to ejaculate, the semen passes into the urethra, which carries it through the penis and out. Urine and semen cannot occupy the urethra at the same time, so the opening for one is turned off as the other makes its way through.

**Secondary sex characteristics** *(margin note)*

## The Woman's Contribution to Fertilization

The woman's external genitals belie the tremendous complexity of her internal reproductive organs. As we see in figure 9.3, the major parts of the female external genitalia are, looking from the front of the body to the rear between the thighs, are the mons venus, the labia major and labia minor, the clitoris, urethal opening, vaginal opening, vestibule, perineum, and the anus.

The mons venus is the hairy, triangular mound at the front of the body, right above the outer lip of the vagina. The labias major and minor

Figure 9.3
**External Female Reproductive Anatomy**

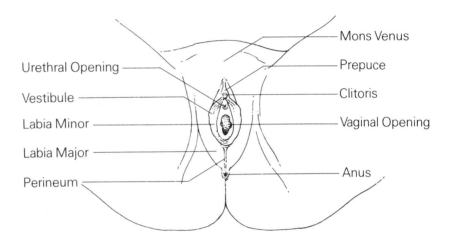

are the outer and inner lips that surround the vaginal opening. The clitoris, a small fleshy structure dense with nerve endings at the junction of the labia minora, is a highly sensitive area in which physical sensation is heightened. Like the penis, the clitoris becomes erect at excitation, and the blood volume inside it increases significantly. But since it is small, this increase is not always noticeable. The prepuce, a small flap of non-sensitive skin, covers the clitoris, preventing it from continual over-stimulation. The vestibule is the area surrounding (and including) the vaginal opening. Between the vaginal opening (the entrance to the vagina) and the clitoris is the urethral opening from which the woman urinates. Behind the labia minora is the perineum, the area between the thighs, extending from the vaginal opening to the anus, and then the anus, through which defecation takes place.

Because these external organs are not clearly visible without careful scrutiny, children and adolescents who have not had an opportunity to learn about them are often confused. There is, for example, a common childhood misconception called the *myth of the cloaca* in which children and young girls especially believe there is only one opening through which urination, defecation, and the birth of the baby all take place. With some lower animals, such as the frog, there is only one opening, which is called the cloaca; and it is from this that the myth takes its name.

A study of the woman's internal reproductive organs, shown in figure 9.4, will help us understand her contribution to the process. The woman's job is much more complex than the man's. She must first provide an egg for fertilization, just as the man must supply a sperm cell. But where his job is finished at that point, hers is just beginning. Next, she has to provide a conducive biological climate in which the sperm and egg, now joined, can become implanted, that is, physiologically connected to her body. Finally, she has to assure that there is a safe and nourishing climate for the many months of prenatal growth ahead. These processes involve the ovaries, the fallopian tubes, and the uterus.

## The Ovaries

The two ovaries are the woman's *gonads,* or sex glands. In a woman of reproductive age, the ovaries are similar in size and shape to small hen's eggs, and they are located at the ends of the fallopian tubes, the "oviducts" that connect the ovaries to the uterus. The female infant is born with almost half a million *pre-ova,* immature egg cells, in her ovaries. As she matures, her ovaries prepare some of these egg cells (singular, *ovum;* plural, ova) for fertilization. From puberty onward, generally only one ready, that is, mature, egg cell is released each month. The ovaries lose their procreative ability during her *menopause,* the time of her life when menstruation ceases, when they no longer respond to pituitary hormone stimulation.

Ovarian hormones

The ovaries, along with the pituitary gland in the brain, work in tandem in secreting the hormones that regulate menstruation and cause the ripening of these eggs. The chief ovarian hormones are *estrogen* and *progesterone.* The fluctuation in the amount of these hormones regulates menstruation as well as prepares the uterus for implantation of a fertilized ovum. These hormones are also thought to be responsible for some of the mood changes a woman experiences at different times of the month. Both the ovary's production of estrogen and progesterone as well as ovulation are controlled by other hormones released by the pituitary gland, which in turn is directed by different centers deep within the brain. A woman may still be capable of reproduction if one ovary is removed. With both ovaries removed, however, she loses the capacity to reproduce because there are no eggs, and her menstruation stops permanently because the hormone production ceases. The surgical removal of an ovary is called an *ovarectomy.*

Figure 9.4
**Internal Female Reproductive Anatomy**

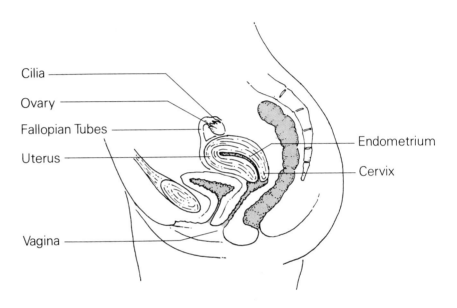

The Fallopian Tubes   The fallopian tubes lie between the ovaries and the uterus. They are narrow, muscular tunnels, lined with tiny hairs, called cilia. After one of the eggs has ripened in the ovary, it drops out. This process is called *ovulation*. The cilia at the end of the fallopian tubes draw the egg into the tube, and other cilia draw it down the tube toward the uterus. It is during this trip, which lasts anywhere from 24 to 72 hours, that the sperm has an opportunity to unite with the travelling egg cell. If the tubes become scarred or damaged, however, there may be a problem in fertility, and the woman may not be able to become pregnant.

The Uterus   The uterus, which is synonymous with the womb, is a pear-shaped organ, the size of a baseball, which rests in the middle of the pelvis. The fallopian tubes are connected to the uterus at one end, and the other end narrows into the cervix, through which the uterus is connected to the vagina. In pregnancy, the fertilized cell will come through the fallopian tube and implant itself in the uterus, where it will grow and develop. Its chief reproductive purpose is to provide an environment for the growing embryo from shortly after conception until birth, when it is expelled.

The walls of the uterus are muscular and able to expand and contract, for they must be strong and flexible enough to hold the growing baby, which develops from a tiny little ball into a six—, seven—, or eight— pound newborn. The uterus does not affect sexual response, which is why when it is removed in a surgical procedure called a *hysterectomy,* the sexual drive is not physically affected (although it may be psychologically affected). But the uterus is involved in the menstrual cycle. This cycle is responsible for getting the unfertilized egg out of the uterus every 28 days or so. Since an unfertilized egg will not implant in the wall of the uterus, it can be expelled from the body. This is done by discharging the *endometrium,* the tissue lining the uterus, along with some blood, which together constitute the menstrual flow. If the uterus is removed, menstruation will cease permanently.

## Pregnancy

*Pregnancy* occurs the moment a woman's ovum is fertilized by a man's sperm. This fertilized cell is called a *zygote.* Fertilization usually, but not always, occurs within hours after intercourse. The man's sperms that have been ejaculated into the vagina propel themselves by means of their own tails through the uterus to the fallopian tube in which, if ovulation has occurred, a ready egg is waiting. The sperm and egg join and float in the uterus for three or four days, where rapid division takes place, after which the zygote becomes implanted in the lining of the uterine wall where it will grow for the next nine months, during the period known as *gestation.*

## Am I Pregnant?

There are several physical signs that indicate a woman is pregnant, signs that appear weeks, and sometimes months, after fertilization. There may be swelling of the breasts, a nauseous feeling in the mornings, an unusual heartburn, as well as internal physical signs that can reveal pregnancy on examination. A woman generally first suspects that she is pregnant when she misses her menstrual period. It is at this point, when her period is about two weeks overdue, that the physician might recommend a pregnancy test to determine if the woman is or is not pregnant.

There are a number of tests available, including home pregnancy

Signs of pregnancy

Pregnancy tests

kits, which have proven to be accurate and reliable. The old tests, such as the famous rabbit test where the rabbit died if the woman was pregnant, have been replaced by a number of new tests that are much faster and cheaper. These tests use a urine specimen to determine the presence of the hormone *HCG (Human Chorionic Gonadotropin),* which is present in urine only during pregnancy. The urine sample is mixed with a special solution, which causes a clumping in normal urine. Thus, if the specimen clumps, the woman is not pregnant. If there is no clumping it indicates that the woman's urine contains a chemical to inhibit the clumping and that she is pregnant. These hormonal tests, especially when they are positive, are very accurate. Negative results, however, are more inconclusive, and the test is typically repeated a week to ten days later.

## The Experience of Pregnancy

During her pregnancy the woman's body undergoes massive physical changes, both within and without, that will bring forth a human life in a matter of months. Her entire system changes to accommodate this growing individual within her. Many of these changes have sociological and psychological dimensions as well. Moreover, we should recognize that the physical, social, and psychological changes are entwined and that it is virtually impossible to consider them totally separately.

Usually the first noticeable signs of pregnancy are about four weeks after conception and these may include morning sickness or swelling of breasts as discussed above. But since these signs are only noticeable to the woman herself, others still do not know she is pregnant. Should she tell her husband? Should she make an appointment with the doctor? What are her feelings about possibly being pregnant?

The developing baby at this time is called an *embryo.* Up through the third month this embryo grows to about three inches in length and weighs about one ounce. At this point, the term *fetus* is used instead of embryo.

During the embryonic period, there are probably no outward signs of pregnancy, and it is relatively easy to conceal, if the woman wants to. During the fourth month, however, the abdomen begins to stretch, and the condition is more obvious. Society affords a special social status to the pregnant woman, but this varies according to many circumstances and among cultures. For instance, in some subcultures the unmarried pregnant woman is looked down upon, perhaps treated poorly, while the married pregnant woman achieves a high level of social esteem. Whatever the reaction, it usually becomes manifest around the time that the pregnancy is obvious.

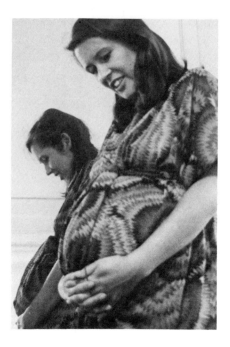

The fetal heartbeat can usually be heard easily at four months. The fetus is said to be "viable" at five and a half months (24 weeks) by medical definition, although its chances of survival at this time are poor. However, by seven months, the majority of infants born prematurely will survive.

Most women have first felt movement by four and a half to five months (called "quickening") and are aware of definite kicks in the sixth month. During the seventh and eighth months, the woman becomes more aware of the baby's movements in the uterus. In addition to kicking, moving around and stretching the walls of the uterus, there may even be hiccupping. The woman may observe ripples of movement on the abdomen as the baby moves around. As the uterus grows larger to accommodate the baby, pressure on the bladder may cause the woman some discomfort and may require more frequent urination. Hemorrhoids are another possible side effect of pregnancy.

As the pregnancy progresses and as the woman's body is more obviously changing and the reality of the expected baby becomes more imminent, various changes may take place in the marital relationship.

Effects on the couple

Couples often become totally involved in the prospect of parenthood, spending all their spare time making plans and preparations for the forthcoming event. For the first child especially, there is so much to do. They may have to paint a room or even find a new apartment. Couples some times fight about the plans involving the new baby, possibly as a way of getting rid of some of the anxiety they feel about becoming parents.

### Fern and Jeff

"When Fern was in her seventh month," Jeff explains, "I think we fought more than we ever did before. And you wouldn't believe about what stupid things. She wanted me to store my fishing gear at my parents, so she could use the hall closet for diapers and blankets, and I became furious. I laugh now; I mean I haven't even had the time to go fishing *once* since Amanda was born."

There are many challenges the pregnant woman and her husband face, especially during the later months of pregnancy. The myriad anxieties of expectant parenthood can put a strain on the most intact marital relationships and may especially interfere with the normal level of sexual functioning to which the partners have become accustomed (Whelan 1978). The partners, if this is their first child, have to prepare for their roles as parents, and this often requires significant changes in their own self-perceptions, as well as in social behaviors. They may "rehearse" parent-role behaviors, either playfully between themselves or in public situations, such as by attending a parenting group given by the hospital. New types of interactions with their respective nuclear families of orientation sometimes cause role confusion.

The ninth month

During the final month, the ninth month, the woman psychologically and socially prepares herself to give birth. There is a clear interaction between the physical, social, and psychological realms of her existence. Her social circle, for example, helps provide sociological definition for her impending change in social roles, as her body begins to prepare physiologically for the experience. About 15 days before childbirth, the head may begin to drop into the pelvic cavity. The uterus moves to accommodate this change. This process is referred to as lightening, and may enable the woman to feel more comfortable during the final days of the pregnancy. Many women feel less fetal activity immediately prior to the onset of labor. This lessening of activity may worry some women, but it is quite normal.

## Social Aspects

Pregnancy is a unique social status. In some social interactions the visibly

The pregnant woman

pregnant woman may be treated condescendingly as if she were handicapped; in other interactions she will be treated deferentially, held in awe. People tend to act overfamiliarly with a pregnant woman: the person standing in a line next to her, for example, will think nothing of saying, "Do you want a boy or girl?" or "When is your due date?" The way she is perceived and treated depends on the situation and on the people with whom she is interacting. But one thing is certain: she will be treated differently than she was before she was pregnant.

To a large extent, the pregnant woman has been socialized for this role from early in life. If she has younger siblings, then she has witnessed pregnancy in the nuclear family of orientation. If she has friends who are or who have been pregnant, she has had many opportunities to discuss it with them. But, as with parenthood, until she is actually pregnant, she has not had opportunities to audition and enact the roles associated with this new status. She may be uncomfortable with the responses she now elicits, since she has not had opportunities to practice her new behaviors in public.

One reality the pregnant woman must deal with is the change in her body image and in her physical stamina. She probably doesn't have as much energy as she did before, and her feelings about herself may change dramatically, along with the shape of her body. This is true in first as well as in later pregnancies. In fact, with each subsequent pregnancy there is an increasing fear of body "mutilation" and more negative attitudes toward the pregnancy (Westbrook 1978). The excitement of the first pregnancy may have worn off, and now pregnancy is viewed more as a chore necessary for childbearing than an exciting experience in itself. The emotional support and nurturance given by her husband is important, as are the attitudes of all the significant people around her.

## Childbirth

The period of pregnancy terminates with *childbirth* when the infant is delivered into the world. Delivery takes place following a process called *labor,* during which the mother, and some helper, such as a midwife, doctor, nurse, or the father, work together to get the baby out of the body in the safest way possible.

The baby, which is fully developed now, somewhere between six and nine pounds, has to make its way through the small opening of the cervix and down the narrow birth canal. It seems so difficult as to be impossible but most of us have done it. For those who cannot make the trip for whatever reason, surgeons can make an insertion in the mother's abdomen, open the uterus, and take the baby out. This process is known as a *Cae-*

sarean section, so named because of the unproven assertion that Julius Caesar was delivered in this way. If the infant is able to get partly out, but not to complete the trip, doctors can also use forceps to pull the baby from the birth canal.

**Stages of labor**

Labor is divided into 3 stages. The first stage is by far the longest, lasting sometimes up to 20 hours, although typically more like 8 to 16 hours. During this stage the narrow opening at the neck of the uterus, called the cervix, must expand, or *dilate,* to allow the baby through. Since the measurement is usually made by inserting the fingers into the vagina, it is sometimes expressed in finger-widths, although more correctly it is measured in centimeters. At first it is fully closed, then gradually it dilates one finger, two fingers, three fingers, four fingers. At about 10 centimeters or four inches, (five fingers), the baby is ready to pass through.

The second stage is from the time of the cervical dilation until the baby actually passes through the birth canal and comes out. This is the stage of labor during which the baby, expelled from the uterus by muscular contractions, makes its way down the birth canal, with the mother actively pushing the baby through. This can last anywhere from half an hour to 90 minutes or more. As the baby's head begins to emerge from the vagina, in what is sometimes called crowning, if it is absolutely necessary, the doctor may use forceps to help the baby complete the journey. The doctor may also make a small incision in the woman's perineum in order for the baby to get out more easily. This is called an *episeotomy,* and in most hospitals is now standard procedure for all deliveries.

Finally, the third stage extends from the birth of the baby through the expulsion of the *afterbirth;* the *placenta,* through which the embryo transported its wastes and received its nourishment in the uterus, along with all the accompanying material, including the roots of the umbilical cord. This final stage of labor usually takes only a few minutes.

## Social Aspects of Childbirth

While the biological process of childbirth is the same across all societies, the actual way it is handled varies greatly from society to society. Throughout history and from culture to culture, Whiting (1974) points out, folk wisdom has adequately governed the procedures of childbirth. Specific rituals define how society expects the participants to act and what conditions are perceived as necessary and desirable for healthy childbirth. Often the social origins of the practices are obscured by the belief that they are medical absolutes rather than what they really are: cultural conventions reflecting the social beliefs of a particular group of people.

The approach to childbirth varies in three areas particularly: where

Hospital deliveries

the baby is delivered, who assumes what responsibilites in the delivery, and some of the specific procedures relating to delivery and childbirth.

In the United States, the large majority of women deliver their babies in hospital facilities. This practice has been considered standard and desirable since the 1930s, when at-home deliveries, which were a common practice before then, came to be viewed as hazardous. If asked, most women will admit that they chose the hospital not only because they thought it a safer environment but because they never thought they had a choice. Danae Brook (1976, p. 50), writer and advocate of natural childbirth methods, points out,

> Part of the reason for this is the attitude which has taken hold, that giving birth is automatically treated as a sickness, that we need the "safety" of medicines and mechanization in order to deliver our children. Our own bodies have ceased to provide a

Figure 9.5
**Infant Mortality in the United States**

Annual rate of mortality per 1,000 living at specific time:

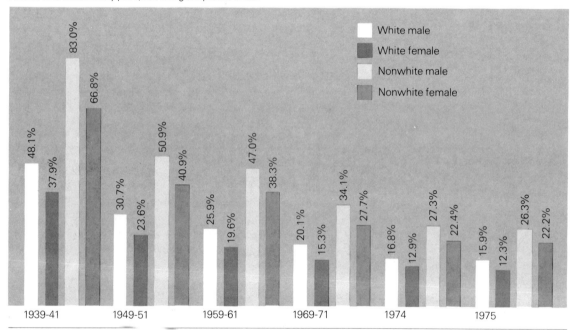

Source: U.S. National Center for Health Statistics

sense of security to most of the people of the second half of the twentieth century.

Such an attitude is a reflection of our general beliefs about the efficacy of the medical profession and the sanctuary of the hospital in particular. Of course, as shown in figure 9.5 contemporary obstetric practices have enabled thousands of mothers and babies to survive who could not have done so otherwise. And, the growing pediatric specialty of neonatal medicine saves many babies today that a dozen years ago would have died within weeks. Still, between 1975 and 1980, at-home deliveries increased significantly, as more women, especially if it were not their first deliveries, chose to stay home and have their babies. This increase may indicate a change of attitudes, one that more nearly reflects the millions of years of human experience with childbirth.

*At-home deliveries*

The second cultural factor is who delivers the baby. If a prospective mother in the United States is asked who will deliver her baby, she will probably without hesitation name her doctor, never considering that for centuries doctors were only called into the delivery situation when there were medical complications. Yet, ''in most societies the mother or mother-in-law plus other older women are on hand from the time a woman goes into labor, and they support, reassure, and advise her during the birth, stay to bathe the infant, and counsel as to when and how to nurse'' (Whiting 1974, p. 10). Today in traditional societies, this concern of older women for young mothers is also an expression of distrust of hospitals:

> Women anthropologists who have had babies while doing research in remote field stations can document both the solicitousness and wisdom of older women in traditional societies. One of the members of our Child Development research Unit in Kenya who is working among the Samburu reports that her adopted mother advised her strongly not to go to Nairobi to a strange hospital and be delivered by an unknown male doctor but to stay where people knew her and cared for her. When the infant was newborn the Samburu surrogate mother walked three miles daily to see that the new mother was caring for herself and her baby properly. Similar advice and counsel is given to parents by the elders of the family during the entire cycle of their grandchildren's development.

*Midwifery*

Midwifery, an ancient profession, has been a common practice. A *midwife* is a person trained in the art of assisting the woman at deliveries. Traditionally the midwife has been a woman, although there are also male midwives now. In the United States, the male-dominated medical

*We now assume that a doctor will be present for the delivery of a baby, but for centuries babies were delivered by midwives.*

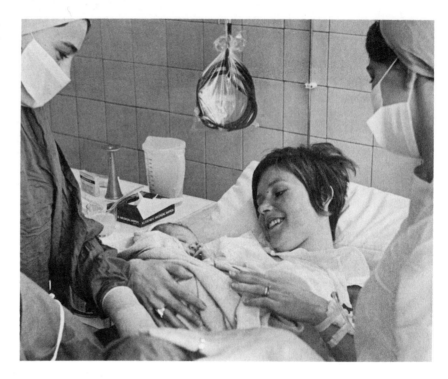

Oxytocin

profession exerted enormous pressures to prevent lay midwifery. Only those who are licensed as nurses or employed by a hospital, in either case under the control of the medical profession, are allowed to assist at deliveries, in the hospital or at home. In California recently, criminal charges were brought against a group of lay midwives who were attempting to help women who wanted home deliveries (Brook 1976, p. 57).

Finally, we come to specific childbirth practices. These practices, of course, are related, directly or indirectly, to the ''who'' and ''where'' discussed above. There are many different ways to give birth, and the method a woman chooses may be strongly influenced by her physician or friends. Rarely does a woman objectively choose what is right for her while recognizing the force of these outside influences.

First, the prospective mother is faced with the question of natural vs. medically directed childbirth. *Natural childbirth* can be defined as a labor and delivery without the use of anesthetic, forceps, or labor-inducing drugs, such as oxytocin. A common form of natural childbirth in the United States is in hospital with doctors and nurses present. In this form, the medical profession may be called upon to ''deliver'' or ''intervene.'' To understand the full implications of what natural really means, it is necessary to understand what in our culture have been the accepted medical procedures used in uncomplicated childbirths. And, it is equally important to understand that many of these practices were not absolute necessities, but had been deemed so by our medically oriented culture!

In order to cope with the pain of contractions during labor, the mother, if she has not chosen to follow certain breathing techniques such as those taught in the Lamaze method, may be anesthetized at some stage during labor. Anesthetics used during labor might include injection of a pain killer (a narcotic), injection of a local anesthetic in the cervix (called a paracervical block), or continuous lumbar epidural (which is a regional, not a local block). The fetus' journey, so to speak, is not made any more or less difficult by any of these practices. Delivery, however, is a different story.

Anesthetics may also be used during the delivery process which occurs after labor (although a laboring mother who has chosen to follow breathing exercises such as those of the Lamaze method may choose not to be anesthetized during delivery). Anesthetics which might be used during delivery include local injections (e.g., directly into the perineum), continuous lumbar epidural (a regional block), or—rarely today—a general anesthetic. A local anesthetic does not interfere with the mother's ability to bear down and push the baby out; a general anesthetic always does.

There has been much discussion concerning the use and abuse of oxytocin. Oxytocin is a natural hormone secreted by the pituitary gland (it is even secreted by the fetus). Currently, oxytocin is used in two ways: to induce or start labor; or to stimulate or speed up a natural labor which is *abnormally* slow (a natural labor is not necessarily a *normal* one). There are pros and cons in any discussion of the use of this substance because it can be (and has been) abused. Too much oxytocin, for example, can make contractions of the uterus occur so frequently that oxygen supply to the fetus can be reduced.

More important, however, than these specific differences is the implicit attitude underlying the natural method. With the medically directed method, the implicit attitude is, "Just leave everything to the doctor who knows what's best." The natural method, however, says, "Only the woman can really know what's happening in her body, and she must therefore become totally familiar with the processes of pregnancy, labor, and delivery. Since the father is a very interested participant—and since he is the father!—he should be there all along, to help the mother, to coach her in her breathing and pushing, and to comfort her and cheer her on."

Where a decade or two ago, the natural method was quite controversial and perceived as a rebellion against established medical practice, nowadays it is much more widely accepted, and many physicians encourage their patients to take the Lamaze natural childbirth course or some variation. Whereas a decade ago, young physicians advocated this method while older, more conservative physicians generally did not, now-

Lamaze method

adays that generation gap appears to have been bridged. The natural method has found wide acceptance in the medical profession, where we find physician, expectant mother, and prospective father all knowledgeably working together for the best possible delivery.

Birth   Cultural factors also play an important role in how we treat the *neonate,* newborn infant, immediately after delivery. In some societies, following delivery the baby was physically separated from the mother, who was not allowed to see or touch it. The baby was exposed to loud noises and harsh lights for a few moments. The baby finally collapsed from shock and was removed to an area some distance from its mother, who was viewed as unfit to touch her baby. Other interested parties could view the baby from some distance, through glass.

This "horrible" society, of course, was our own some years ago. The practices discussed were standard hospital hygienic practices, which had become widely accepted since women began relying on hospitals for delivery. Some aspects of these practices have changed, rapidly.

Our attitudes about the birth experience are in the process of undergoing important changes. Early psychologists, such as Freud and Otto Rank, emphasized the trauma of birth, arguing that it was such a difficult experience that its aftereffects would actually last one's entire lifetime. But while this attitude told us how difficult a process it was, it told us little about how to improve it. Anthropologist Ashley Montagu points out a

The trauma of birth

*The Lamaze method of natural childbirth has found wide acceptance among physicians and expectant parents.*

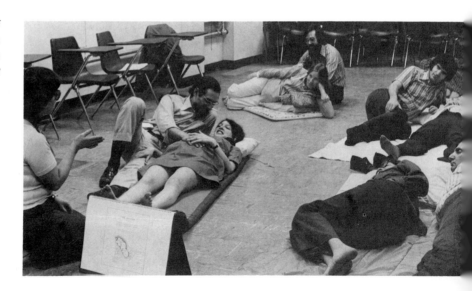

changing social trend in our perception of birth, one that does help us make it a less traumatic experience for the newborn. Where we used to think of birth as the end of the period of gestation and the beginning of independent functioning, ''we are now coming to see more and more clearly . . . that a newborn child is almost as dependent on his mother as he was before he was born'' (Montagu 1965, p. 232). This realization is influencing our view of how to deal with the child immediately after birth. Specifically, we try to minimize the immediate separation.

Leboyer method

The revolutionary concept of birth without violence was introduced by the French obstetrician Dr. Frederick Leboyer whose book *Birth Without Violence* has had a wide social impact. His basic argument is that the first few minutes of life are critically important and that since the newborn baby is hypersensitive to the new extrauterine environment, it should be born in a quiet, inobtrusively lighted, pleasant environment. More significantly Leboyer and others advocate strongly that at birth the baby be placed right by the mother, right next to her, so that she and her new baby can begin to get used to each other. This view is directly contrary to the practice of separating mother and child at birth, but this innovative practice is receiving increasing acceptance today.

More and more mothers, even those who are not using the Leboyer method for their deliveries, now expect to have contact with their baby at birth. The practices of mother-child interaction at birth, once viewed as medical decisions, are now being considered more appropriately as culturally, rather than medically, determined.

## Birth Control: Biological Aspects

*Birth control* is the intentional act of preventing live births. Birth control includes practices such as abortion and infanticide, as well as contraception, which is a direct procedure for preventing fertilization. *Abstinence,* not engaging in sexual relations, is the most direct method of all. But since for the most part this situation is not viable and hence cannot be relied on, a large number of other contraceptive methods that allow for nonreproductive intercourse are used.

Decisions and choices

Today, especially, decisions about birth control are of increasing importance, as couples explore their own feelings about having children. Once there was little choice—''nature took its own course''—or the marital role expectations were too inflexible for choices to be seen. Things have changed dramatically.

# Contraception

Most methods of *contraception* work quite simply. They prevent the sperm from reaching the ovum, thereby preventing conception from taking place. Thus, they are called contraceptive methods, that is, against conception. Some forms of contraception are available over the counter and some only by prescription. Contraception may be the individual responsibility of the man or of the woman or it may be a joint responsibility.

Active vs. passive

We can divide the methods into two basic types: the active and the passive methods. The active methods are those that require some conscious participation at the time of intercourse. The passive methods are decided upon once and do not require further decisionmaking each time the individual has intercourse.

## Active Methods

The active methods of contraception include a variety that ranges from the simple, based on the human body alone, to the more complex and more effective. Each requires thought each time a couple has intercourse.

*Coitus Interruptus*  *Coitus interruptus,* or withdrawal, is probably the oldest method of birth control. The man withdraws his penis from the vagina before ejaculation. Theoretically, he then ejaculates outside the vagina. This method is cheap and always available. But, it is also the least

Ineffectiveness

effective method. It fails for a number of reasons. Sperm may leak out before the man feels the ejaculation, or in the heat of passion the man may not be able to remove his penis in time.

Rhythm Method  The *rhythm method* is also readily available and costless but not quite as simple. The idea is to avoid intercourse at the time of the month when the woman is fertile. Technically, this period lasts only about three to six days per month. But which three to six days? That is the big question. The rhythm method is only as effective as the accu-

Accuracy of determination

racy of the determination of whether the woman has ovulated or not. If her menstrual periods are used as guides and if it is assumed that the woman ovulates right in the middle, on the fourteenth day, there is great possibility for error. The success rate of this method is then no greater than that of coitus interruptus.

However, there is a more sophisticated way of using the rhythm method. Immediately after ovulation there is a slight increase in the body temperature. A woman can use a special thermometer that measures such slight increases to determine with a high degree of accuracy when she is ovulating. She must take her temperature daily, every morning upon awakening, and keep an accurate chart. It is the same process she would follow in order to increase the likelihood of fertility, if she were having trouble getting pregnant. By knowing exactly when she ovulates, she substantially increases the success of the rhythm method. However, since many factors other than ovulation may cause slight changes in a woman's daily temperature, even this refinement does not render the rhythm method sufficiently safe for many women.

Condom   A *condom* is a thin sheath worn over the penis during coitus in order to prevent the sperm from entering the vagina. A good condom must be strong and free of physical defects in order to be effective. But it must also be thin and conductive enough to allow skin sensitivity so that the partners can freely enjoy the sensual experience with each other. Condoms may be made of synthetic rubber materials or with the natural membranes of animals. They may also be lubricated in order to decrease their friction and to allow for greater sensitivity.

Figure 9.6
**Advantages of Condoms as Seen by Men and Women Respondents to CU's Survey**

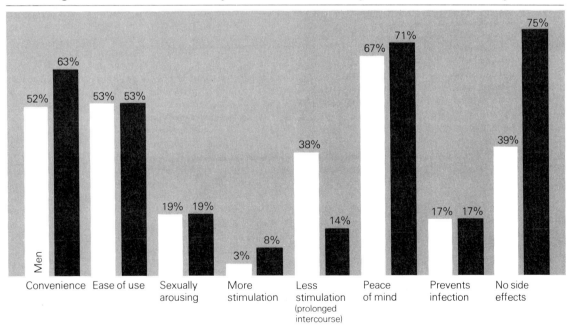

Note: Multiple responses were possible.
Source: *Consumer Reports*, October, 1979, Volume 44, No. 10, p 583. Reprinted by permission of Consumers Union.

Figure 9.7
**Disadvantages of Condoms as Seen by Men and Women Respondents to CU's Survey**

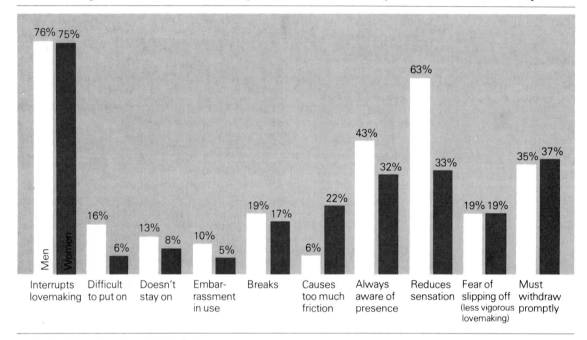

Note: Multiple responses were possible.
Source: *Consumer Reports*, October 1979, Volume 44, No. 10, p. 585. Reprinted by permission of Consumers Union.

**Advantages and disadvantages**

Condoms have some advantages and some disadvantages as contraceptives (see Figure 9.6). They are relatively easy to use, inexpensive, and very portable. They can be carried around by the man and are thus available to him whenever he is expectedly or unexpectedly about to have intercourse. As effective contraceptives, they are only as good as the care taken in manufacturing them and in using them. They have to be placed over the penis correctly, not too tautly or too loosely, with a little bit of slack at the end to collect the semen and they must be removed correctly to be really effective.

There are some practical disadvantages to this method (see figure 9.7). If the condom is not used during foreplay and if the couple becomes passionately involved without thinking rationally, they may have intercourse without first putting the condom on. Or the very fact of having to stop to put on the condom may break the momentum of passion that has been built up. A condom may also break or slide off during intercourse.

And if it is not removed properly, sperm may drip into the vagina, live there for some time, and then finally fertilize the egg even though both partners think that the condom has been successful.

## Spermicide
*Spermicides* are chemical agents that kill sperm. They are available over the counter. The woman inserts the spermicide all the way back in her vagina by the cervix, prior to intercourse. Spermicides

Variety and application

come in the form of spray foams, jellies, dissolving tablets, suppositories, and creams. Some spermicides are inserted directly, and some are placed up against the cervix by means of an applicator. The *douche,* which is also used for cleansing, may contain a spermicidal wash designed to rinse the sperm from the vagina after intercourse. This contraceptive method is particularly ineffective since by the time the douche is used a large proportion of the ejaculated sperm have already travelled beyond where the spermicidal wash can reach effectively.

As with condoms, the use of a spermicide, which is an active contraceptive procedure, varies in efficacy with the intelligence of its use. The greatest error in the use of spermicides is the application of them too early, thus rendering them useless against the sperm they are supposed to kill. One other major disadvantage with spermicides is that many women find them irritating, so that the sensitive wall of the vagina hurts after intercourse, even for days or sometimes weeks.

## Diaphragm with Spermicide
Considerably more effective than the use of a spermicide by itself is the use of a *diaphragm,* which is used with the spermicide. The diaphragm is a rubber or synthetic equivalent cup with a springlike metal ring around its circumference. It is flexible and can be bent in half to be inserted in the vagina. As it reaches the cervix the spring releases and it pops back to its original shape, covering the cervix. It is measured for each woman to adequately prevent the entrance

Correct fitting

of sperm into the cervix. Though the fit is by no means airtight, if the woman is correctly fitted, the diaphragm by itself should act as a physical barrier to the sperm. Along with the spermicide it is doubly effective.

For the diaphragm to be most effective, it must be used properly with the spermicidal jelly or cream. It is recommended that the diaphragm and spermicide not be inserted any more than two hours prior to intercourse, and to be fully effective it should not be removed until six or eight hours after intercourse, since it may take this long for all the living sperm to die. A diaphragm with spermicide is a generally effective contraceptive if it is fitted properly by the physician, if it is inserted properly before coitus, if it is not defective, and if it is left in long enough after coitus to destroy the viable sperm.

## Passive Methods

The above are all *active* contraceptive methods. Each requires that one or both partners make a specific decision or take a precaution before or immediately after each act of intercourse. Consequently their general risk factor is higher, since clearly if the partner does not make the decision these methods fail to work. At the other extreme are the passive methods, where one partner makes a decision and need not make a decision each time intercourse occurs.

### The IUD
While most methods work to prevent the sperm and egg from meeting, the IUD works on a different principle. The *intrauterine device,* commonly called the *IUD* or sometimes the *IUCD,* intrauterine contraceptive device, is a soft plastic or metal device that comes in different shapes and sizes. It is implanted in the uterus by the physician. No one knows exactly how the IUD works, and there are several different theories. One is that the IUD does not interfere with the fertilization of the egg but rather it interferes with the motion of the fallopian tubes so that the egg is not transported properly to the uterus thus preventing the implantation of the egg in the uterus, thus preventing pregnancy. Another is that the IUD causes the cervical mucous itself to become spermicidal. A third theory says that because the IUD is a foreign body it causes inflammation of the endometrium making it hostile to implantation of the fertilized egg. However it works, it is a relatively effective passive contraceptive device: once the woman has it implanted she will, theoretically, remain infertile as long as it is in place.

Theories

There are several problems with the IUD, however. Because it is essentially an irritant, many women experience discomforting physical symptoms, including vaginal bleeding, cramps, or other problems, such as infection or puncturing of the uterus, that require the removal of the IUD. Or, especially in the case of young women without children, it can spontaneously fall out, without the woman realizing it, thus making her fertile while she thinks she is protected. Although modern technology has gradually reduced this problem, some recent studies have suggested the possibility of a 25 percent rejection rate. Also, if the woman does accidentally become pregnant while the IUD is still in place there is a far greater likelihood of complications leading to abortion.

Drawbacks

### Sterilization
*Surgical sterilization* is in the process of becoming an increasingly popular contraceptive method in the United States. The man or woman can be rendered sterile through surgery. This is a relatively minor procedure for the man and considerably more major for the woman. It is regarded in both sexes as a permanent procedure, although in some instances it can be surgically reversed.

*Those who know where and how to obtain contraceptives now have a choice about parenthood.*

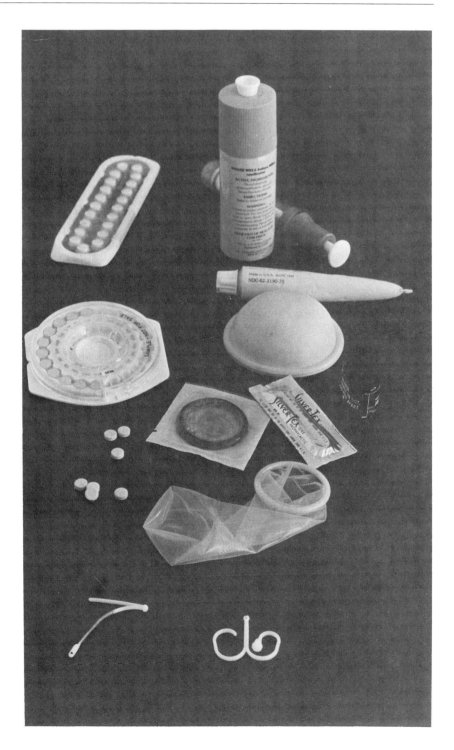

For the man the surgical procedure is called a *vasectomy.* An incision is made in the scrotum and the vas deferens, the ducts in which the sperm are carried, are tied. The man may experience swelling and discomfort for several days, but then there is a return to normal sexual activity. The procedure is generally simple enough to be done in the doctor's office.

For the woman the procedure is more major, although not more complex. In a procedure called a *tubal ligation* the abdomen must be opened and the Fallopian tubes tied. This requires a hospital stay of several days. A more recent procedure, called the *laparoscopy,* requires only two small incisions in the abdomen and a hospital stay of a day or two. But it is still a more serious surgical procedure than the man's.

Despite the popularity of the vasectomy for the man, sterilization in the US is not primarily a male phenomenon. Among whites it is 50/50 male-female, and among blacks it is predominantly a female phenomenon, especially among the poor. Although sterilization is virtually 100 percent effective and is of course totally passive, there are several disadvantages. First, compared to other contraceptive practices, there is a high initial cost, usually several hundred dollars. Second, it is considered permanent, so that the man or woman must feel completely certain that he or she will not want children in the future. Finally, there is sometimes a psychological side effect in which the sterilization causes the individual to feel a loss of sexual competence: a feeling that has no basis in biology. Among the advantages to the married couple is that the confident elimination of reproductive risk can relieve a pressure in the relationship. In fact, Maschoff, Fanshier, and Hansen (1976) found that following vasectomies, there was improved stability in the areas of marital and sexual satisfaction.

The Birth Control Pill    Finally, we come to what is probably the most controversial form of contraception, the birth control pill, also known as the *oral contraceptive.* In terms of category, it is somewhere between active and passive contraception. As long as the woman takes the pill regularly each day for the designated twenty or twenty-one consecutive days each month, she is protected all month and no decision need be made each time she has intercourse. But if she forgets to take it one day it could affect her even a week or two later, rendering her ripe for pregnancy.

The pill works by introducing a hormone or hormones into the woman's system, which interferes with normal ovulation. Most pills on the market today contain a mixture of a synthetic progesterone derivative and estrogen. Research has indicated that for some women there may be some serious side effects, correlated with their smoking habits and their ages. Side effects include clotting, bleeding, painful abdominal cramps, depression, and in some cases endrocrinologic and metabolic changes. There is also believed to be a higher risk of some forms of cancer. However, the dangers of the pill are statistically far less than the risks associated with abortion.

## Abortion

A couple may choose other than contraceptive methods for controlling family size. In fact, the most widely used method of birth control in the world is not contraception or abstinence—but abortion! If unwanted pregnancy occurs, there is always the possibility of abortion, an issue charged with emotional overtones and political debate.

The term *abortion,* technically, refers to the spontaneous or induced expulsion from the womb of the fertilized egg in any stage of development before it can survive on its own. A spontaneous, that is, involuntary, abortion is commonly called a *miscarriage.* The induced, that is, voluntary, abortion, in which the prospective parent or parents consent to terminate the pregnancy, is the controversial one. When an induced abortion is performed to save the life of the mother, it is called a therapeutic abortion.

The time factor

There are several standard methods of abortion. The choice of method depends largely on the condition of the mother and the stage of the pregnancy. The earlier the abortion, the easier and safer it is. During the first trimester, the suction method and scraping are typically used. The suction method involves inserting a suction aspirator through the vagina and removing the thickened lining of the uterus in which the fertilized egg is implanted. Dilation and curetage, commonly called ''D and C'' or scraping, involves dilating the cervix and curetting, or scraping, the wall of the uterus.

After the third month, abortion is a more complex and dangerous procedure, generally requiring a brief hospital stay. Injections of abortion-inducing drugs, such as salt solution, into the uterus are used, although these can be dangerous. An abdominal *hysterotomy* may be performed, in which the abdomen and uterus are opened and the fetus and amniotic sac removed.

Until the landmark Supreme Court ruling in 1973 that said, in effect, that during the first trimester of pregnancy the State cannot prohibit a woman from having an abortion, there was a high mortality rate from illegal abortions, usually performed under less than sterile conditions. Now, abortion during the first three months is legal in all states, and in many states it is legal in later months also. See table 9.1 for the number of abortions performed in the United States from 1973 through 1975.

There are problems when we look at abortion as a method of birth control. A woman who finds herself with an unplanned, unwanted pregnancy may not be in a position to make a realistic decision about what to do. She may be overcome by powerful emotions or in a state of crisis in which her decisionmaking abilities may be impaired. And, since time is essential in decisions about whether or not to have an abortion, it places additional pressure on the couple, who are forced to make this decision quickly. As Smith (1972) points out: "Women confronted with this crisis may decide to terminate the pregnancy without considering other alternatives or discussing their feelings about the situation" (p. 67).

Kalmar (1977) has also pointed out that the abortion decision can never be viewed *in vacuo,* but must always be approached within the legal, economic, social, political, and religious contexts in which the critical decisions are inevitably made. Despite the wide range of research on the emotional effects of abortion, she points out, "there is a wide discrepancy, from those findings which indicate that abortion yields little or no negative consequences to those which reveal it to be a traumatic and damaging experience" (p. 1).

Table 9.1

**Legal Abortions in the United States 1973–1975**

| Year | Number of abortions | Rate per 1,000 women* | Ratio to 1,000 live births* |
|---|---|---|---|
| 1973 | 742,500 | 16.5 | 239 |
| 1974 | 899,900 | 19.6 | 282 |
| 1975 | 1,034,200 | 22.1 | 331 |

*Computed per 1,000 women 15–44 years old.

Source: Adapted fom E. Weinstock, C. Tietz, F. Jaffe, and J. Dryfocs, "Abortion needs and services in the United States, 1974–76." In Alan Guttmacher Institute, *Family Planning Perspectives,* vol. 8, No. 2, 1975.

Figure 9.8
**The Birth Rate**

Births expected in the lifetime of a U.S. woman
of childbearing age, based on current rates.

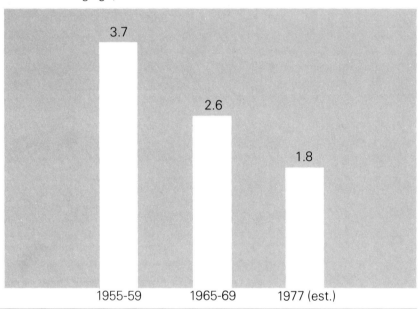

Source: *Newsweek*, May 15, 1978, p. 67

## Social and Psychological Dimensions of Birth Control

We have looked mainly at the biological aspects of birth control. But clearly, there are also important social and psychological dimensions to be considered, when we examine the complex issue of the individual's attitude toward family planning and choice of birth control. As Howard (1978) points out:

> Parenthood, for the first time in human history, is optional, at least for those who know where and how to obtain contraceptives or abortions. One baby was aborted for every five born in the United States in 1975. Nearly five million American men have volunteered for vasectomies. Ten percent of the world's couples have been sterilized. . . . Many educated people of childbearing

age are deciding not to raise families at all, or postponing parent-hood until it is too late. The more education you have, the smaller the family you are likely to raise. Maybe you won't raise one at all.

**Decreasing family size**

Howard's point is well borne out by the data on the decreasing size of families and the increasing number of couples who are remaining child-less. Many factors have been indicated as relevant to the decision about family size and choice of contraception (see figure 9.8). Social class, gen-der, and religious orientation have consistently been identified as impor-tant determinants. Rainwater (1965), in his classic study of family de-sign, found that in addition to these three determinants, couples made individual decisions based on their views of the functions of large and small families and their assessment of the advantages and disadvantages of each. As Rainwater suggests, "A central problem for any given couple in arriving at an optimum family size is that of selfishness versus responsi-bility." He also points out that it was often viewed as irresponsible for couples to have larger families than they could afford to support. Yet, the data also suggest that poorer people tend to have larger families than do people in the middle class and the upper class. These data suggest that there is some inconsistency between verbalized beliefs and behaviors. How do these decisions affect society? Does social pressure encourage or discourage the use of contraceptive methods? What factors influence in-dividuals who wish to use contraception in making their personal choices about what method to use? Can different methods of contraception affect the enjoyment of sex, its frequency, its attitude toward childbirth?

## The Social Interest

Society clearly has a vested interest in the contraceptive and birth control practices of its members. Since the birth rate is a key factor in affecting the perpetuation, growth, and direction of the social order, the recogni-tion that there are direct ways of controlling the birth rate encourages society to promote implicit values and to formulate explicit policies on this subject. In examining a society's views on this topic, Stycos (1974) points out, however, "one must first distinguish between the family and society . . . between population control or population planning on the one hand, and birth control or family planning on the other." He explains the differences between them this way (p. 1):

> Population control or planning is defined as deliberate manipu-lation of the size, composition, or rate of growth of a relatively large collectivity (a clan, an ethnic group, a community, a nation, or the world). . . . Family planning is defined as the deliberate manipulation of the size, composition, or rate of growth of a rela-

The Creation of Families

tively small co-resident unit, united by blood ties (nuclear family, extended family, most households).

*Population control* is more a direct expression of social policy, while *family planning* is the result of the individual's or family's decisionmaking.

Population policy

Of course contraception is only one of several ways a society has for controlling the birth rate, and a very personal one at that. Other ways, using population policy, include encouraging or discouraging through laws and customs the incidence and age of marriage by making it financially advantageous or disadvantageous to marry, providing financial incentives for having children or not having children, and almost all other "areas of domestic government concern—fiscal policies, housing, health, agriculture, transportation . . ." (Fawcett 1974, p. 31). For instance, where a society makes it financially lucrative through its tax structure, couples who are living together on a tentative basis may be encouraged to marry and to have children. Or, if society wants to lower the birth rate, they may make this option unappealing. In both cases these are moderate to long-term devices since there is often a considerable time lag between such societal action and the effects of individual decisions.

Fertility control

In terms of contraceptive usage, the society acts in three ways to affect population through fertility control. First, the development and availability of contraceptives depends to a large part on how much support research and dissemination efforts receive from the government, from charitable and social agencies, from the media, and from other representatives of societal interests. In India, where lowering the birth rate is a major social priority, the government not only pays for the manufacture and insertion of IUDs but also rewards the woman financially for having one inserted. Likewise, the man is given a transistor radio for agreeing to sterilization. In the United States, publicly supported family planning clinics have been demonstrated to be "highly effective" in providing contraception and lowering the incident of unplanned pregnancies (Okada and Gillespie 1977). Such institutions as Planned Parenthood or the Margaret Sanger Foundation, which are active in providing contraception to hundreds of thousands of young people, could not possibly prosper to the degree that they have without large-scale public support.

Secondly, society directly influences the use of contraceptives by its laws. If a state, for example, outlaws the sale of all contraceptives, the rhythm method and coitus interruptus, the two methods that cannot be outlawed, and two of the least effective, would be used more frequently. And the number of unwanted pregnancies would increase. Likewise, if the society rules that insurance programs must pay fully for the cost of voluntary sterilization, there would be an increase in this permanent, highly effective method. Thus, the legal basis of contraception has an important practical consequence.

Finally, every society puts subtle social pressures on its members. The social movement toward Zero Population Growth, for example, has influenced many young couples in their family planning (Lindert 1978). Having large families is no longer ''in,'' although popular shows like *Eight Is Enough* do counteract the preponderance of programs featuring small families. Through the mass media couples see models whose behaviors may be imitated, according to whether they are shown as good or bad, as healthy or unhealthy, as happy or unhappy. The media can have an important effect, even on young people's decisions about what kind of contraception to use. During the late 1960s, for example, the sophisticated and liberated young woman was shown using the birth control pill, in such movies as *Prudence and the Pill.* But then, in the late 1970s, as the hazards of the pill became known, such unabashed use of the pill in the mass media became less common.

*Media influence*

## The Couple's Decision

To each person the decision to use contraception and the type to use is important. Generally, when an individual is a partner in a sexually active continuing relationship, the decision is made jointly. Downs (1977) has shown, however, that in marriages surveyed, wives were more dominant in deciding on contraceptive measures, which seems to reflect the tendency of women to take control of their own bodies, especially since they risk pregnancy.

*Choice of method*

A number of questions are weighed in deciding what type to use. How much can we afford the risk of unwanted pregnancy? When there is some willingness to assume some degree of risk, this of course affects the decision, the riskier methods may be used. Do we ever want children? Townes (1977), among others, in trying to explain how people make their decisions, has suggested a *utility theory* to explain the choice of contraceptive in terms of effectiveness, risk, and benefit. The more beneficial it would be for a couple to have children, this theory asserts, the more likely it is that pregnancy will occur. On the other hand, where there is minimum benefit, there is less likelihood for pregnancy to occur, and contraceptive choices are made accordingly. A middle-aged couple with three children in college, according to this point of view, may decide that they definitely would never want any additional children. Pregnancy would be of minimum benefit to them. They may therefore opt for sterilization. But the parents of one child who think at the time they do not want any more children may not opt for sterilization for fear that something may happen to their child, that they may separate, or that for some other reason they may change their minds about having more children. They choose a less permanent—and less secure!—method, since the benefit of having the option to change their minds is greater than the risk involved in choosing a less secure method of contraception. At the present time, sterilization is the "method of choice among couples married a decade or more, as well as among couples who have all the children they want" (Westoff and Jones 1977).

Socioeconomic and educational factors have also been associated with the choice of contraceptive method, as well as with birth rate. Traditionally, the lower the socioeconomic status, the higher the birth rate has been and the less contraceptive procedures have been used. Also, as Rainwater (1965, p. 208) points out,

> Middle and lower class people differ in the ways they think about the effectiveness of family planning. Middle class people tend to have high confidence in some methods (condom, diaphragm, pills) and to have a low expectation of method failure. They seem to believe that most people have accidents either because they are too ignorant to use effective methods or because they do not use effective methods correctly. In other words, middle class people tend to differentiate methods rather sharply in terms of effectiveness and to differentiate users in terms of competence. In the lower class these distinctions are very much blurred. There is a greater tendency to see the more effective methods as subject to failure, and also a greater tendency to see the less effective ones as perhaps proving adequate "if you're lucky."

Rainwater goes on to point out another difference affecting the choice of a contraceptive method. Couples, he found, choose a method in relation to how segregated or joint their marital relationship is—how much or how little they share social responsibilities and labors with each other. Couples who have highly segregated role relationships, that is, who divide the labors separately and don't interact much with each other, tend to choose less effective methods, leaving their chances to "luck," while couples in low segregated relationships tend more toward the effective methods.

Religious factors may also affect the individual's decision. Some religions prohibit the use of certain forms of contraception, and a practitioner of such a religion may be motivated by conscience in his or her choice. There is also the psychological mechanism of denial. Many people deny their sexual tendencies and refuse to use any kind of contraception. For instance, people may tell themselves that they won't be having relations and believe it. But suddenly they find themselves in love and in bed—unprotected. These deniers are the very people most likely to become pregnant by "accident." Since they don't want to admit that they may find themselves in sexual situations, they refuse to think about contraception until it is too late.

**Psychological effects**

The choice of contraceptive, it should be pointed out, may have a number of marked psychological consequences. Sterilization, for instance, has been noted to have the psychological, though not biological, side effect of reducing some people's sexual interest because they feel less sexually competent. The use of a condom may intrude on the spontaneity of the sexual encounter, making it less pleasant. On the other hand, the use of oral contraceptives may lead to more spontaneous and uninhibited sexuality. Thus, both social and personal considerations enter into the frequency and effective use of different types of contraceptives. Birth control is not solely or even primarily a biological matter; it includes social, ethical, practical, and religious considerations.

## Summary

1. In the first stage of human reproduction, a sperm cell which has been emitted by the male unites with an egg cell inside the female. This union results in fertilization.

2. During pregnancy the fetus develops inside the woman's uterus. The woman undergoes massive physical and psychological changes, many of which also have sociological dimensions.

3. Pregnancy is a unique social status. To a large extent, the pregnant woman has been socialized for this role from early in life. But, as with parenthood, until one is actually pregnant, one has not had opportunities to audition and enact the roles associated with this new status.

4. The period of pregnancy terminates when the infant is delivered into the world. Delivery takes place following a process called labor, during which the mother and a helper work together to get the baby out of the body in the safest way possible.

5. While the biological process of childbirth is the same across all societies, the actual way it is handled varies greatly from society to society. This variety is especially visible in three areas: where the baby is delivered, who assumes what responsibilities in the delivery, and some of the specific procedures relating to delivery and childbirth. Cultural factors also play an important role in how we treat the newborn infant immediately after delivery.

6. Birth control is the intentional act of preventing live births. Birth control includes practices such as abortion and infanticide, as well as contraception, which is a direct procedure for preventing fertilization.

7. There are active and the passive methods of contraception. The active methods are those that require some conscious participation at the time of intercourse. The passive methods are decided upon once and do not require further decisionmaking each time the individual has intercourse.

8. Society has a vested interest in the contraceptive and birth control practices of its members. Since the birth rate is a key factor in affecting the perpetuation, growth, and direction of the social order, the recognition that there are direct ways of controlling the birth rate encourages a society to promote implicit values and to formulate explicit policies on this subject.

9. The decision to use contraception and the type to use is an important decision for each individual. Generally, when an individual is a partner in a sexually active continuing relationship, the decision is made jointly. Factors that affect the decision include social values, religious values, and psychological factors.

## Key Terms

The following terms were introduced and defined in this chapter. Definitions also appear in the glossary.

| | |
|---|---|
| abortion | laparoscopy |
| abstinence | luteinizing hormone (LH) |
| afterbirth | menopause |
| birth control | midwife |
| Caesarian section | miscarriage |
| childbirth | myth of the cloaca |
| coitus interruptus | natural childbirth |
| condom | neonate |
| contraception | oral contraceptive |
| diaphragm | ovarectomy |
| dilate | ovulation |
| douche | ovum |
| ejaculation | placenta |
| embryo | population control |
| endometrium | pregnancy |
| episeotomy | pre-ova |
| estrogen | progesterone |
| family planning | rhythm method |
| fertilization | semen |
| fetus | spermatogenesis |
| gestation | spermatozoa |
| gonads | spermicides |
| HCG | surgical sterilization |
| hysterectomy | testosterone |
| hysterotomy | tubal ligation |
| intrauterine device | utility theory |
| IUD | vasectomy |
| labor | zygote |

**Discussion
Questions**

1. Describe the reproductive structures of man and woman indicating the function of each of the following in procreation: penis, corpora cavernosa, scrotum, testes, spermatozoa, testosterone, semen, vagina, clitoris, prepuce, ovaries, gonads, pituitary gland, luteinizing hormone (LH), ovum, fallopian tubes, uterus, and endometrium.

2. Ask women who are now or recently have been pregnant to describe the reactions of others to them during their pregnancies. What does our society communicate to pregnant women? Is it supportive, nurturing, or insensitive? How do social factors influence the period of pregnancy and childbirth? Do you notice any trends in changing attitudes about deliveries and at-home childbirth?

3. List all the methods of contraception discussed in this chapter, briefly describing how each one works and its relative advantages and disadvantages.

4. What factors influenced or would influence your choice of a contraceptive method? Would you say that physical, social, or psychological factors were most important in making this choice?

5. What are your personal feelings about abortion? What social factors do you think affect general attitudes and laws regarding abortions? What do you think is the interrelationship between frequency of abortion and contraceptive availability in a society?

6. Visit a Planned Parenthood or similar clinic or facility and bring to class some of the free educational literature provided. What does this literature tell you about the needs of the community served and about the services that are provided. Also, what are some of the social attitudes and values reflected in the literature? Are these consistent with what you and your peers believe?

7. From your reading of this chapter, describe specifically how cultural values and social factors affect the following: pregnancy; childbirth; fertility control.

## Suggested Readings

1. Leonard Benson. *Fatherhood: A Sociological Perspective.* New York: Random House, 1968.

A fairly comprehensive summary of sociological knowledge about the changing role of the father in the family. It is easy to read and will serve the novice well.

2. Ronald Freedman, P. K. Whelpton, and A. A. Campbell. *Family Planning, Sterility and Population Growth.* New York: McGraw-Hill, 1959.

A good example of an important study of family planning, intentions, practices, and problems of a representative sample of over 2,500 married women.

3. Paul Gebhard et al. *Pregnancy, Birth and Abortion.* New York: Harper, 1958.

This is the third volume from the Kinsey group and draws upon detailed interviews with over 7,000 women about their reproductive histories, including frequency of spontaneous and induced abortions. There is also an appendix on the abortion problem in other countries around the world.

4. The various studies by Kantner & Zelnick or Zelnick & Kantner, which appeared in *Family Planning Perspectives,* 1972, 1973, 1977.

Kantner and Zelnick have a continuing research program on human sexual behavior. The results of various aspects of these continual surveys generally appear in several journals, particularly in *Family Planning Perspectives.*

5. James Leslie McCary. *Human Sexuality* (2nd ed.). New York: Van Nostrand Reinhold, 1973.

A comprehensive textbook for courses on human sexuality that is stronger on the physical and physiological aspects than the psychological or the sociological.

6. Lee Rainwater. *And the Poor Get Children: Sex, Contraception and Family Planning in the Working Class.* Chicago: Quadrangle, 1960.

A beautifully written, sensitive study of the sexual and family planning attitudes and practices of almost a hundred working-class men and women.

7. Lee Rainwater. *Family Design: Marital Sexuality, Family Size and Contraception.* Chicago: Aldine, 1965.

Another sensitive analysis by Lee Rainwater of family, sexual and reproductive practices which builds upon the 1960 work by adding approximately 300 interviews, including a middle-class sample.

8. SIECUS. *Sexuality and Man.* New York: Scribners, 1970.

A compilation of study guides on different aspects of human sexuality by the Sex Information and Education Council of the United States, an important national, voluntary non-profit organization devoted to the promotion of up-to-date information about human sexuality and its responsible integration into human activities.

# Chapter 10

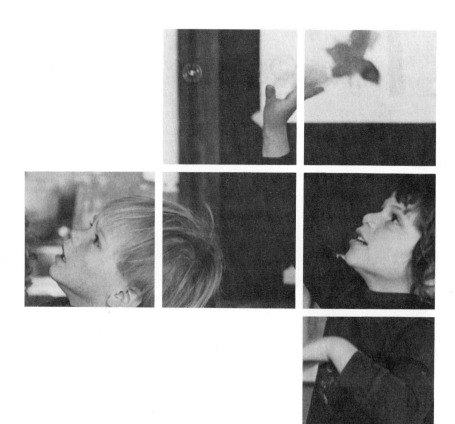

# The Transitional Years of Family Life: Bringing Up Children

## Chapter Aims:

1. To look at the complex of social and cultural factors that affects child-rearing practices.

2. To view the differing styles of childrearing and methods of discipline.

3. To explore the primary and secondary socialization of people for the role of parenting.

4. To outline ''clusters'' of parental attitudes and values.

5. To evaluate the effects of birth order on socialization and personality development.

6. To consider the implications of the single-parent family and the working mother.

## Overview

What determines what kind of parent you will be? The relationships people had with their own parents, their socioeconomic status, and ongoing influences in the external world, such as books and the media, socialize people toward certain styles of childrearing. These and the unique personalities of all parents affect the way they view their own parental roles.

Socializing influences on children include these cultural, social, and personal factors. The interactions with parents and siblings—based on whether one is a firstborn or a later-born—add to the uniqueness of each person's socialization. Also important are the effects of a mother working and whether one or both parents are living at home.

## What Are the Guidelines for Childrearing?

If you ask some friends who are parents of young children why they are doing certain things in raising their children, they will probably be able to tell you a host of logical reasons. "Little Mary has to learn not to be spoiled," they may explain, taking away a piece of candy she has picked up off the table. "If you spare the rod you will certainly spoil the child," they say to justify a spanking. Likewise, if you ask friends about their parents they will probably have many opinions on how well or how poorly their parents raised them. "My parents were too strict," or "My parents didn't understand my needs" are common complaints. Individual parents differ widely in their ways of childrearing. However, in terms of what they teach their children and how they teach it, there is a common denominator within any given society that reveals beyond question the powerful social influence in childrearing.

Childrearing practices have many social and cultural determinants of which most people are generally unaware. Although the general norms of childrearing are socially and culturally determined, these normative behaviors are filtered through the prism of parents' own experiences in their nuclear families of orientation. The resulting behaviors with respect to their children, therefore, represent a mixture of social and psychological determinants.

## Cultural Influences

Bringing up children is not necessarily something that comes naturally to everyone. Rather, childrearing is something that most people have to work at. In our complicated, industrialized, urban society, which is rapidly changing, raising children requires many complex decisions. Childrearing is not simply a personal expression of the parents' beliefs and values but involves cultural guidelines and social restraints. In response to this need, there is a growing movement in the schools toward teaching parenting skills.

In style, in substance, and in goals, the role of the parent is almost

Cultural norms

entirely culturally determined. There is virtually no empirical science of how to bring up a child with which everyone would agree. There are also few, if any, universal rules. In practice, the way children are raised and the way they ultimately develop represent a mixture of biological, psychological, and social "forces in their lives—from genes to government policies, from life in the womb and cradle to experiences with family, teachers, and friends" (Segal and Yahraes 1978, p. 3). This mixture includes many of the parents' own personality characteristics blended into the normative social fabric.

We should not minimize the importance of the possibly natural parental tendency for the preservation and the protection of one's own children. But cultural norms, embedded in the parents' own socialization when they were children and transmitted through their secondary socialization as they were being taught how to parent, shape the way parents bring up their children.

An interesting example of how cultural differences affect childrearing is found in a recent study of Navajo and Caucasian mothers' differing perceptions of children's social behavior. Guilmet (1978), observing that Navajo children in a California day-care center were considerably more reserved and apparently more reluctant to express themselves than the Caucasian children, decided to find out why. He showed a group of Navajo and Caucasian mothers videotapes of some children playing. He then interviewed the mothers about their perceptions of what the children were doing and asked them to rate the children's behaviors as desirable or undesirable. To the Navajo mothers, who expected the children to act less aggressively, excited behavior was viewed as mischievous, while the Caucasian mothers had more positive attitudes toward the same behavior. Guilmet concluded that Navajo mothers discouraged very active speech and behavior because they considered it discourteous and undisciplined. Caucasian mothers, on the other hand, did nothing to discourage such behavior, since they didn't perceive it negatively.

What are some of the questions and problems for which parents seek answers in these cultural norms. There are four main areas of concern:

1. *Discipline:* How strict or liberal should I be in bringing up my children? How many rules should children be taught to obey out of a sense of duty, and how many can they learn on their own through experimentation?
2. *Family Interactions:* What kinds of contact and interactions with other family members are permissible and desirable, and what should be discouraged or prohibited?
3. *Education:* What are the best types of educational experiences, inside and outside the home, for my child? What can I do, for example, in choosing a community in which to live or in selecting

a school, to see that my child gets the best possible educational experiences?

4. *Physical Health:* What can I do to prevent illness, to provide the best diet for my children, and to offer an environment that will promote the highest level of physical functioning?

Of course, within these categories are virtually thousands of specific questions and problems that have to be dealt with on an almost daily basis. Parents learn to work out these problems by knowing the capacities and responses of their own children, by looking back on their own childhood experiences, by asking friends and professional acquaintances, by considering folk wisdom that is handed down, and by relying on printed manuals and primers—books that provide advice for parents.

## Parenting Manuals

Manuals of advice on how to raise children have been available to parents since ''the invention of printing in the West'' (Stewart, Winter, and Jones 1975). But it is only as societies have become more industrialized, more urban, more scientific, and presumably more enlightened that reliance on printed manuals has become especially important as a cultural source of parental advice, supplanting folk wisdom as the primary source of information on childrearing (Whiting 1974).

*While some cultures perceive it negatively, our culture encourages activity on the part of children.*

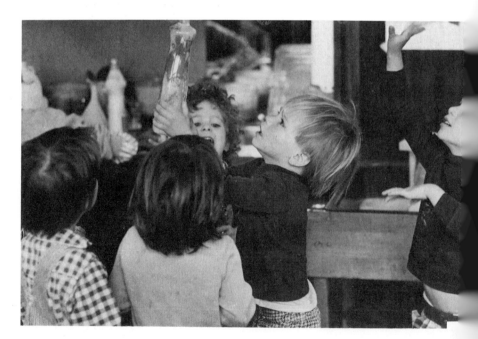

Dr. Benjamin Spock

By far, the most popular parenting manual ever published—in fact, the most successful book of all time except the *Bible*—is Dr. Benjamin Spock's *Baby and Child Care,* which has sold over 28 million copies since its publication. Virtually, two entire generations of Americans have been raised in accordance with Dr. Spock's ideas, which, incidentally, have changed with the times, sometimes dramatically. For instance, in the early editions of the books, childrearing ideas for little girls were highly sex-stereotyped, while in later editions the socialization of boys and girls was treated identically.

It is fascinating to see how ideas about childrearing do change. See table 10.1 for how they changed from the sixteenth to the nineteenth century in England.

In addition to the redoubtable Dr. Spock's book, there are dozens of other popular primers, ranging from psychologically oriented books such as Hiam Ginott's *Between Parent and Child,* to task-oriented books on toilet training and discipline, such as Arnold Lazarus' *Toilet Training Your Child,* to such general childrearing programs as *Parent Effectiveness Training* (PET). A more recent book, *How to Influence Children* (Schaefer 1978), attempts to relieve parental ''stress'' by explicating 69 specific ways to influence one's children with what the author calls ''child management skills'' and ''child guidance skills.''

How important are these parenting manuals? How accurate are they? A comprehensive survey and analysis by University of Chicago psychologist Alison Clarke-Stewart (1978) found that almost all parents in the United States today read at least one book on childrearing and most parents read more. Articles in popular magazines provide another source of authoritative advice on how to raise children. Parents are more likely to rely on books and articles with the first child than with later children. Clarke-Stewart found that most parents are extremely eager for what they consider expert advice and typically they regard someone who has published a book as an expert. The implication of her work is that the authors of these guides have become the spokespeople for our culture, offering to parents the advice and guidance that in another age and culture may have been provided by religious leaders, community sources, or folk wisdom.

## Parenting Modes and Methods of Discipline

All parents are faced with a challenging range of specific decisions in the course of raising their children. What values should I try to teach my child?

Table 10.1

## How Have Childrearing Practices Changed over the Centuries?

Changes in the Significant Issues in English Child-Rearing Manuals, Sixteenth–Nineteenth Centuries[a]

*Sixteenth Century*
Mother and father both encouraged to be co-rearers.
Father described as the ultimate authority.
Corporal punishment is advocated, and the child's obedience is supposed to precede the parents' love.
Virtues: Obedience, silence, patience, reverence.
Vices: Rudeness, disobedience, noisiness, talkativeness.

*Seventeenth Century*
Increased emphasis on obedience, and decreased emphasis on reverence as virtues.
Fewer vices mentioned (especially rudeness, noise, and talk).
Slight increase in the importance of early learning.

*Eighteenth Century*
Slight decrease in all issues associated with nursing.
Mother seen as the primary rearer, with some anxiety expressed about this.
No mention of which parent is the ultimate authority.
Some advocacy of sex-differentiation.
First (and strong) mention of encouraging independence.
Fewer vices mentioned.
Restrictions on corporal punishment.
Manners de-emphasized.

*Nineteenth Century*
No mention of nursing issues.
Mother seen as the primary rearer, without anxiety.
Strong differentiation of children by sex, in all areas.
Increased emphasis on independence and creativity, and decreased emphasis on obedience and mildness as virtues.
First mention of aggression as a vice.
Reward and love (vs. punishment) as motivators.

[a] This appendix is to be read downward, cumulatively: The sixteenth-century description is given, and then each following century changes from the previous one in the ways mentioned.

Source: Stewart, Winter, and Jones (1975), p. 701.

## Childrearing Styles

How should I use discipline? How free or rigid should I be in providing direction and guidance in my child's life? Baumrind (1971) has identified three overall styles of childrearing, which vary in terms of parental attitudes and methods of discipline. These have been shown, in subsequent research, to affect the child's social and personality development. She calls these the authoritarian, the permissive, and the authoritative approaches.

The *authoritarian method* describes parents who are detached, controlling, restrictive, and overly protective. Such parents discourage their children from asking questions, exploring, taking risks and doing things on their own initiative. Authoritarian parents also impose rigid rules that are not explained but are enforced coercively, by punishment.

### My Old Man

"My old man, he used to kick my butt if I didn't do what he said to do. Of course, he wasn't an S.O.B. or nothing like that . . . he always taught me things for my own good, I mean. You know, he said I was a stubborn cuss all the time. I remember one time, my old lady was downstate visiting the family, and he told me to clean up the kitchen before he went to work. I was busy or something so I forgot until he came home, and, man, when I saw the face on him I knew I better get that kitchen cleaned up real quick. But before I could even lift a finger, he had his belt off and he was after me, boiling mad, I tell you. Jesus; I got the hell out of that house before you could say Jack Robinson."

Social ramifications

One of the most interesting examples of the social ramifications of widespread authoritarian childrearing is the pronounced effect it has had on our Anglo-American culture, where for many years this was *the* method of correctly raising children. Historians "have long recognized that subduing the willfulness of stubborn children was considered the first and foremost task of religious parents" (McLoughlin 1976). One of the most dramatic examples of how this approach works is found in a letter published anonymously in *The American Baptist Magazine* in October 1831. The letter, as we now know, was written by the Reverend Francis Wayland, a nationally known clergyman, author, teacher, educational reformer, and the President of Brown University (McLoughlin 1976). The following passage is from the letter, which is reprinted in its entirety in McLoughlin, and offers us an unforgettable picture of authoritarian childrearing:

### Reverend Wayland and His Son

I put him into a room by himself, and desired that no one should speak to him, or give him any food or drink whatever. This was about 8 o'clock in the morning. I visited him every hour or two during the day, and spoke to him in the kindest tones, offering him the bread and putting out my arms to take him. But throughout the whole day he remained inflexibly obstinate. He did not yield a hair's breadth. . . . He went to bed supperless. It was now twenty-four hours since he had eaten anything.

He woke the next morning in the same state. He would take nothing that I offered him, and shunned all my offers of kindness. He was now truly an object of pity. He had fasted thirty-six hours. His eyes were wan and sunken. His breath hot and feverish, and his voice feeble and wailing. Yet he remained obstinate. He continued thus, till 10 o'clock A.M. when hunger overcame him, and he took from me a piece of bread, to which I added a cup of milk, and hoped that the labor was at last accomplished.

In this however I had not rightly judged. He ate his bread greedily, but when I offered to take him, he still refused as pertinaciously as ever. I therefore ceased feeding him, and recommenced my course of discipline.

He was again left alone in his crib, and I visited him as before, at intervals. About one o'clock Saturday, I found that he began to view his condition in its true light. The tones of his voice in weeping were graver and less passionate, and had more the appearance of one bemoaning himself. Yet when I went to see him, he still remained obstinate. You could clearly see in him the abortive efforts of the will. . . . All I required of him was, that he should come to me. This he would not do, and he began now to see that it had become a serious business. Hence his distress increased. He would not submit, and he found that there was no help without it. It was truly surprising to behold how much agony so young a being could inflict upon himself.

About three o'clock I visited him again. He continued in the state I have described. I was going away, and had opened the door, when I thought that he looked somewhat softened, and returning, put out my hands, again requesting him to come to me. To my joy, and I hope gratitude, he rose up and put forth his hands immediately. The agony was over. He was completely subdued. He repeatedly kissed me, and would do so whenever I commanded. He would kiss anyone when I directed him, so full of love was he to all the family. Indeed, so entirely and instantaneously were his feelings towards me changed, that he preferred me now to any of the family. As he had never done before, he moaned after me when he saw that I was going away.

McLoughlin (pp. 21–23) goes on to point out,

> It would appear that evangelical children underwent a profound psychological experience when, at a very early age, they were forced to submit to their fathers' wills and give up their own. Freudian psychologists might see this as a ''reaction formation'' in which feelings of reverence and dependence were unconsciously substituted for those of anger and hostility in order to resolve the intense conflict. . . . Children raised under such patterns of paternal discipline probably spent their lives trying to act consistently within them and looked to their fathers' approval long after they had reached maturity. Moreover, having repressed their own hostility toward their fathers, such evangelicals, when they became fathers, doubtless felt threatened by any refusal of their children to submit to their will.

While the authoritarian style provides tight external controls, it may inhibit the development of integrated values that promote self-control.

The *permissive method* involves some features that are in diametric opposition to the authoritarian method. Permissive parents have a warm but laissez-faire attitude. They are noncontrolling, nondemanding, and nonpunitive toward their children. But this noninterfering approach means that children are not encouraged to explore, achieve, and try new things. They are deprived of guidelines against which they can evaluate their competency and the appropriateness of their behavior.

The *authoritative approach* combines the best aspects of the authoritarian and the permissive approaches. It is found among parents who are warm and caring; who encourage achieving, independent, and exploratory behavior; and who provide rules that, although enforced with mild punishment, are explained and are subject to change depending upon the children's reactions to them. The following shows how a young woman remembers the warm behavior of her father and the effect it had on her.

Mild punishment

*The* authoritative ap-
proach *to discipline is
found among parents
who are warm and caring
and who provide rules
which are explained.*

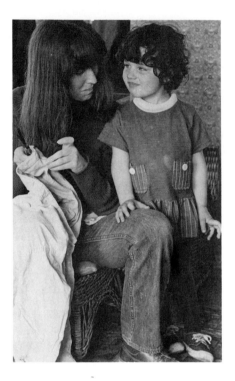

### My Pet Frog

''I can remember the time when, I don't know, I must have
been four or five, and I had this pet frog I was very attached to,
what was its name again. . . . Anyway, I came home one day
and the frog had been run over by a car. So my parents were
there, looking very grave, very serious. . . . I thought my
grandma had died, and then they told me about the frog. Well,
the reason I bring this up is that I'll never forget how, after I
was upset and cried and talked to them about it, my father took
my hand very gently, and we walked into the woods near the
lake looking for another frog. I think I remember this because I
see it, at least in retrospect, as the beginning of my being what
you called 'resourceful.' ''

One question that is surely of interest as we look at these childrearing
styles is what predisposes a parent to one style of childrearing rather than
another. While this question is not easily answered by any single factor,
Melvin Kohn (1959) sheds a great deal of light on it in his extensive re-

Table 10.2

**What Parents Consider the Most Highly Desirable Characteristics for Their Children**

| Characteristic | Middle-class Mothers* | Working-class Mothers* | Middle-class Fathers* | Working-class Fathers* |
|---|---|---|---|---|
| Honesty | 44% | 53% | 52% | 58% |
| Happiness | 46% | 36% | 37% | 22% |
| Considerateness | 39% | 27% | 35% | 14% |
| Obeys parents well | 20% | 33% | 13% | 39% |
| Has self-control | 22% | 13% | 20% | 6% |
| A good student | 15% | 17% | 7% | 9% |
| Curiosity | 18% | 6% | 13% | 8% |

*Percentage who select each characteristic as one of three "most desirable" in a ten- or eleven-year-old child.

Adapted from: Kohn, M. L. Social class and parental values. *The American Journal of Sociology,* 1959, 64, 337–351.

Socioeconomic status

search on social class and parental values, as shown in table 10.2. Kohn found, as we mentioned briefly in chapter 3, that parents' behaviors toward their children are class related. We find, moreover, when we look at his data that parents' attitudes toward childrearing and what characteristics they value as most desirable in their children are directly related to socioeconomic status. For example, when we look at a certain trait, such as curiosity, we see pronounced class differences. While 37 percent of the mothers of the highest socioeconomic status value this as one of the most desirable characteristics for their children, only 3 percent of those in the lowest group consider it important. Thus, mothers from the higher socioeconomic class are more likely to develop a childrearing style that will encourage curiosity, that is, a permissive style, and to avoid a childrearing style that will thwart the child's curiosity: the authoritarian style.

To cite another example, while 22 percent of the middle-class mothers and 20 percent of the middle-class fathers thought it was important that the child have self-control, only 13 percent of the working-class mothers and 6 percent of the working-class fathers considered this characteristic highly desirable. Thus, working-class parents are more likely to subscribe to a childrearing style, such as authoritarian, that does not attempt to foster self-control than to one, such as authoritative or permissive, that combines external controls with internal self-controls.

Moreover, while certain characteristics such as honesty, considerateness, happiness, obedience, and dependability were highly valued by all parents, regardless of social class, Kohn points out that the ways parents interpret these characteristics and the way they believe they can best be cultivated vary from class to class. This insight, combined with our earlier discussion of how middle-class parents emphasize internal standards, shows how childrearing styles may develop, at least with respect to parents' social class.

Discipline   Parental rearing patterns, we should emphasize, differ not only with respect to the overall approach, but also in terms of the type and degree of discipline used to control socially undesirable behavior. The

Curbing misbehavior

disciplinary philosophy of the authoritarian, permissive, and authoritative approaches are obvious. We mentioned earlier the social-class differences noted by Kohn, with working class parents more prone to physical discipline than their middle-class counterparts.

By analyzing the findings from 11 studies dealing with parental disciplinary practices and conscience development in children 4 to 13 years, Hoffman (1970) identified the following types of disciplinary control that mothers and fathers use to curb their children's misbehavior: (1) *power assertion,* the use of punishment, including physical punishment or deprivation of privileges, and threats of punishment; (2) *love withdrawal,* the use of psychological punishment, such as ignoring or scorning children or telling them that they will be unloved and unwanted as long as they misbehave; and (3) *induction,* avoiding both physical and psychological punishment and explaining that certain behaviors, not the children themselves are undesirable because of the adverse effects of these behaviors on the well-being of the children or of others.

Both power assertion and love withdrawal appear to be techniques associated with authoritarian parents, whereas induction is the preferred technique of the authoritative parent.

Social class, ethnic identification, and religious affiliation have all been identified as factors that correlate with the parental styles of discipline. Bronfenbrenner (1961), for example, found that a working-class parent was more likely to be permissive with the opposite-sex child and more punitive with the same-sex child. In an upper-class family, on the other hand, there is a greater degree of equal treatment of boys and girls. It has also been found that these class differences in parental permissiveness and discipline are related to the observed differences in intellectual development and inceased socialization between classes (Radin and Epstein 1975).

To a large extent, the success that parents have as socializing agents

Reciprocity

depends upon the mode of discipline they use and the consistency with which they use it. Moreover, as we pointed out in chapter 3, child socialization is a recriprocal process, in which the child indirectly or directly influences the behavior of the parents at the same time that they are influencing the child. This parent-child reciprocity has been identified as far back as early infancy, were Brazelton (1978) suggests that the infant and parent ''reward and guide'' each other into appropriate behaviors. Many other childrearing attitudes, it has also been suggested, are directly related to the child's personality and its effects on the parents (Seth and Khanna 1978).

Research also suggests that when parents are inconsistent, children perceive them as unreliable and link the receipt of punishment with their moods and not to the behavior. When parents consistently discipline undesirable behaviors and reward desirable ones, the child learns to distinguish socially approved from socially disapproved behaviors. Consistent behavior, of course, facilitates the socialization process. Let us then examine factors involved in this socialization process.

Induction *avoids the use of physical or psychological punishment. Undesirable behavior is explained to the child.*

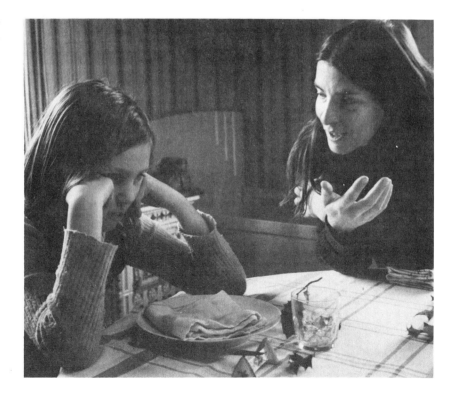

## Socialization Factors

Every society provides explicit and implicit guidelines for the rearing of children. As Mechling (1976) points out, "the rearing of children is a task-problem which all human societies must solve" (p. 48). This is accomplished through the processes of primary and secondary socialization: the former in the parent-child relationship and the latter through subsequent learning, as in the educational system, the media, and parenting manuals. Actual childrearing practices then represent a combination of three things: how the parents were raised, what they have learned subsequently, and the circumstances in which they find themselves.

As we discussed in chapter 3, the behaviors, attitudes, feelings, and beliefs of the parents are the first and primary socializing influence on the child. If children are influenced by their parents' actions, then it is important for us to understand what these actions are and how they are communicated to the child. We noted in chapter 3 how important the maternal environment is in socialization and personality development. One of the big problems in attempting to discuss the parents' attitudes throughout the childrearing years is how to categorize the many and diverse attitudes a parent has into some comprehensible framework. To do this, we do not need consistency among all the parents' attitudes in different areas of parent-child interaction, but we would expect broad patterns of behaviors and values to emerge. These help us understand the process by which parents socialize their children.

## Parents' Views of Their Own Roles

Parental attitude clusters

Sims and Paolucci (1975) propose "clusters" of parental attitudes and values. Each of these clusters represents a set of related and interacting attitudes and beliefs about childrearing. They are taken from a widely used test called *The Parental Attitude Research Instrument,* in which a parent surveyed might strongly agree, agree, disagree, or strongly disagree with certain statements about parents and children. By looking at these clusters, we can see that the children learn some definite patterns of beliefs from their parents' implicit and explicit attitudes. We will use eight of these points of view to examine some areas of parental decision-making. Ask yourself, as you look at these, how you think your parents would respond and how you would respond to each of them.

### Parents Are All-Wise   "Whenever a parent tells a child something, the child should always listen for his own good." Parents who

agree strongly with this point of view will be more likely to insist that their children listen to them unquestioningly. They will also expect their children to accept parental opinions as superior to their own insights, since parents are all-wise. In terms of decisions, the parent would communicate, "If I tell you to do this, then just do it because I say so." This position might stifle curiosity and the free exploration of values by children.

## Children Should Be Treated as the Equals of Parents

This position says that "the child has a right to speak as freely to his parents as they do to him." Parents who ascribed to this point of view would have an egalitarian relationship with their children. Their children would be allowed to express their dissatisfaction with their parents as readily as parents would express their dissatisfaction with their children. Moreover, children would not be expected to accept their parents' beliefs without question or challenge just because they were the parents' beliefs.

## Children Should Trust Only Their Parents   The child's confidence and belief in the parents is a result of the trust the child has. Parents who agreed with this viewpoint would argue, "If a relative tells your child something bad about you, the child shouldn't believe it under any circumstances." Such parents would be likely to discourage the child from challenging anything the parents say since the parents' word should be accepted on trust.

## Unquestioned Loyalty   "A child should never say anything bad about his parents to anyone." This position is related directly to the attitude above. Loyalty is the key word: it combines the quality of trust with an attitude of respect.

## Deception   It is not necessary that parents always be completely truthful with their children. The parent who agreed strongly with this viewpoint would argue that, "sometimes a child has to be temporarily misled to do something that is for his own good." It sees deception as a legitimate part of teaching children the realities of life.

## Homemaking   Some mothers feel that "it's basically impossible to get anything done while taking care of children." Or a mother may say, "I never get out of the house anymore unless it's to do chores for the family." These feelings affect the way these mothers socialize their children, in that they view childrearing responsibilities as a limitation of their freedom. Mothers who strongly agreed with these positions would be less likely to take a job outside the home, less likely to seek paths of devel-

opment outside childrearing. Such a mother would also be more likely to feel isolated from the outside world.

### Children Are Demanding!

Parents who agree with this position recognize that it does not always require a specific reason for a parent to be upset with his or her child. "A parent can easily lose her temper with her child just because of the general strain the child places on her." Such parents are more likely to recognize some of the natural strain inherent in the parent-child relationship and are probably willing to accept their angry feelings more than a parent who does not acknowledge this dimension of childrearing.

### Frequent and Occasional Dissatisfaction

This viewpoint varies by degrees from "Sometimes a parent gets so annoyed she just wants to get away from her children" to "Children are generally very annoying, demanding, and unappreciative of what their parents do for them." Generally, however, it points to the levels of dissatisfaction and irritation a parent feels in response to the demands of the children. It also has a direct effect on the parents' feelings about childrearing.

Role configurations

These clusters, while they are certainly not exhaustive, do represent a wide sample of the way that parents express their attitudes in the socialization of their children. They also show us the different ways that parents conceptualize their roles and the roles of their children. An understanding of parental role is essential in understanding parental behavior. Wood, Bishop, and Cohen (1978) have suggested four major role configurations that account for most parent-child interaction patterns. There is the "potter," who sees the role of the parent as shaping and molding the child into the adult figure he or she is expected to become; the "gardener" who provides the nutrients and climate for the child to grow; the "maestro," who orchestrates growth by direction but allows some flexibility; and the "consultant," who is less authoritarian and guides his or her child with solicited advice. The parent's view of his or her role has important underlying implications in the attitudes that are articulated and in the resulting behaviors and learned role expectations of their children.

### Other Attitudes

Several social psychological factors influence parents' attitudes toward their children.

Sex of the child

The sex of the child definitely has an effect on the way the child is socialized, as we discussed briefly in chapter 3. Moreover, parental preference for a son or daughter may affect the parents' attitudes about the child as well as influence their style of parenting. The bulk of studies have clearly revealed that in the United States there is a "slight boy preference especially for firstborns, [a] desire for one of each sex [if possible], and [a] preference for a predominance of boys over a predominance of girls if a balanced number of each was not chosen'' (Williamson 1976, p. 63). The parents may not overtly favor their boy children; but because of these preferences, it is possible that the attitude is subtly communicated that ''It is better to be a boy than a girl.''

''Accidental'' pregnancy

The parents' consensual decision to have a child as opposed to ''accidental'' pregnancy may also affect their feelings about the child. Birth order and family stability also play a part.

The parents' social class and income level has also been related to a number of childrearing attitudes and behaviors. The Kohn study discussed in chapter 3, where different childrearing attitudes were revealed between working-class and middle-class parents, is one classic example. Over the years, more than 200 published studies have indicated a relationship between social class and the style of mother-child interactions. Wandersman (1973) has carefully documented and analyzed the bulk of evidence and points out as a conclusion,

> Small but consistent trends appear throughout the research of class difference in mother-child interaction: *lower class mothers interact using more authoritative, coercive and physically assertive techniques, while middle class mothers interact using more egalitarian, guiding and verbally orienting techniques.* The stylistic difference is suggested to be rooted in the greater emphasis of middle class mothers on responsiveness and reciprocation in interaction (italics ours).

This, again, is consistent with Kohn's earlier findings. We should emphasize that this in no way implies that lower-class mothers do a less competent job, but merely that they have a different ''style'' of dealing with their children and that this style is transmitted from generation to generation, especially if there is little or no social mobility and if there are no opportunities to learn new behaviors.

Such socialization factors as we have discussed are not alone in exercising influence over a child's development. Another major factor which we will now discuss is birth order.

## Birth Order and Relationships with Siblings

We mentioned at the beginning of this chapter that cultural influences combine with other factors in the raising of children. One variable that has been the subject of much attention in recent years is *ordinal position in the family:* the birth order of a child with respect to his or her siblings. As we look at this subject we will see some intermixing of cultural, social, and personality factors in childrearing.

There is some evidence to indicate that the child's ordinal position in the family structure has an influence on the child's socialization and personality development. However, the evidence at this time is still confusing and far from conclusive on any given factor. But since sibling relationships and birth order variables are likely to influence the child's socialization, it is helpful for us to be sensitive to the impact of birth order and sibling relationships on social development and maturity.

Adler's personality theory

The first important discussion of the effects of birth order on personality was put forth by pyschiatrist Alfred Adler, who made ordinal position an integral part of his personality theory. Adler argued that the positions children occupy in their families influence various aspects of their personalities. He noted, for example, that the oldest child is likely to develop leadership qualities later in life but, because he or she has been dethroned as a child by the arrival of the second-born, is also likely to feel insecure and develop problems relating to this insecurity later on. The second or the middle child "may resist the authority asserted by the older child and develop a rebellious nature. He may become uncooperative in the presence of authority. Such oversensitivity to authority may retard adjustment to group life" (Garfinkle, Massey, and Mendel 1976). Because the youngest child never experiences being replaced by another sibling, he or she may become the "spoiled" child of the family (Garfinkle, Masser, and Meude 1976, p. 80).

Adler's work, although it has enjoyed a pervasive influence, was more speculative than scientific. In the years since his ideas appeared, however, many empirical studies have been conducted, some of which support his theory, some of which are quite different, and some of which refute his main points. Stanley Schachter (1959), investigating factors related to gregariousness and conformity, by chance produced one of the definitive studies of the effects of birth order on socialization. He found that the firstborn child tends toward group values and is more likely to be a conformer than the child born later (p. 87). Firstborn children also tend

IQ scores

to have higher IQ scores than children born later, probably because parents pay less attention to any one child when there are many children present. Although a number of studies have persuasively argued that the firstborn is more adult-oriented than later-born children (Bradley 1968; Bragg and Allen 1970), it has been pointed out that while there may be some truth to this assumption, other factors besides birth order are primarily responsible for the differences. Some of the "other" factors commonly cited are: sex of the child, sex of the siblings, social class, maternal attitude and expectation, father presence or father absence, and size of the family.

**Second-borns**

Although firstborns have been more extensively studied than children born later, there is also some research on the latter group. McGurk and Lewis (1972) found, for instance, that second-borns sought more adult help and more adult approval than did either firstborns or later-borns. Moreover, second-borns, they point out, "also spent more time in individual activity . . . were generally more talkative . . . and expressed more negative affect than other subjects" (p. 366). One of the important conclusions of this study, in regard to the middle child, is that "the effects for birth order are more revealing and highlight the second-born as different from his firstborn or later-born siblings. Second-borns, for example, showed more dependency behavior (seeking help, approval, and affection from adults) than siblings from the other two ordinal positions" (p. 366).

An advantage of being the youngest child that is often cited in the literature is that having older siblings increases opportunities for early socialization. Having an opportunity to "model" himself or herself after the interactions of older siblings offers the youngest child opportunities to explore avenues of social interaction in the home environment that were not available to the oldest child. In one interesting study, Collard (1968) investigated firstborn and later-born infants' responses in unfamiliar situations. The purpose of this study was to determine if later-born infants, who had opportunities to interact with older brothers and sisters, as opposed to firstborns, whose interactions were limited to the parents and usually to the mother, would be less fearful of strangers. An experimenter, with whom the infant was not familiar, placed a toy on the table in front of the infant, who sat on the mother's lap. The time it took the infant to pick up the toy was judged to be related directly to the infant's anxiety over the presence of the "strange" experimenter. On the average, firstborns took about fifty-five seconds to pick up the toy and later-borns took about eight seconds: a significant difference. Moreover, in analyzing the data, it was found that not only was ordinal position important but also the degree of age difference between the later-born and his or her older sibling.

Infants with widely spaced birth orders, whose older sibling was more than 6 years older, responded the way firstborns did. They apparently lacked the opportunities to socialize that are available to more closely spaced later-borns. "The firstborn and widely spaced infants made significantly fewer responses to the toy than did the later-borns matched to them. . . . Firstborn and widely spaced infants made significantly more negative social responses such as fussing and crying than later-born infants did" (p. 172).

There are several important implications from this study that transcend the birth order question and have profound implications for understanding socialization in the family. Collard (p. 173) concludes in part:

**Later-born children**

Infants receiving social stimulation from few persons will tend to show more fear of strangers than will infants receiving stimulation from a variety of persons. Compared to later-borns with preschool siblings, firstborn and widely spaced infants tended to make fewer exploratory and play responses to a novel toy and to respond more slowly to the strange person and toy. . . .

Variability among infants in degree of acceptance of strangers is probably determined by a number of factors, including (a) the number of persons the infant is exposed to and their variety in terms of appearance and behavior, (b) the frequency and duration of exposure to different persons, and (c) the infant's developmental level at the time of exposure to others.

The implications of these findings are also relevant in understanding the child's level of socialization with his or her peer group and in the school environment.

Sibling socialization

An important distinction between the socialization role of siblings in industrial and preindustrial societies has been pointed out by Whiting (1974; see also Whiting and Whiting 1974). Generally, the less industrialized the society, the more opportunities children have to take care of their younger siblings, acting during the day as surrogate mother. The effect of this on ordinal position differentiation, according to Whiting (1974, p. 11) is that

the characteristics reported peculiar to elder children in families in the United States are only present in the [New England] sample in the six culture study. In the other five societies where we have samples of children's behavior in naturalistic settings there are no significant differences in our measure between the behavior of oldest and middle children—only the youngest child is significantly different.

This finding is consistent with Collinge's research, insofar as the youngest in these societies receives the most stimulation.

What does this research show? Without overemphasizing the role of ordinal position as a factor in social development, we can say with reasonable certainty that the child's exposure to others during the early years facilitates socialization; later-born children, who have an older brother or sister close in age, will tend to be the most social children, the most comfortable in interpersonal and social interactions.

Clearly, the bulk of evidence on ordinal position does not strongly support any single theory or point of view. One of the main difficulties in drawing firm conclusions is the fact that other variables interact with birth order and it is difficult, if not impossible, to separate them in research studies. To say, ''The firstborn child is . . .'' or ''The middle child is . . .'' or ''The youngest child is . . .'' must always be a reasoned guess rather than a valid statement. Variables such as the sex of the child, sex of the siblings, number of years' difference in age, maternal environment variables, socioeconomic class, and so forth, are all vital factors that interact with ordinal position in the normal course of socialization.

Now, let us turn our attention to a question in childrearing that has come under much attention in recent years, particularly as the sex-linked roles of ''mother'' and ''father'' have been undergoing rapid changes: What are the effects of the single-parent family on the children?

# Children in Single-Parent Families

## Effects of the Parent's Absence

While parenting primers and general cultural values do indeed influence childrearing practices, another factor of considerable importance is the home situation. There are some practical differences between the single-parent and two-parent home situations, and these differences are coming under greater scrutiny as the number of children from single-parent families increases dramatically. Educational statistics show that more children from single-parent families, usually with the father absent, are currently enrolled in the schools than in any other period of American history! In this section, we shall examine some of the effects growing up in a single-parent family has on the developing child.

Single- vs. two-parent

Herzog and Sudia (1973) provide the most comprehensive review and analysis of the literature, although their work is unfortunately limited to the children of fatherless families. Moreover, the studies they examined evaluate the effects of father absence on boys, which reflects the general trend of research in this area, where for the most part girls have been sorely neglected. In summarizing the findings of over 120 studies, Herzog and Sudia (1973, p. 214) concluded:

> Despite the ambiguity of the results, the review does provide sufficient basis for some firm conclusions that apply to all three areas (school problems family problems, and antisocial behavior), and probably to any research on the effects of the father's absence.
> 1. However inconclusive present evidence may be, there is a firm basis for rejecting blanket generalizations about the consequences of father's absence. Its behavioral and psychological

effects are probably much less uniform and much less uniformly handicapping than is widely assumed.

2. The impact of father's absence on a boy is conditioned and to a large extent mediated by a complex of interacting variables and probably cannot be explored fruitfully as a discrete, critical variable in itself.

3. More specifically, the impact on a boy growing up in a fatherless home is strongly affected by the elements that were presented before the father's absence.

4. The number of parents in the home is likely to be less crucial to the child's development than the family functioning of the present members—which is far harder to assess. Family functioning would include the mother's role and coping ability as well as the general family climate.

5. Family functioning is determined not only by individual characteristics and the interactions of its members but also by the circumstances and environment of the family unit.

**The child's feelings**

These are broad conclusions, drawn from a wide range of studies conducted over many years, using different methodologies, different assumptions, and attempting to answer different types of questions. Such studies rarely touch upon the child's deeper feelings, which may include feeling "different from other children" or angry at the absent parent. Or, as some studies have shown (Baker et al. 1967), the child may develop an image of the father based on information and attitudes received from the mother.

Studies often prove inadequate in answering questions about the child from the single-parent family, because the absence of a parent is only one of the many different factors affecting the child, and "absence of parent" per se tells us little about the family condition. Recognizing this problem, Nass and Nass (1976) have surveyed over one hundred studies on this subject. They pinpoint seven "variables which contribute to the differences in the children of split and intact families," and these help us considerably in understanding the child's social and psychological situation. Nass and Nass (1976, p. 319) list the following variables:

(1) the age at which the child is deprived of the parent;
(2) the sex of the single parent who rears the child;
(3) the family attitudes and social values of the parent in charge of the household;
(4) the economic consequences of the split household;
(5) the circumstances which deprive a child of either parent (i.e., death, divorce, separation, illegitimacy, military leave, etc.);

(6) the race and cultural norms of any particular one-parent household; and,

(7) the sibling composition of a one-parent family.

Single-parent problems

Beyond these seven variables, there are a number of practical problems which also have to be taken into account. The single parent who is dating may experience conflicts between childrearing duties and the demands of an active social life. Also, friends of the dating parent may, if they are childless, lead a very different lifestyle. Economic problems of single parents are generally greater than those of intact-parent families, and these may cause some intrafamily pressures.

Much has been discovered on the differences between father absence and mother absence, including the effect of a full-time working mother of small children on the intact family and on the single-parent family.

## The Role of the Father

While it is with the mother that we usually form our earliest strong attachment, we also form attachments to our father during infancy, particularly if he participates in our care, as many modern fathers do, bottle feeding the baby, rocking the baby at night, among other things (Burlingham 1973; Kotelchuck 1976; Lamb 1976). However, father's role is usually less significant than mother's during infancy and only gradually becomes of increasing significance at age two or three when we have more opportunities to interact with him. Indeed, a study by Lynn and Cross (1974) of children aged two through four indicates that, if we are boys, we prefer to play with father more than mother beginning at age two and continuing through age four. If we are girls, at two years we also show a greater preference for playing with father; but, beginning at three years, our preference reverts to mother, perhaps because of our beginning sense of gender identity and, consequently, our identification with her as a female.

Sexual identity

Father also contributes to our sense of sexual identity, and the absence of father, therefore, may affect the development of gender identity. Some research indicates that father-deprived boys tend to be passive and dependent during early childhood years and then hyperaggressive and bullying during preadolescence, perhaps as a defense against feelings of masculine inadequacy (Biller 1974; Crumley 1973; Hetherington and Deur 1972). Recent research has attempted to pinpoint specifically some behavioral and emotional characteristics that result from father absence on boys and girls. Hoffman (1971), for example, investigated the effects of father absence on conscience development in seventh-grade children.

He found that "father-absent boys obtained lower scores for all the moral indexes [and] were also rated by teachers as significantly more aggressive than father-present boys. *No differences between father-absence and father-presence were obtained for girls*" (p. 400, italics ours). In general, the evidence of the effect on girls is less clear-cut.

Some research suggests that father-deprived girls have a less clear feminine gender identity and a less positive feminine self-concept by adolescence (Hetherington 1972). On the other hand, a recent study of female college students reared in a metropolis indicates that father absence during childhood need not be associated with a negative feminine identity and self-concept during adulthood (Hainline and Feig 1978). Such disparate findings may be traced not only to the differing populations of fatherless girls who were studied but also to variations in several factors that influence the impact of father neglect or absence on a female's self-image and gender identity. The effects are least adverse (1) if the father absence stems from something unavoidable, such as business trips, illness, or death, rather than desertion, separation, or divorce; (2) if the father absence occurs during middle rather than early childhood; (3) if mother speaks well of father; and (4) if father surrogates are available (Biller 1971; Lynn 1974; Oshman and Manosevitz 1976).

## The Working Mother

Children from intact families may experience some parallels to the child of the single-parent family if the child's mother works outside the home. While years ago it was relatively rare for the mother to work, modern perspectives on womanhood as well as changing financial realities have made the working mother a common phenomenon. It is no longer unusual for a child to have a mother who works full time.

Why should the working mother be of particular concern to the child's socialization? If we examine the research on this subject, we find that although many years ago certain antisocial behaviors and psychopathologies, as well as lower school performance, were associated with children of working mothers, this is no longer the case. In a 1960 study, Stolz found that teachers rated the children of working mothers as lower in intellectual achievement than children of nonworking mothers. Hoffman (1961), in a paper written around the same time, points out that the working mother may tend to overprotect the child out of a sense of guilt and this may have an adverse effect on the child's performance in school. Times have changed, however, and recent research leads to entirely different conclusions.

Williamson (1970), for instance, found no differences in IQ between students of working and nonworking mothers. Black (1974, p. 51), in an even more cogent paper, reviewed the vast literature and concluded:

> How a child does in school is not in any major way affected by whether or not the mother works. . . . There has also been concern over the possible adverse effects of maternal employment upon the personality or behavioral problems. However, such a statement represents a finding about averages; it appears that sometimes family situations and children's reactions become worse when the mother works, sometimes there is no change, and sometimes things become better. . . . Two major factors determining a child's reaction are *the age of the child when the employment begins and the nature of the child care arrangements made.* (italics in original)

Apparently, then, factors other than the mother's working or not working are relevant to the child's socialization, psychological adjustment, and performance in school.

## Effects of Day Care vs. Home Care

As the number of young mothers entering the work force has increased, one question that has taken on particular social significance is how the socialization of the child is affected by a working mother. This question has taken on important significance in determining government policy and public spending with regard to child care, as well as by raising some important questions (Marver and Larson 1978) that affect mothers' potential employment status. Does a ''good'' mother have to stay home to care for her child and forsake all possibilities of finding some fulfillment in the working world? Do children do worse, as well, or better when their mothers are out of the home working for a good part of the day? How does the child learn to socialize outside the mother-child dyad? What factors directly or indirectly influence the children's socialization?

What all these issues often come down to, in practice, is the basic question of what effect being enrolled in a day-care facility as opposed to being raised in a home-care environment has on the child.

There are many variables including the age of the child, the type of day care, and so on. This question has been explored in detail during the past ten years as the number of young mothers entering the work force has risen dramatically. According to Lynn (1976) in 1950 women with children under 6 years of age made up about 12 percent of the work force, while in 1975, ''the participation rate for women with children un-

*Findings show that* quality *day-care provides as
good socialization as
home-care does.*

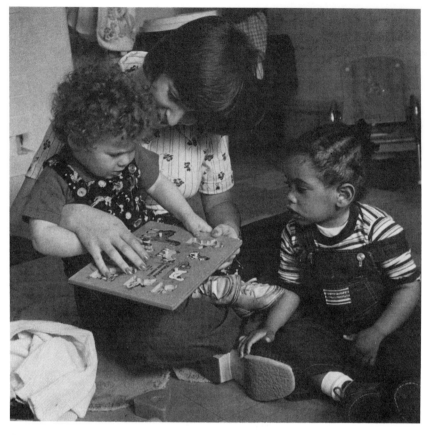

der three years was about 33 percent, approximately double the 1960
rate for this group.'' These figures reflect in part contemporary woman's
view of herself as not only full-time mothers, but as professionals or workers in the labor force too.

Types of day care

Of course there are different kinds of day care, in terms of setting, the
adults held responsible, and the quality of care. Prescott (1978) identifies
the three most common types as: care in the child's own home (61 percent); family day care (31 percent); and out-of-home center care (8 percent).

Within these types there are many different arrangements. The family day-care setting, in which children from different families may take
turns staying at one house one week and another house the next offers a
middle range of possibilities between at-home and out-of-home-care settings. The out-of-home setting, widely used by lower-income, working
mothers, has been scrutinized as a possible agent for early child socialization.

There are also different caretakers, ranging from relatives to teachers to aides to other mothers. In the child's home, for example, the caretaker may be a grandparent, aunt or uncle, sibling, or hired babysitter. These variables have some effect, to be sure, but it is impossible to pinpoint any single one as the most critical. Prescott points out too that the closer a day-care center comes to the model of a good home, the better it is for the child. Goodman and Andrews (1980) have shown the advantages of family day care for the preschool child's cognitive development.

The research results of the effects on the child of day care vs. home care has generally been encouraging for those parents who want to avail themselves of day-care facilities.

Day- vs. home-care

Findings have consistently shown that quality day care provides as good socialization as home care does and that it does not adversely affect the child's relationship with the mother. Doyle (1975) found, for example, that in terms of socialization and overall development "high quality day care for infants is an acceptable alternative child-care arrangement" (p. 656). Cornelius and Denney (1975) too found no major differences between children attending a day-care facility and those experiencing home care, except that home-care girls showed slightly higher levels of dependency than home-care boys did. They go on to point out that "since dependency is one of the dimensions on which sex differences are frequently found [see chapter 2 of this book], the results suggest that day-care children may be *less* sex-typed than home-care children" (p. 575). Of course, this conclusion is very tentative, but the important point is that day care produces no adverse effects.

The mother-child dyad

In terms of the mother-child relationship, it is clear that after the first two years of development, during which the child needs the mother's direct contact most, there is little or no adverse affect upon the relationship when the child is placed in day care. For instance, in a recent study, it was again reaffirmed that day care initiated at three years of age or later "does not affect the child's relationship with the mother" (Moskowitz, Schwarz, and Corsini 1978), and this seems to be the prevailing view.

We can conclude that the socialization of the child is not adversely affected by day care and in a certain sense may even be facilitated by increased exposure to other children and earlier play interactions. It is almost like having many brothers and sisters to play with all day.

## Summary

1. The role of the parent is almost entirely culturally determined. In practice, the way children are raised and the way they ultimately develop represents a mixture of biological, psychological, and social forces. This mixture includes many of the parents' own personality characteristics blended into the normative social fabric.

2. Baumrind has identified three representative styles of childrearing: the authoritarian, the permissive, and the authoritative approaches. Socioeconomic status may be related to the style of childrearing chosen by a parent.

3. Parents also differ in the type and degree of discipline they use with their children. The methods of discipline tend to be related to the style of childrearing that the parents use as well as their socioeconomic status.

4. There is some evidence to indicate that ordinal position in the family has an influence on the child's socialization and personality development, although the evidence at this time is still confusing and far from conclusive on any given factor.

5. Every society provides explicit and implicit channels for socialization into the role of parenting. This lifelong process encompasses the tandem processes of primary and secondary socialization: the former in the parent-child relationship and the latter through subsequent learning, as in the educational system, the media, and parenting manuals. Actual childrearing practices represent a combination of three things: how the parents were raised, what they have learned subsequently and the circumstances in which they find themselves.

6. In order to see how parents view their own roles, one can use the "clusters" of parental attitudes and values proposed by Sims and Paolucci. Each of these clusters represents a set of related and interacting attitudes and beliefs.

7. There are some practical differences between the single-parent and the two-parent home situations. There are also a number of variables, such as gender and age of child, gender of remaining parent, and the economic situation, that affect the child in a single-parent home.

8. Children from intact families may experience some parallels to the child of the single-parent family if their mothers work outside the

home. While years ago it was relatively rare for the mother to work, modern perspectives on womanhood as well as changing financial realities have made the working mother a more common phenomenon.

9. There is evidence to support the theory that quality day care may not have adverse effects on the socialization of the child.

## Key Terms

The following terms were introduced and defined in this chapter. Definitions also appear in the glossary.

authoritarian method of childrearing
authoritative method of childrearing
induction
love withdrawal
ordinal position in the family
permissive method of childrearing

## Discussion Questions

1. Although it is difficult with such matters to be fully objective, attempt to describe your own parents attitudes about childrearing in terms of the "clusters" described in this chapter. How do you think these sets of attitudes affected your socialization into adulthood? In what ways would you raise your children differently than the way you were raised?

2. Looking at your ordinal position in the family, with which findings from the literature on the effect of birth order on personality and socialization do you agree? With which do you disagree? Informally survey your classmates to determine what generalizations you can support about ordinal position, family size, and personality. Are there any clear-cut patterns about which the majority of class members can agree?

3. With the increasing number of single-parent and working-mother families in the United States today, it is not uncommon for children to

meet challenges that were relatively rare years ago. Using the single-parent families with which you are familiar, what would you cite as the major problems and challenges that the children of the family face? What enables some children to meet these challenges, while other children experience many difficulties?

4. From your reading of this chapter, list *in order of importance* what you believe were cited as the main factors affecting socialization for parenthood. Specifically, what do parents do or not do and what family factors influence how we learn to be parents?

5. Using the "clusters" mentioned above, what cultural values are reflected in the different kinds of parenting styles? What attitudes toward children are explicitly or implicitly expressed in our culture?

**Suggested Readings**

1. Evelyn M. Duvall. "Conceptions of Parenthood," *American Journal of Sociology,* No. 52 (November 1946), pp. 190–192.

A classic empirical study of mothers' views of parenthood. Duvall examined differences in the conception of the parental role by race, social class, and age of children. She found more traditional ideas of the appropriate parental role among lower class women, black women, and mothers of older children—though some role conceptions were common among all categories.

2. Daniel F. Hobbs, Jr. "Transition to Parenthood: A Replication and Extension," *Journal of Marriage and the Family,* No. 30 (August 1968), pp. 413–417.

A good example of the need to replicate social research findings. In this case, careful research suggests that while parenthood is initially stressful, the stress is not quite as severe as earlier studies had concluded.

3. Louis W. Hoffman and F. Ivan Nye. *Working Mothers.* San Francisco: Jossey-Bass, 1974.

A nicely done review of the existing sociological and psychological literature of the effect of the mother's employment on the family. The authors provide useful interpretive summaries of the sociocultural context within which maternal employment takes place.

4. E. E. LeMasters. *Parents in Modern America: A Sociological Analysis.* Homewood, Ill.: Dorsey Press, 1974.

A thorough-going, sociological analysis of the social role of parenthood. The basic starting point of this book is that parenthood is a difficult and complex role that requires greater thought and understanding than it is often given.

5. Daniel Miller and Guy Swanson. *The Changing American Parent.* New York: Wiley, 1958.

An analysis of childrearing practices that emphasizes the effects of the increasing bureaucratization of American life on the goals and methods of parenting. Although there has been some methodological criticism leveled at this work, it did serve to highlight the importance of examining empirically the effect of large-scale social change on family life in America.

6. Robert R. Sears, Eleanor E. Maccoby, and Harry Levin. *Patterns of Child Rearing.* Evanston, Ill.: Row, Peterson, 1957.

An important empirical study by a team of social psychologists on the patterning of childrearing practices and their relation to the family social background.

7. Alan Roland and Barbara Harris (Eds.). *Career and Motherhood: Struggle for a New Identity.* New York: Human Sciences Press, 1978.

With the increasing number of women who are combining motherhood with a long-term career commitment come a number of controversial and challenging questions. In this book, recognized authorities examine the historical and psychological forces that have shaped women's attitudes and roles in the past and ask how contemporary women are now overcoming this legacy.

# Chapter 11

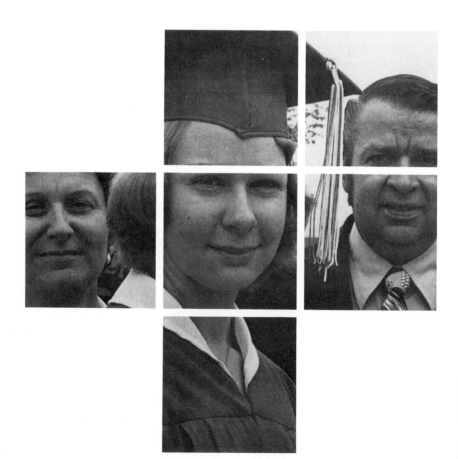

# The Mature Family: The Middle Years and Old Age

**Adults: Who Are They?**
Stages of Adulthood
Crises
**Challenges of Middlescence**
Children
Sexual Adjustments
Career
The Middle-Aged Woman
The Middle-Aged Man
**Challenges of the Mature Years**
Residence Choices
Attitudes Toward Older People
Career and Health
**Happiness in Adulthood**

## Chapter Aims:

1. To look at the sociopsychological characteristics and problems of middle age and old age.

2. To view the challenges of the ''empty nest'' syndrome, sexual adjustment, and new career options in middle age.

3. To view midlife as it affects women and men.

4. To discuss the challenges that confront the mature person: where to live, what to do after retiring, and how to adjust to the status of older person.

## Overview

There are several unique developmental challenges associated with the adult years. While childhood is a period of foundation learning both emotionally and socially, and adolescence is a time in which new social behaviors are explored and new perceptions integrated into a coherent self-image, adulthood—by far the longest period—comprises many vastly different stages of development. During these years the individual takes on major new roles and develops new responsibilities. From the role of child one may assume the roles of head of household, parent, and ultimately grandparent. A career, a vocational, or a nonvocational lifestyle is established during these years, as is growth and development in interpersonal relationships.

Middle age and old age present individuals with opportunities for growth as they respond to the conflicts and challenges in their lives.

## Adults: Who Are They?

As the children near the end of adolescence and their need for parental supervision and guidance wanes, the family enters a new phase of development and often of change. We can call this period of family life that begins approximately when the youngest child reaches high-school age and continues until that youngest child leaves the home to get married or to live on his or her own the *middle years of family life.* Following this period the parents are by themselves, a pair, alone with each other as most were at the beginning of their marriage.

We will use the term *middlescence* to describe the period typically characterized by midlife change and often crisis. It begins approximately when people are in the mid to late forties and lasts through the mid to late fifties or even into the early sixties. We will use the term *mature years* to describe the years following the resolution of the middlescence period, from about 55 years of age onward. These periods differ from person to person, and the ages we have mentioned are merely averages.

*Increasing numbers*

These years deserve a great deal of attention since there are increasing numbers of people in the United States in these age groups. We know that "the fraction of the population aged sixty and over rose from less than four percent in 1830 to fifteen percent in 1976" (Clark and Spengler 1978, p. 8). The middle-aged person, between 45 and 65, now constitutes about 20 percent of the population; so between these two age groups, we are speaking of about 35 percent of all people in the United States.

## Stages of Adulthood

Erik Erikson (1963) has tried to look at the psychosocial development of the human being over the entire life cycle. He views psychosocial development as a lifelong process, which he divides into what he calls the

*Middlescence is that time of life when parents are by themselves again as they were at the beginning of their marriage.*

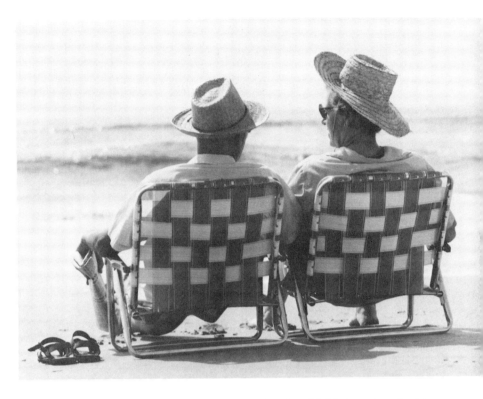

"Eight Ages of Man"

"Eight Ages of Man." These stages, which begin with birth and end with old age, are sequential and continuous. The final two stages can help us conceptualize the adult years. We will point out briefly the characteristics of the first six stages, up through early adulthood, which together provide the context for understanding the two final stages that describe challenges and goals of the middle and mature years of life.

In the earliest phase of development, according to Erikson, infants develop feelings of "Basic Trust vs. Basic Mistrust," depending upon the care afforded the child by the primary caretaker. These feelings of trust and mistrust affect one's relationships with others throughout life. Children then move on to the stage Erikson calls "Autonomy vs. Shame and Doubt." Here, children see themselves as independent creatures, capable of choosing from options within the environment. While children may require some external control and parental restraint during these early years, they must at the same time be allowed outlets to grow as independent, autonomous creatures.

During the next stage, "Initiative vs. Guilt," which extends from about three years of age to the end of kindergarten, children extend the autonomy of the second stage into initiative, the willingness to contemplate and execute new actions on their own, the emergence of an individual identity, derived from but also differentiated from the parents' identities. During late childhood, the period that immediately precedes puberty, children enter what Erikson calls the stage of "Industry vs. Inferiority." Here, children's independence increases in several ways. Greater cognitive capabilities allow more challenging of the adult's point of view; there is an increasing growth in critical thinking and in questioning about cause and effect. New social awareness gives a balance to the previous dependency on the parents, and this makes the peer group more influential. The ability to concentrate is increased, and children spend more time mastering difficult tasks. This, according to Erikson, is the time when children begin to develop a sense of industry, to try to perform complex tasks, to understand how things work.

Erikson sees the basic developmental challenge of the adolescent period as the individual's search for self-identity. He calls this stage "Identity vs. Role Confusion." It is through this search that adolescents come to see themselves as unique individuals, different from all other people. Failure to establish identity during these years leads to what Erikson calls "role confusion," and this may be responsible for many of the conflicts of adolescence. Often, the term "identity crisis" is used to describe the adolescent in transition, who is unable to feel secure with an identity.

"Intimacy vs. Isolation," stage 6, immediately follows the adolescent period, in which a sense of identity is acquired. In stage 6, "the young adult . . . is eager and willing to fuse his identity with that of others. He is ready for intimacy, that is, the capacity to commit himself to concrete affiliations and partnerships and to develop the ethical strength to abide by such commitments, even though they may call for significant sacrifices and compromises" (p. 58). Individuals who are not able to achieve intimacy during this period, who find themselves cut off from others, suffer from "a deep sense of isolation and consequent self-absorption."

Stage 7, "Generativity vs. Stagnation," refers to the conflict between the drive to prepare future generations, directly or indirectly, versus the tendency to become overabsorbed in self and unable to foster growth in others. In its broader sense, according to Erikson, generativity means not only bringing children into the world, but also such productive things as creativity. Creativity, as it is used here, does not only refer to artistic creativity, but also to the individual's ability to find new and different ways of growing, personally and along with other family members. During this stage, which would take in most of the middle-age period, individuals seek to fulfill themselves through creative, productive living as well as through satisfaction in childrearing. Some of the family troubles of this period, such as the provider-spouse who no longer wishes to expend the energy needed to make a living that the family has become accustomed to, are associated with the following conflict: "Do I have to give up my identity to maintain my family?"

Finally, there is stage 8, *Ego Integrity vs. Despair.* ''Only in him who in some way has taken care of things and people and has adapted himself to the triumphs and disappointments adherent to being, the originator of others or the generator of products and ideas—only in him may gradually ripen the fruit of these seven stages. I know no better word for it than ego integrity'' (p. 206). With these words, Erikson sums up what is perhaps the highest point of human development: the knowledge that we have contributed to our families, the world, to future generations, and to humanity. This can produce an enormous feeling of personal satisfaction in old age as one looks upon his or her children and grandchildren and sees their lives and growth, and recognizes that in part the family life that was established by the grandparents has endured generation after generation.

## Crises

What are some of the practical problems and challenges of these stages? Is there such a thing as a midlife crisis, and, if so, what are its implications in terms of the family organization and marital relationship? There are several life crises characteristic of these stages: health catastrophes that affect the entire family structure; children and grandchildren may be asked to provide supportive resources that inconvenience them; or unplanned and unwanted changes in career or economic status. All of these crises relate to our roles as parents, children, and spouses. Kimmel (1976) has suggested three common crisis points in adult life that help us understand adulthood better, and each is related to some aspect of family life.

Validation

The first one he calls, *''Where Did We Go Wrong?''* This is a conflict of late parenthood, where parents ''are tempted to look to their children's success and accomplishment—or lack of it—for validation of their own success as parents and, to an extent, for validation of their sense of generativity'' (p. 104). Whenever parents discover that their grown children did not turn out the way they wanted them to, this crisis can come about. Often, of course, it represents a failure to get from their own lives what they wanted; they may then transfer their own disappointments to their children.

*''I Hate Putting Mother in There!''* is the second common midlife crisis. Nowadays, it is not at all uncommon for grown children to place their aging parents in retirement homes or nursing homes. ''Many adults,'' Kimmel points out, ''face the difficult choices of having the parents move into their homes, trying to find support services for their parents in the community, or placing them in a nursing home'' (p. 106). This is a common conflict, one for which the increasing life expectancy and the loss of extended family structures are primarily responsible.

Finally, one of the most poignant conflicts: *''How Can I Go On?''* The

*In late parenthood, parents are tempted to look to their children's accomplishments as validation of their own success as parents.*

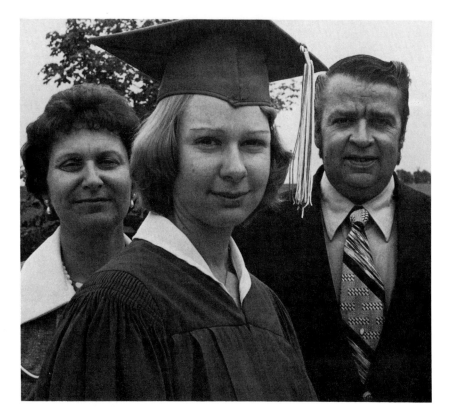

loss of a loved one, especially a spouse, results in a grief crisis, which we discuss in chapter 14.

## Challenges of Middlescence

There are several social and developmental difficulties associated with the middlescence period. As the number of years without dependent children has increased, people see possibilities for new careers. There is marital role strain, or learning to function socially as an older married person. There may be changes in health that require minor or major adjustments in lifestyle. As the changing biologies of the partners as well as the potential for conflict with their adolescent children bring pressures to bear on marriage and on family relationships, there are new psychological challenges to be met. Still some couples are able to experience what we call a "second summer," in which many of the feelings of pleasure and excitement that were with them at the beginning of their relationship are able to blossom anew.

"Second summer"

## Children

### Childrearing and Self-Image

Raising children presents many challenges to the parents. As they are socializing their children with the energy and effort that that task requires, they are being challenged by the children to see things differently. The parents must work together to make the marriage and family strong and to deal with the economic realities of life. As the children become older and more independent, they develop new attachments outside the family, and the parents may feel a sense of loss, a disruption of what they saw as the unity of the family. Furthermore, during the adult years aging is viewed much more detrimentally than it is earlier in life. Children and adolescents often lie about their age by making themselves a bit older; with the adult, just the opposite occurs. Seeing one's body age, especially as one approaches the forties and fifties, is to those who have been socialized to adore youthfulness a frightening, disheartening experience. And this change in one's appearance may occur at the very time that the children are growing in physical strength and attractiveness.

*Changes in appearance*

### Is There a Generation Gap?

One phenomenon that has been cited often by sociologists and psychologists is the *generation gap,* in which the middle generation loses touch with the younger generation over almost all basic values. Although there are some differences in values, the idea of a gap has not been borne out by the research. The value differences are actually surface ones, more associated with aspects of public presentation, such as dress, style of language, and peer-influenced taste in music and films, than with entrenched beliefs, including morality and life goals (Goodman 1969). Research generally indicates that generations agree basically about values related to roles and that they are in even closer agreement about goals (Mahoney 1976). The evidence indicates that the concept of generation gap, at least as the term is typically used, is, if not actually a myth, grossly exaggerated. In fact, on matters of public policy and personal morality, differences between social classes may be greater than those between generations (Yankelovitch 1969, 1974). Still, the differences that do exist, superficial though they may be, can become a source of conflict within the family.

### When the Children Leave Home

There have been dramatic changes in the timing of the family cycle over the past few decades. Neugarten (1977) points out that children leave home at an earlier age. The life span has lengthened because of the advances in medicine and the growing availability of health care. These changes have led to an extended postparental interval in which the husband and wife are the only members remaining in the household.

**Postparental interval**

After the period of family life in which rearing a child or children was of primary importance, the sudden absence of children in the home can be difficult to adjust to. Just as early in marriage there is an adjustment to the new role of parenthood, so too, later in life, there is an adjustment to no longer having this role. The term *"empty nest" syndrome* is used to describe the difficulties that parents may have at this time.

### Mrs. Pynchon

"When Gilda left for college, " Mrs. Pynchon explains, "Charlie and I were alone in the house for the first time in about twenty-five years. I remember when Chuck left for service and then when Pauli got married, how their room seemed so empty. We made it into a little den but never used it. But we still had Gilda at home then. With her out of the house now, there's kind of an empty feeling. Maybe we're getting bored with each other. We don't have anything to talk about or even to argue about."

On the other hand, research by Pineo (1961) and by Rollins and Feldman (1970), though subject to some methodological problems, suggests that marital satisfaction increases at this time. Many couples feel more pleased with each other after the children have left the home. Thus, the empty nest apparently offers both challenges to be surmounted and opportunities for a couple to recapture the feelings they had for each other prior to the complications of parenthood.

**Becoming grandparents**

For many, the difficulties of adjustment are eased somewhat if the parents can assume the role of grandparents. This role gives them a feeling of purpose and continuity in seeing the perpetuation of the family line and in once again experiencing the pleasures of holding an infant and of teaching a young child. There is a social prestige to be enjoyed as well, as they interact with their peers, trading stories about their grandchildren and looking at the latest photos.

## Sexual Adjustments

As people change, it may be necessary to make sexual adjustments in their relationship with each other. As Gadpaille (1975, p. 423) points out in his excellent study, *The Cycles of Sex,* where he examines individual and interspousal sexual development over the lifespan,

Society's expectations

Foremost is the task of coping with one's own and society's expectation that sex should retain little interest for those past reproductive age. That this is patently false is demonstrated by the high frequency of middle-aged sexual flings and remarriages. . . . Our Christian and Victorian heritages have steadfastly influenced the association of sex with reproduction, with the quite explicit exclusion of sex in the premarital and post-reproductive years. A discouraging number of vital middle-aged people accept as true that they should lose their interest in sex, and their expectation becomes a self-fulfilling one.

For many years the sexual expectations of married couples in middlescence were consistent with the myth of less sexual activity. Therefore, they were not, at least superficially, troubled by the decline in their marital sex life. But things have changed, middle-aged couples now have greater sexual expectations, but they may find themselves confused about their new roles and the "new norms" of middle-age sexuality. As Cleveland (1976, p. 235) points out,

Middle-age sexuality

During the past few years there has been a growing trend which is essentially a reversal of the traditional norms defining aging as a-sexual. . . . Post-parental couples are urged to develop a "second honeymoon" marriage. They are encouraged to read marital enrichment manuals, to learn new sexual arousal techniques which will make their sex lives as exciting as they had been in the early years of marriage. Rather than defining aging as a-sexual, the new norms imply a continuation of sexual behavior throughout life.

Cleveland goes on to suggest that to some extent these new norms may be just as unrealistic as the old ones, and they may place just as many social pressures upon couples to conform to values they do not feel comfortable with personally.

The important point is that sexuality in the mature marriage can still contribute to its satisfactions or to its difficulties, but it cannot and should not be taken for granted. It requires as much thought and attention as do other aspects of the marital role that are changing over the life cycle.

## Career

As the adult's life expectancy has increased and with it the promise of healthy physical functioning well into the later years, the vocational options available to the adult have changed dramatically. As Rebelsky (1975, p. xix) points out,

Vocational options

This longer life brings with it new potentials and problems. For example, a forty-year-old professor, teaching for ten years, could learn an entire new field at age forty and devote more time to the new field than he gave to the first one. Women who have opted to stay home until their children are grown are now able to be ready for entire new careers at an age when, at the turn of the century, mothers were dead or still having babies.

Career options, therefore, are an important part of the new challenges of this period.

Because of their sex-stereotyped socialization, there are considerable differences in career expectations, challenges, and adjustments between men and women in middle-age or maturity. Typically, it is the man's career—its successes, failures, rewards, and stresses—that exerts the most profound effect on the family. Some of the ways the family may be affected by the provider's career include: the need for mobility (where the family as a unit may be forced to uproot and move so that the man can rise in his profession); the requirement of maintaining certain social relationships advantageous to occupational advancement (entertaining the boss and his wife); demonstrating certain social attitudes and beliefs to which one may not really ascribe (belonging to the "right" church or club). The man's career can also contribute to a family mid-life crisis, especially where he feels he has not succeeded at accomplishing what he set out to do when he first entered his profession. Such a man may look now, after many years of relative disinterest, to finding new satisfactions in the family. But it is often a family that has learned to get by without him; the children are either leaving or have left and his wife is now looking outside the family for personal satisfaction. Thus, the husband's and wife's expectations at this period are different, and while the man is looking inside for fulfillment, the woman is seeking new fulfillments outside.

While the woman's career has not traditionally been as important a factor in affecting the family, this is changing somewhat. Now, many older women, having raised their children are eager to enter or reenter the job market. Still, an older woman may face many frustrations when she finds there is no place for her in the job market, that she has no contacts, that her skills are no longer needed. She may resent the younger women who are working, or she may mobilize her resources and try to develop the skills and contacts necessary for job survival.

## The Middle-Aged Woman

In a recent television interview, actress Lauren Bacall, when asked how she felt about aging, suggested that it has not been as much of a problem for her as for many women because she was able to afford to maintain a lifestyle consistent with what she had when she was younger. Moreover, she was still attractive, still famous, and still socially desirable. In her fifties she was receiving the same social recognition that a young starlet would.

But for some women in the age group of 45 to 65, unfortunately, this is not the case. Women during this age period, aside from experiencing some biological changes, often feel neglected by their husbands and not needed by their children. In addition to a biological menopause, some women experience a *psychological menopause,* in which they come to question the values that have remained unchallenged since adolescence.

**Increased satisfaction**

On the other hand, a survey of 100 women aged 43 to 53 from working-class and middle-class backgrounds revealed that the post-parental stage rather than being a stressful time for women, as the researchers had expected, is associated with a higher level of satisfaction than is found among younger women. Evidently, Neugarten (1977) says, caring for children at home is more taxing and stressful than having children who are married and launched. Another surprising finding of the survey was that overall, these women held relatively favorable views of the menopause and did not regard it as a major loss of feminine identity, no matter how severe their physical symptoms had been. Middle-aged women, then, are assuming new social roles, more active and quite different than the ones they had been enacting for generations.

**Continuing education**

More and more middle-aged and older women today enroll in college to continue or to begin their education during or after raising their children. Educational opportunities for older women have generally been well received. Laden and Crooks (1976) studied a group of representative mature women who went back to school to determine what influenced their decision. They found that these women were seeking self-fulfillment and personal growth and that the college experience was, on the whole, a boost to their self-esteem. Significant others, such as their children and spouses, reacted positively to their choice, although many husbands' initial enthusiasm during the spouse's first year began to lessen during the second year. Laden and Cross suggest that this decrease in enthusiasm may be "as a consequence of the woman's increasingly liberalized perception of her roles and the likely loss [to the husband] in traditional services. . . ." (p. 34).

## The Middle-Aged Man

Important research on the middle-aged man's psychosocial development has been conducted in recent years by Levinson and his colleagues at

Yale University (Levinson et al 1977). They have attempted to develop a comprehensive view of male development, from the end of adolescence to the middle forties, and Levinson himself has presented these ideas and others in a worthwhile book called *The Seasons of a Man's Life* (Levinson 1978).

Levinson and his colleagues studied 40 men representing 4 occupational groups: blue- and white-collar workers in industry, business executives, academic biologists, and novelists. After observing them for a total of from 10 to 20 hours over 2 years, the researchers constructed a five-stage theory of adult male development in the age span of about 20 to 40. These stages explain how the man's socialization has prepared him to continue developing in a fairly predictable pattern.

**Five stages**

The first stage, *leaving the family* (LF), is a transitional period between adolescence and entry into the adult world, covering roughly the ages 16 or 18 to 20 or 24. It is a transitional stage because the person is usually half in and half out of the family. He is making an effort to separate from the family and to develop a new home base, but he still maintains many deep attachments to his nuclear family of orientation. This stage usually begins at the end of high school and ends when the family balance shifts and some independence is attained. It ends, therefore, when a young man has in fact separated from the nuclear family of orientation and has begun to make a place for himself in the adult world.

The second stage, *getting into the adult world* (GIAW), begins when the center of gravity shifts to the person's new home base. This stage starts in the early twenties and extends until about age 27 or 29. It is a time of "exploration and provisional commitment to adult roles, memberships, responsibilities and relationships." According to the investigators, the overall developmental task of the GIAW period is to "explore the available possibilities of the adult world, to arrive at an initial definition of oneself as an adult and to fashion an initial life structure that provides a viable link between the valued self and the wider adult world" (p. 51).

**Settling down**

The third stage is *settling down* (SD). This period ordinarily begins in the early thirties. The man now makes deeper personal commitments, gives more of himself to his work, his family, and to a set of highly valued interests. It is during this stage that he makes and begins to pursue long-range plans and goals. This period extends until the late thirties or early forties, when various internal and external changes bring on new developments.

The fourth period is called *becoming one's own man* (BOOM), and it occurs in the middle to late thirties. The investigators see this as the high point of early adulthood. A key element is that no matter what he has actually accomplished to date, the individual feels that he is not sufficiently his own man. He feels overly dependent on the people who have authority over him or who exert great influence on him, such as his superiors at work or someone, such as a teacher, adviser, or protector, who has played the role of mentor to him until this point. The final giving up of mentors usually occurs between the ages of 35 and 39. This is the period in which a man tries very hard for a crucial promotion or other form of public recognition, such as writing a best seller or being recognized as a scientist or becoming a full professor.

Midlife transition

The fifth period is called the *midlife transition* (MLT). In this period, which may or may not involve considerable turmoil, the person asks himself if whether what he has gained up to that point is really what he wants. To Levinson and his colleagues, it is ''a matter of the goodness of fit between the life structure and the self'' (p. 57). A man may achieve his goals but find his success hollow. He has a midlife crisis if he questions his life structure and decides to modify or change it drastically. During this period, there is a sense of physical decline, the feeling of not being as young as one used to be, and a recognition of one's mortality, a sense of being old rather than young. The MLT reaches its peak in the early forties, after which there is an important period of restabilization, in which a new life structure begins to take shape. This stage, which is the outcome of the midlife transition, is currently being studied by this research team, who view it as a period with great developmental possibilities as well as a period of potential threat to the individual and the family. Some well-known men, such as Gandhi, Freud, and Jung, made great personal and professional strides during their forties, whereas others, such as Dylan Thomas and F. Scott Fitzgerald, could not manage the crisis and destroyed themselves in it.

Although the Yale team has provided a useful addition to our understanding of adult men, it should be clear that its generalizations need not be accepted unconditionally and that it is a single study using a small, selected sample.

## Challenges of the Mature Years

As people grow into the mature years, they are faced with new challenges. Often they must find new places to live. They must adapt to the way people treat them in their new status and the way they perceive themselves. There are also the conflicts and challenges associated with retirement and changes in health.

*Congregate housing offers older people opportunities to enjoy themselves together, free of the responsibilities of maintaining a home.*

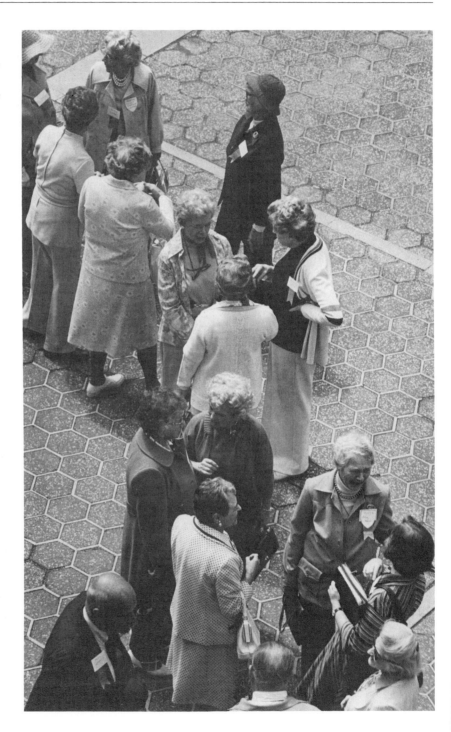

## Residence Choices

One of the major problems facing the older person or couple is where to live. Too often the apartment or home in which the family was raised is no longer appropriate to the needs of the older person or couple. This is especially true in large cities and their suburbs, where maintaining a house or renting an apartment is too great a financial burden for the older person, especially a retiree living on a pension. Even where the house is owned, the cost of heating it and the job of taking care of it may be more an effort and cost than the older person is capable of or willing to make.

Moving in

There is sometimes the option of moving in with one's grown children and their families, but this can cause conflicts and result in a generally uncomfortable living situation. Where the older person once enjoyed the role of parent and authority or head of the nuclear family, he or she is now a "guest" in the child's home. This change requires quite a bit of adjustment.

Retirement homes

Retirement homes in special communities are another option for those who can afford it. Here, while there are opportunities to socialize with one's peers, there is invariably a tendency to lose touch with the outside, multigenerational world. At the very point when interactions with young people could stimulate one's own drive and change one's perceptions and expectations of life, the retirement community cuts off the youthful world, along with its potential for important later-life socialization.

The recent concept of *congregate housing* has been receiving some attention. Congregate housing works something like a college dormitory, where elderly people share the common facilities, but have their own one-bedroom or efficiency apartments. The advantages of congregate housing are that people are not institutionalized as they would be in an old-age home and living there does not require the time, energy, and responsibilities that living on one's own in a retirement community would. It also facilitates companionship and provides many opportunities that would otherwise not be as readily available. Rosenfeld (1977) has shown how particular living arrangements of the elderly influence how they choose to dispose of their material and symbolic resources through their wills. Those who live with their families are more likely to include their families in their wills, while those who live in other arrangements are more likely to leave their resources to extrafamily persons and organizations. This may be taken as a sign that the elderly person who lives with his or her family feels a continuing sense of attachment, commitment, and responsibility.

## Attitudes toward Older People

The attitudes our culture expresses directly and indirectly about older people not only influence how older people are treated and their status but also how they feel about themselves.

Social perceptions

A number of studies have been made over the years to find out how older people are perceived by the young and by the older people themselves. These studies have focused also on whether there are differences in these social perceptions depending on the class and educational level of the respondent. Several formal questionnaires have been developed; one of the most popular is Kogan's Attitudes Toward Old People Scale, which measures some of these attitudes.

Respondents who had higher levels of education generally showed more positive attitudes toward older people (Thorson, Hancock, and Whatley 1974). However, race and social status have not been found to be significant in how older people are perceived by others (Thorson 1975).

Age discrimination is a constant problem for the elderly. Recently, federal legislation has attempted to deal with the most flagrant cases, but more subtle forms, in a society that still venerates youth, generally abound. As the elderly become an increasing proportion of the population and acquire more social and political force, it is likely that even these subtler forms will be reduced if not eliminated. And increasing the educational level of the population may also serve the same function (see Thorson, Hancock, and Whatley 1974).

## The Older Woman

"The older woman in our society," Payne and Whittington (1976) point out, "is socially devalued and subject to a number of harmful, negative stereotypes that picture her as sexless, uninvolved except for church work, and alone." In their investigation of some of the more common stereotypes, they found some supportive and much contradictory evidence when they actually examined the available research data on women in their late forties through late sixties. Table 11.1 displays some of their findings.

## Career and Health

Difficult adjustments

What prove to many older adults to be the two most difficult adjustments are retirement and poor health. The person who has for so many years worked to build a career and with it a sense of self-esteem and worth now faces the possibility of retirement and potential loss of these roles. Later there is the ever approaching prospect of poor health and of death. One may see one's contemporaries die and lose people one loves.

Table 11.1

**Stereotypes of the Older Woman**

| Stereotype | Research evidence |
| --- | --- |
| Older women are usually either widowed or have never been married. | While most older women are widowed (53%), a relatively large number (38%) are married and only about 9% have never married or are divorced. |
| The older woman is both sexually inactive and sexually uninterested. | Research clearly demonstrates that there is no reason the older woman cannot and should not be sexually active, although the extent of her activity is determined by the availability of a partner and by the partner's sexual capacity. |
| The older woman is a pleasantly plump granny, who spends her time in a rocking chair knitting or sewing. | Women have been socialized to enjoy limited types of activities and this small field of interest may persist into old age. Also, "most older women still prefer the activity they enjoyed most five years ago." |
| Women are more religious than men at every stage of the life cycle and particularly so in old age. | The stereotype is generally supported, at least insofar as religion is typically the most meaningful value in older women's lives. But church attendance begins to decline with advancing age, perhaps because of the physical difficulties of getting to church. |

Adapted from Payne and Whittington (1976).

*Today many mature women are enrolling in college to continue or begin their education after raising children.*

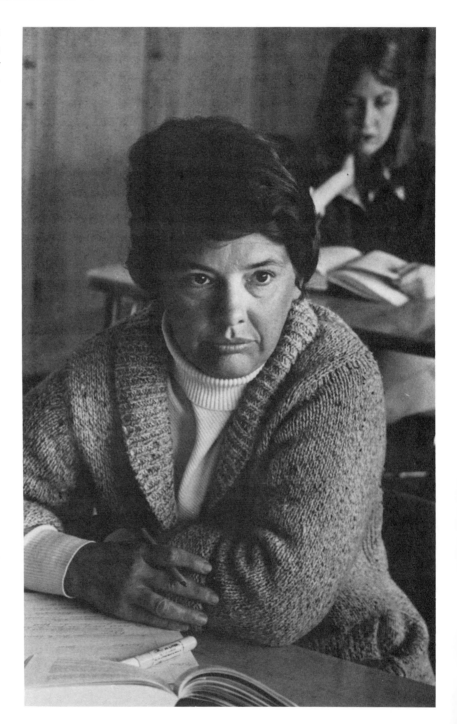

Older adults do not so much face acute disease as they do chronic illness, which results in severe and frequent restrictions on their ability to do what they want to do. Increasing health problems compound the other difficulties of old age. For example, much of the dependent behavior of the elderly is in large part attributable to the disabling effects of health problems. However, architectural and environmental considerations can considerably reduce the problems faced by older adults.

These problems may seem overwhelming, but for many there are exciting possibilities for growth during these years. People may be relieved that they have an opportunity to retire and to spend time pursuing other interests. They may be able to travel, to pursue volunteer possibilities, to paint— the possibilities are as numerous as there are retired people. Also, with the wisdom older persons have gained through their lifetimes, they may be able to relax and enjoy these later years as they achieve the ego integrity described in Erikson's stage 8.

## Happiness in Adulthood

One issue that has generated much interest is whether the middle and later years are happy years in life. We know that the suicide rate is very high after 60 years of age, but what does that tell us? Bradburn (1969), in his classic study of psychological well-being and happiness tried to investigate this question. He and his colleagues found that after 60 years of age there was a sharp increase in the number of people who described themselves as "not too happy," but it seemed that many of these respondents were affected by physical illnesses. So, we can't conclude from this that after 60 is an unhappy time of life. However, Bradburn did find that in general, at all age levels, married people tended to be happier than unmarried people, and "there is an association between overall measures of psychological well-being and measures of marriage happiness" (p. 179). In other words, if during the middle and mature years the couple is able to find fulfillment in their marital relationship, it is likely they will experience psychological well-being and a sense of happiness with life.

There is controversy about the levels of happiness one can achieve during middle age and old age. However, a recent poll of readers of *Esquire* and *Redbook* magazines sheds some interesting light on this question. Sheehy (1979) plotted the results of responses from 2 thousand men and 52 thousand women about happiness at various stages of life. As shown in figure 11.1 both men and women were perceived as experiencing higher levels of happiness later in their lifetimes than they had experienced earlier in their lives. Most interestingly, we see that the low-

Figure 11.1
**The Life-Happiness Graph**

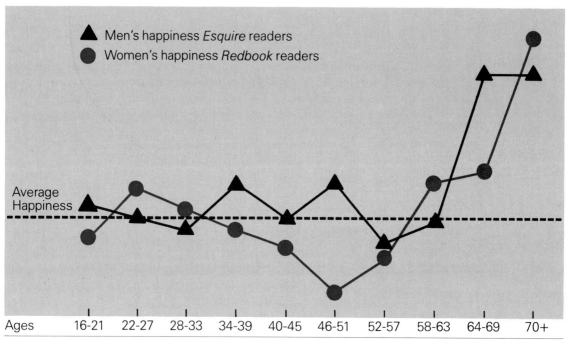

Source: Gail Sheehy, "The Life-Happiness Graph," *Esquire*, October 1979, p. 33.

est point of reported happiness in this poll is around the age of 50 and that after 60 the level of happiness rises steadily. This is not consistent with other studies that show the postsixty period to be one of trouble and unhappiness. There are several ways we can interpret these data. We could say that the respondents, who are readers of *Redbook* and *Esquire,* are atypical of the population. Or, we could note that there are increasing educational and recreational opportunities for the retiree which were not available in the past. Combined with better health care, more social services, and a more enlightened attitude toward the elderly, it may be possible now to enjoy a period of life that years ago was rife with difficulties. Perhaps we are witnessing the beginning of the end of old age stereotypes which have persisted through the years. Of course more research will be needed before we can fully understand what it takes to make the later years of life happy years.

## Summary

1. There are increasing numbers of people in the United States in middlescence and in their mature years.

2. Erik Erikson designates three stages of his ''Eight Ages of Man'' as characteristic of adulthood: intimacy vs. isolation, generativity vs. stagnation, and the final stage of ego integrity vs. despair.

3. According to Kimmel, some of the problems and questions people have to deal with as they reach the middle and the mature years are: Have we been successful as parents?; What do we do about our aging parents?; How do we deal with the death of our loved ones?

4. There are several social and developmental difficulties associated with the middlescence period.

5. Childrearing presents many challenges to the adult. As the needs of the children change, parents must adapt to these changes. Ultimately, when the children leave home, some parents experience the ''empty nest'' syndrome as they attempt to adjust to being alone together again. Many find greater marital satisfaction at this time.

6. As people change and grow older, it may be necessary for members of a couple to make adjustments in their sexual relationship for their mutual benefit.

7. Career options are an important part of middlescence as life expectancy and possibilities for good health increase.

8. While some middle-aged women may feel neglected and useless, there is evidence that many find satisfaction in these years as they accept new challenges and roles.

9. Levinson and his colleagues have developed a comprehensive view of male development from the end of adolescence to the middle forties.

10. As people move into the mature years, they are faced with new challenges: where to live, how to view themselves, what to do after retiring, and how to deal with their physical conditions.

11. Men and women report that they achieve high proportions of happiness later in life as shown in the life-happiness graph plotted by Gail Sheehy in *Esquire.*

## Key Terms

The following terms were defined and introduced in this chapter. Definitions also appear in the glossary.

congregate housing

empty nest syndrome

generation gap

mature years

middlescence

middle years of family life

psychological menopause

## Discussion Questions

1. Who are the people over 65 most significant in your life now? What observations about them and about their lifestyles are consistent or inconsistent with what you have read in this chapter? How would you imagine your life would be when you are that age? How would you like it to be?

2. Conduct an informal survey of the percentage of student population at your school that are middle age, about 45, or older. Ask some of the older students what made them decide to attend college at this time in their lives. What differences do you note between younger and older students in terms of their motivations, educational expectations, and graduation goals?

3. Is there a generation gap? Using yourself and your classmates from another generation, that is, younger or older by 15 years, compare attitudes on these subjects: premarital sex for men and women, availability of abortion on demand, extramarital relationships, whether aging parents should live with their married children and families.

4. From your reading of this chapter, what would you cite as the main developmental challenges of the middle and later years of life? Divide these into areas of personal growth and areas of marital and family functioning.

5. What are the contradictions between popular stereotypes of older women and the research findings? Why do many of these stereotypes persist?

**Suggested
Readings**

1. Vern Bengston. *The Social Psychology of Aging.* Indianapolis: Bobbs-Merrill, 1973.

The importance of this volume is that it integrates social and psychological perspectives, pointing out how the individual and the family are affected by the cultural implications of aging, as well as by psychological changes.

2. Zena Smith Blau. *Old Age in a Changing Society.* New York: New Viewpoints, 1973.

A nice blending of a review of modernization trends in contemporary society with an analysis of relevant research that critically assesses earlier views that disengagement is an important part of aging. Blau argues that old age should be an active period in one's life and also it is important to train individuals to plan for the changing role commitments that come with age.

3. Jack Botwinick. *Aging and Behavior: A Comprehensive Integration of Research Findings.* New York: Springer, 1973.

An excellent review and integration of the research literature on aging. The dividing of chapters along major topics relevant to the aging process makes this book an excellent resource both for students as well as practitioners working with the aged.

4. Elaine Cumming and William E. Henry. *Growing Old: The Process of Disengagement.* New York: Basic Books, 1961.

A theoretically oriented study of growing old by a sociologist and psychologist who define aging as a process of disengagement from and alteration of earlier social roles. This book became the focal point for much of the discussion and research of social gerontology during the 1960's and '70s.

5. Matilda White Riley, Ann Foner, and Marily Johnson. *Aging and Society* (3 Vol.). New York: Russell Sage Foundation, 1968.

An extremely ambitious attempt to pull together the research literature on social gerontology and to place it within a sociological framework which makes it more useful to those who work with the aged.

6. Irving Rosow. *Socialization to Old Age.* Berkeley, Calif.: University of California Press, 1973.

A theoretically oriented book about the socialization process of aging which suggests the lack of both social norms defining the importance of the elderly in society and appropriate role models for the aged. Rosow suggests the establishment of age-segregated communities, a view that has generated considerable controversy over the last few years.

7. Carl Eisdorfer and M. Powell Lawton (Eds.). *The Psychology of Adult Development and Aging.* Washington, D.C.: American Psychological Association, 1977.

This book, a product of the American Psychological Association's Task Force on Aging, is probably the most comprehensive outline of the subject to date. All areas of adult developmental psychology are covered, reflecting a social psychological orientation, and the book clearly points to the directions of future research.

# Part FIVE

# Family Troubles and Social Problems

We know from experience that life requires many adjustments to external demands and that even the best of lives have their share of tragedy, turmoil, and failure. In this part of the book, we will look at some of the troubles that are commonly a part of marital relations and of family life. These will range from minor problems to the dissolution of the family to the reestablishment of a new family, a second family, formed from one or from two earlier family units. We will also see that family dissolution and remarriage are increasingly common in the United States.

We will deal with a number of important issues in this part of the book, many of which one cannot fully appreciate until having experienced these kinds of profound difficulties:

- What are the chief sources of spousal conflict in married life? What can be done to minimize the effect of these conflicts on marriage?
- When marital partners are no longer able to resolve their own adjustment difficulties what can they expect from marriage counseling or family counseling? What are the goals of marriage and family counseling?
- What is the extent of intrafamily violence in the United States today? What have been identified as its main causes? What social supports are available for victims? For the prevention of violence? For the treatment of perpetrators?

- How common a phenomenon is divorce in the United States today? Does the divorce rate indicate that marriage is a failing institution?
- What is the social status of a formerly married person following a divorce? What is required to adjust to this new status? What supports does society offer the formerly married?
- When a family unit is disorganized or dissolved by the death of a member what type of intrafamilial adjustment is necessary? What is meant by "grief work"? What social supports are offered, and how do these differ from postdivorce social support?
- When a new family is formed from two dissolved families, what have been identified as some of the potential problem areas?

These key issues will be divided into three chapters. In chapter 12, "The Difficulties of Married Life: Conflict, Adjustment and Counseling," we will look specifically at the types of conflicts that produce marital discord and can eventually lead to family disruption and divorce. We will focus too on some of the patterns of marital adjustment and consider the option of family counseling, when a family is not able to work out its problems without objective professional help.

Then, in chapter 13, "Crises in the Family: Violence, Alcoholism, Divorce," we will focus on the more extreme cases and on actual dissolution following unresolved conflicts. Specifically, we will look at family violence, at the shattering effects of alcoholism, and at the emotionally difficult processes of marital separation and divorce. Finally, in chapter 14, "Reestablishing Equilibrium: Readjustment and Remarrige," we will, on a more optimistic note, see how, even after social turmoil and emotional devastation, many people are able to readjust and start over, often creating new families in the process.

# Chapter 12

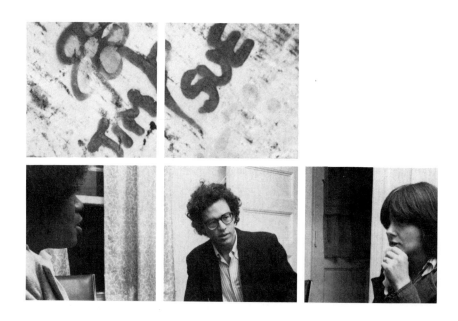

# The Difficulties of Married Life: Conflict, Adjustment, and Counseling

## Chapter Aims

1. To consider some of the chief areas of marital conflict, including jealousy, money, childrearing, and sex.

2. To look at adjustments in marriage and some of the variables that affect levels of marital satisfaction or dissatisfaction.

3. To outline the purpose and method of marriage and family therapy, thereby providing some case material to show how it helped a family in conflict.

## Overview

Stresses and changes that occur during marriage bring challenge and conflict. Jealousy, money, children, and sex are among the most common fields of battle. Factors helpful in maintaining a successful marriage are mutually satisfying marital roles and ongoing communication. People's needs and expectations change with regard to many things, including sex, and it is important, therefore, that communication be a continuous process.

When there are difficulties in marital adjustment, the couple may seek the help of a counselor, who can aid the family in defining the problems and in learning new methods of problem solving.

## Marriage: Commitment through Change

If two people entering marriage intentionally planned to maintain their happy relationship for a limited period of a year or two, there would be little need to worry about resolving conflicts, adjusting to varied new circumstances, and working out complex role transformations. Their romantic love and the adventure of a new marriage would in all probability carry them along over the year or two, and then they would part friends, each merrily on his or her own way.

Stress in marriage

However, most people enter marriage with the expectation of its being a lifelong commitment, even though statistically the odds are stacked against such an outcome. Moreover, unlike the relationship limited to a year or two, so many momentous and highly stressful events happen during the course of a typical marriage that the stresses and strains are greater than most normal people can cope with without a good deal of resourcefulness and support.

What are typical things that happen to most of us? Just to name a few, if a couple has been married ten years or more, probably most of the following have occurred at one time or another:

- change of job for one or both spouses (36)
- death of a parent (63)
- death of a friend (37)
- pregnancy (40)
- birth of one or more children (39)
- moving from one apartment to another (20)
- trouble with in-laws (29)
- sexual difficulties (39)
- personal injury or illness (53)
- marital separation (65)
- business readjustment (39)
- change in financial state (39)

The number next to each event is very significant. It is called a *life change unit* (LCU), and it indicates the relative stress that events place upon people. The higher the number the greater is the stress. Therefore, pregnancy (40) is more stressful than moving from one apartment to another (20). These numbers are part of a scientifically devised measurement system developed by Holmes and Rahe (1967). They developed a test called the *Social Readjustment Rating Scale* (SRSS), which consists of a 43-item checklist of common situations that require a change in adjustment. Using this test, several subsequent studies have shown that the higher number of stress units, the more likely a person is to become ill, depressed, or to lose the ability to function.

With all the stresses in marriage, is it possible to maintain a successful marital relationship over a period of years? The answer is yes, but a qualified yes in the sense that the two marital partners have to be willing to work at it in an intelligent, goal-directed way. They have to become adept at marital adjustment.

## Conflicts in Marriage

As we mentioned in chapter 7, maintaining a functional marriage essentially involves the ability of two people to adapt to compatible role situations. You have in any marriage two individuals who are unique personalities, each with certain set beliefs, values, and expectations, in a situation that to some extent is always changing in response to internal and external forces. While in the course of living and growing, the members of the paired relationship change, they do not necessarily change at the same time and rate as does the relationship. Problems occur in all marriages; successful marriages are those in which these problems are met and dealt with. As a team, the partners have to cooperate to play out and reinforce each others' roles. When one partner, however, feels some behavior is within his or her role and the other doesn't, a conflict may arise.

### Elaine and Lee

Elaine and Lee have been having a lot of difficulties lately in their relationship. Elaine complains that Lee is not understanding enough, that he doesn't listen to her "legitimate complaints." Lee, on the other hand, says that Elaine has become a "whine," a "nag," always complaining, complaining, complaining. We find, as we look at the situation in more depth, that Elaine's complaints are totally compatible with her perceived role in the relationship. "A woman," she says, "should be able to complain to her man, and he should be willing to listen, should be sympathetic." She views this as a masculine-feminine distinction. Lee, however, sees the role of the woman as representing a totally independent person, even more independent than a man, and he views the complaining as a sign of dependency. In this situation there is a conflict between the two partners' perceptions of the role of the wife.

**Sources of conflict**

Marital conflicts may occur over virtually anything. Couples fight about who takes out the garbage, in-law problems, and career vs. marriage. Some areas that can lead to severe difficulties are jealousy, money, childrearing, and sex. However, despite the specific issue over which a battle is fought, the basic source of most difficulty is that marriage is an intimate, interpersonal relationship between two separate individuals who are not only themselves constantly changing and not always jointly in the same direction or at the same rate, but who also live in a complex and shifting social environment that is often beyond their control. For example, war, inflation, recession, illness, or a car accident can occur and put a severe strain on a marriage. While the courtship and mate selection process often reduces personal and social background differences, it does not eliminate them. These other surface issues, such as who takes out the garbage, become the concrete manifestations of the difficulties of intimate pair living. They are important in themselves, but they must also be seen in the proper context.

## Jealousy

When jealousy becomes firmly entrenched in a relationship it can be a vicious enemy, chipping away at the very foundations of trust and love that hold the two partners together. As a married couple conflict when one or both partners are jealous, it is very difficult to resolve the problem, since any explanation is turned away as untrue and the jealousy becomes even stronger.

What does jealousy really mean? How does it survive in a relationship? What part does it play? In our society by far the single greatest reason for jealousy is the standard of sexual exclusivity in monogamous relationships. Most *jealousy* centers on the belief that the other person is sexually interested in or involved with someone else. It may be a general belief that the other person is carrying on, or the jealous party may feel that his or her partner is involved with someone in particular. In most jealousy situations, one partner acts as the accused and the other as the accuser. Sometimes each partner may play a role alternately, but typically each plays the same role in every jealous encounter. As the situation

**Sexual exclusivity**

*Jealousy can chip away at the foundation of love and trust that holds two partners together.*

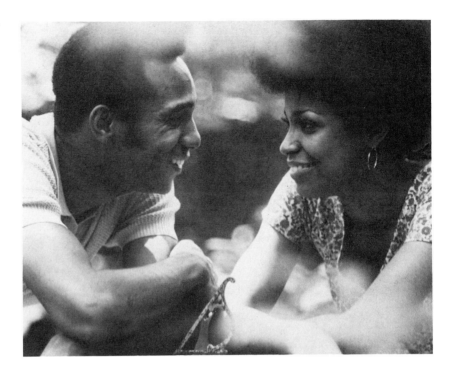

continues over a period of time, the partners may become accustomed to playing their roles.

Or jealousy may sometimes be of a nonsexual quality. The accuser may feel that someone else is overstepping his or her role and providing for needs of the accused that should be provided within the relationship. Generally, anything that threatens to weaken the relationship bond can become a possible cause for jealousy (Clanton and Smith 1977). For instance, even though he doesn't feel sexually threatened, a husband may become jealous when his wife has an intellectual discussion with another man. The fact that she is having some of her needs met by someone else weakens the bond between them.

There are a number of scenarios about jealousy that can be acted out in a relationship. In some cases the jealousy becomes pervasive and provokes fighting in all related and tangential areas. "We just can't get along about anything because of this one thing," a partner may complain. Sometimes the jealousy represents a more deeply imbedded conflict, and the partners are in effect denying the deeper conflict by emphasizing the jealousy. Sometimes jealousy may be positive although caution should always be taken. Even where Jane says, "Douglas is kept on his toes because he always thinks either I'm interested in some other guy or some other guy is interested in me," seeds of discord are planted by the presence of the jealousy.

Partners don't always act to minimize the level of jealousy in a relationship. On the contrary, there may be an intentional game to increase the amount of jealousy. Jane feels more important, more sexual, more desired precisely because Douglas is jealous. Were he not to be jealous or not show it, she would think that he wasn't interested in her, that he didn't find her attractive and couldn't possibly imagine any other man being interested in her.

*Minimization of jealousy*

## Fighting over Money

One of the main areas of marital conflict is money. There may be disagreement about how to spend the money available, that is, a dispute about priorities, or angry exchanges about the fact that there is insufficient money to meet the couple's needs.

Clearly, it does not matter significantly how much money is objectively available: rich people fight about money just as much as poor people. What is important is whether or not the couple's expectations and assignment of roles about who makes spending decisions, how they are made, and what takes priority has been implicitly or explicitly worked out.

*The traditional breadwinner*

A number of cultural factors have an influence here. Traditionally, in our culture, the man has been the chief breadwinner, the one who "brings home the bacon," as the old adage states. In recent years this situation has been changing dramatically as we pointed out in chapter 7. More and more women have been entering the work force as at least secondary breadwinners. However, these two-paycheck couples have not necessarily worked out more satisfactory ways of dealing with the sharing of financial responsibilities or the division of their monies. In fact, sometimes when both partners are earning a living, there are more intense conflicts at home about how the money should be spent. Caroline Bird (1979), in her book *The Two-Paycheck Marriage*, points out that the working wife's new status has changed the entire family configuration, including the delegation of power, sex roles, childrearing responsibilities, and more. These changes can actually encourage money conflicts for a number of reasons.

Money Is Power!   Throughout history wealth has been recognized as a source and a sign of power. Moreover, when a person has money, he or she *feels* powerful. Expressions like "Money buys power" or "Every person has a price" reflect this recognition.

Part of the power struggle in a marriage, therefore, may be waged over money.

### Adrienne and Mort

Although Adrienne earns as much as Mort, he feels that some of the decisions about how to spend the money should fall primarily on his shoulders, because, as he puts it, he ''is more knowledgeable about the economic facts of life.'' Adrienne and Mort had a big fight recently when she wanted to invest in a piece of property and he did not think it a wise investment. He said that what he particularly resented was that she made the decision without consulting him. ''But it's my money,'' she insists. ''I earned it.''

''That's not the point,'' he rebuts, failing to state what the point is.

In fact, the point is that Mort feels undermined, that his ''masculine'' power has been eroded because Adrienne makes decisions about money without consulting him. There is also a sexual bias here too. Mort doesn't feel women know enough about how to handle money and therefore feels they shouldn't make important money decisions without consulting a man. He wouldn't say this aloud for fear that his sex-stereotyped views would appear ''old-fashioned,'' which he hates to admit he may be. However, his sexist attitude does pervade his thinking, and his wife knows it. In one way, her spending the money on her own reflects her attempt to gain power over him to show him that she can handle things quite well on her own.

Money Is Love!   Early in life we learn to feel appreciation and love when our parents give us presents. Love and presents become associated in the mind because the giving of parents is interpreted as the concrete

A manifestation of love   manifestation of love. Many people, no matter how much they are given, still feel deprived in some areas. Later, when they begin to earn money, they use this new mercantile commodity to buy things in order to make themselves feel good. For instance, when people are depressed, they may go out and buy some presents for themselves. These may be clothing, hobby equipment, jewelry, or just a frivolous indulgence that they would not ordinarily spend money on.

When the person you love, therefore, is telling you that you don't deserve things and that you shouldn't be spending so much money, you may feel that that person is saying to you: ''You don't deserve to be loved. I don't want to give this to you.'' This reaction can provoke deep feelings of hurt, resentment, and isolation, feelings that the other person really wants to deprive you of love.

## Derek and Linda

Derek resents it terribly every time Linda yells at him about the money he is spending on his hobby: fixing up old cars. She just can't understand, he tells his friends, how important this is to him. On a deeper level, he feels very hurt because it is as if his wife were saying, "You don't deserve to have that fun. I don't want you to have that pleasure in life." But from Linda's point of view, she resents the time Derek spends on his cars. She considers it foolish and sees it as taking time away from her. It's not so much the money to her as it is the time. And yet, neither spouse can fully communicate his or her feelings to the other.

Self-esteem

Money Is Status!  It is unfortunate but true that in our society people are often judged by how much money they have. Thus, one's self-esteem can be tied in with one's finances. Fighting over money, in the marital relationship, may be a way of symbolically fighting about self-worth. For example, when Derek insists on spending the money for his cars, he is saying, "I want this prestige among my friends. I don't want to be viewed as a person who doesn't deserve to pursue his hobby."

## Fighting about Childrearing

Another potential source of conflict in a marital relationship is children. The conflicts may begin even before the child is conceived, at the point when a couple cannot agree whether or not to have children at a particular time. Then there may be areas of conflict about how large a family to have. Questions regarding discipline, education, and expectations of what the child should do may also become potential sources of conflict. Abramowitz (1977) has pointed out that many of the parents' anxieties arise because they cannot see how trends in economic development and large-scale social conditions are affecting their childrearing attitudes. For example, the effects of poverty, inflation, and job discrimination may bring pressures to bear on raising children.

The first child

The arrival of a new child, especially the first child, invariably puts a strain on a couple. As two people learn their new parenting roles, they may be giving less attention and less time to each other. There may also be significant changes in their sexual functioning, as well as changes in the lifestyle to which they have become accustomed. As Nass and Weidhorn (1978) point out, "One may discover, as more and more couples are doing nowadays, that although one likes children, one does not like them enough to put up with a cramped lifestyle'' (p. 95).

When a child is having some problem—either physical, emotional, or intellectual—the parents, in addition to being concerned for the child, may begin to blame each other for what they perceive is the problem. No parent wants to feel that he or she has created a ''deficient'' child. Araoz (1977) makes the interesting point that within the family context, very often the ''disturbed'' child, who has not fulfilled the parents' expectations of what they want their child to be, becomes the ''disturbing'' child, as the stability of the marital relationship is disrupted in irrational counterattacks of blame.

**The disturbing child**

One other area of childrearing that tends to lead to conflict occurs as children reach adolescence. Because they are now at a period where some rebellion against their parents is commonplace, this can lead to an invisible but persistent tension in the home, which can precipitate fighting between the parents and make it even more difficult to help the child adjust to his or her situation.

**Adolescence**

## Fighting about Sex

Sex is such an integral part of the marital relationship that it inevitably becomes a source of heated conflict, either directly or symbolically. Sex is sometimes used as a weapon, to be withheld as punishment or offered to force compliance of the partner. It is also a source of many arguments. When the partners are dissatisfied sexually, they may take it out on each other, and this conflict in turn makes the hope of sexual reconciliation even less likely. It is a vicious cycle. Edwards and Edwards (1977) studied 110 married couples over a three-month period. They found that there was a functional relationship between arguing and sex: that ''couples who engaged in sexual intercourse at a higher rate than they argued described their marriage as 'happy.' Marriages with rates of argument higher than rates of intercourse described their relationship as 'definitely unhappy' '' (p. 187).

**Use of sex**

These findings should not be interpreted as implying that marital satisfaction or dissatisfaction rests primarily on how well or how poorly the couple is functioning sexually. Rather, the conclusion of the study may stem from the fact that a successful, enjoyable, satisfying sexual relationship involves a series of intimate communications between spouses, requiring great subtlety, a warm feeling, and considerable cooperation between the two partners—in fact, those same interpersonal characteristics that are also required for general marital satisfaction. In effect, the sexual relationship may be conceived of, in part, as a barometer of the overall marital relationship.

*After the arrival of chil-*
*dren, couples must make*
*adjustments to the pre-*
*parental lifestyle to which*
*they were accustomed.*

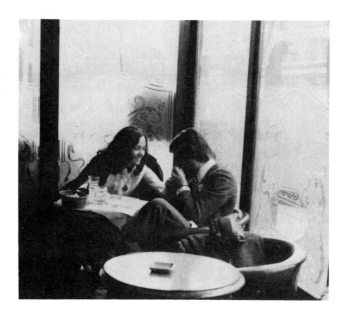

## Other Areas of Potential Conflict

In-law problems

The specific areas of conflict we have covered are but a fraction of the things that couples fight about. In-law problems are common areas of conflict. The long process of separating from one's nuclear family of orientation and the attachment to one's mother or father may involve jealousy or competitiveness on the part of the spouse. Also, a spouse's parents' attempts to intervene in the marriage—for example, in giving gratuitous advice about childrearing, where to live, or how to keep the home clean—can foster a great deal of resentment.

### Nina and Fred

"It's not that I hate Fred's mother," Nina insists, "although she is a pretty hatable person if there ever was one. What I resent is that Fred, who is, or should be, above all, my husband and the father to our daughter—what I resent is that he would do something she'd tell him instead of something I'd tell him. He thinks his mother knows everything, especially about how to raise our daughter."

One last point should be mentioned. Many conflicts are the result of small differences that multiply as a consequence of poor communication or incorrect perceptions. For example, Kleinke (1977) has found that hus-

*The arrival of children puts a strain on couples who must adjust their way of relating to each other to accommodate the child's needs.*

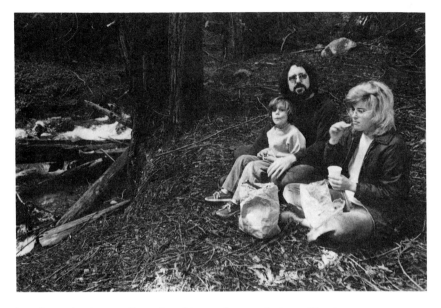

bands and wives still assign blame for marital conflict by stereotyping: blame in the area of housekeeping conflict is assigned to the wife and blame for economic conflict to the husband. It is getting beyond this point that leads us to the subject of marital adjustment.

## Marital Adjustment

Because many marriages do work, with one or both partners experiencing relatively high levels of marital satisfaction, we can infer that there are ways of adjusting to and resolving the conflicts that crop up in marriage. There have been dozens of studies of marital satisfaction, from the classic 1939 work *Predicting Success and Failure in Marriage* (Burgess and Cottell, 1939) to more sophisticated statistical analyses of marital role competencies as indicators of satisfaction (Nye and McLaughlin 1976). Mari-

An ongoing process          tal adjustment is an ongoing process made necessary because there are two different individuals who, although paired, are probably developing at different rates and, on some matters, even in different directions. All of this personal change occurs within a continually changing social context, only a part of which is under their control. Hence, marital adjustment is a complex psychosocial process that involves a high level of partner cooperation.

Blood and Wolfe (1960), in their comprehensive study of husbands and wives, investigated some of the factors that contributed to marital satisfaction. Some of their findings revealed interesting social, cultural, educational, and other factors associated with marital adjustment. Table 12.1 shows, for example, that education is closely related to marital satisfaction. The higher the educational level, the greater is the satisfaction. Occupation and income, which are often thought to be associated with levels of satisfaction, basically are not.

The number of children too affects marital satisfaction, as we see in table 12.2. ''Children are a source of strength in marriage provided there are not too many of them,'' Blood and Wolfe (p. 85) point out. ''Both by the number of children ever born and by the number currently living at home, three is the magic number'' (p. 86).

Coping with stress

But beyond specific factors such as these, what is most important to marital satisfaction over the course of a marriage is the ability of the partners to adjust to a variety of changes and to cope with a number of stresses.

## Role Competence

In general, it is believed that marital satisfaction depends largely on the ability of the marital partners to define and enact mutually satisfying

Table 12.1

**Marital Satisfaction, by Husband's Occupation, Income, and Education**

| Marital satisfaction by | | Blue collar | | White collar | |
|---|---|---|---|---|---|
| Husband's occupation: | | Low | High | Low | High |
| | | 4.61 (155) | 4.61 (165) | 4.85 (81) | 4.80 (155) |
| Husband's income: | | Under $3,000 | $3,000 —4,999 | $5,000 —6,999 | $7,000 —9,999 | Over $10,000 |
| | | 4.32 (57) | 4.75 (165) | 4.80 (185) | 4.61 (82) | 4.72 (54) |
| Husband's education: | Some Grade School | Grade School Graduate | Some High School | High School Graduate | Some College | College Graduate |
| | 4.29 (62) | 4.42 (78) | 4.56 (124) | 4.90 (182) | 4.96 (55) | 5.04 (51) |

Adapted from: Blood & Wolfe (1960).

Table 12.2

**Marital Satisfaction, by Number of Children Ever Born and by Number Presently in Family**

| Marital satisfaction | Number of children | | | | | |
| --- | --- | --- | --- | --- | --- | --- |
| | None | One | Two | Three | Four | Five+ |
| By number ever born | 4.50 | 4.77 | 4.78 | 4.93 | 4.60 | 3.90 |
| | (80) | (140) | (171) | (96) | (43) | (29) |
| By number presently in the family | 4.32 | 4.67 | 4.86 | 5.16 | —4.86— | |
| | (164) | (132) | (147) | (76) | (37) | |

Source: Blood & Wolfe (1960).

Role-competence theory

marital roles, as we examined in chapter 7. Nye and McLaughlin (1976) have developed a role-competence theory of marital satisfaction that is based on the notion that "the greater the role competence of a role player (as reported by his or her spouse), the greater the marital satisfaction of the role enactor's spouse" (p. 119). In other words, a husband or wife is satisfied to the extent that he or she feels the spouse is satisfying certain role expectations. As shown in figure 12.1, Nye and McLaughlin go on to propose that when we break down marital roles into the categories we presented earlier in the book—namely, the therapeutic, child socialization, child care, recreation, housekeeper, provider, and sexual roles—we can assign relative values to each one in terms of the importance of role competence in that area to overall marital satisfaction. Specifically, Nye and McLaughlin (1976, pp. 198–99), point out,

> Some roles predict marital satisfaction much better than others. For both husbands and wives, effectiveness in the therapeutic role is the best predictor of male and female satisfaction with marriage. Competence in child socialization also predicts male and female marital satisfaction about equally for both sexes.
> . . . The other roles have quite different relationships to marital satisfaction. For wives, the husbands' competence in the recreation role predicts satisfaction as well as does the child socialization role but wives' competence in it has no value for predicting satisfaction of the husbands. It might be remembered that these women have one or more young children at home. They may be grateful to have a man competent in organizing materials and schedules for recreation outside the home.

Figure 12.1

**Husband-Wife Evaluations of Competence and Marital Satisfaction**

How important are the evaluations of the husband or wife of the *other's* competence in certain role areas in terms of their marital satisfaction?

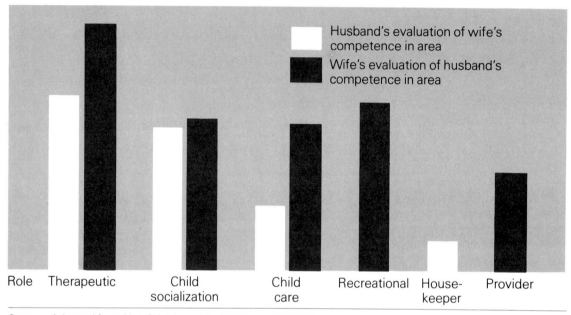

Source: Adapted from Nye & McLaughlin (1976, pp. 198-199)

In other words, when we look at marital satisfaction through the role-competence perspective, we are actually asking how well or poorly each partner is enacting the roles that the other considers most important. And, we note that these important roles may differ between husbands and wives.

## Communication

Change in
expectations

In chapter 7 we explored the ingredients of effective interspousal marital role communication. We should only add two things at this point. First, since both spouses' role expectations change during the course of the marriage, especially in response to conflict situations, it is necessary that they communicate to each other their new role expectations and how these can be enacted. Insofar as communication is used as a basis for this adjustment, there is a reciprocal socialization process occurring, in which each spouse becomes ''a strong socializing agent for the other'' (Cronkite 1977). In other words, through communication each partner is socializing the other as he or she is changing, in order to allow the change or the adaptation to it to be mutual.

### Nancy and Bruce

When Nancy first went back to work, she took Cary and Linette to school in the morning before rushing to catch the 8:11 to the city. She never thought of asking Bruce to take the kids, even though his work schedule was more flexible, because it had been her responsibility for years. But as this arrangement became too straining, she brought up the matter with Bruce, who at first said it would be *better for the kids* if their mother took them, but then admitted that he didn't really believe that. As they discussed it, Bruce began to realize that Nancy was a working wife now and that he was the husband of a working wife. These roles would require new duties and expectations— in short, some new social learning. Through their communication, they were able to socialize each other for their new roles.

The second point we want to add here is that communication styles differ among classes. We noted earlier how childrearing and other socialization skills are class-related, so too are the way spouses communicate with each other. Hawkins, Weissberg, and Ray (1977), for example, found several social-class differences in the way messages are communicated not only in content but in tone as well.

## Sexual Adjustments

As the sexual needs and interests of one or both of the partners change, there are two options. One is to remain secretive, embarrassed, and ashamed and not communicate these new feelings to one's spouse. The other is to speak frankly and forthrightly, telling one's husband or wife what is now desired and expected. Sex researcher John Money (1977) has even suggested ''it would be very good for us if we could make a detailed and explicit contract of what it is we expect to give and get from one another. But we seldom do. Instead we vaguely assume that she or he will want what I want and I will want what she or he wants.'' These assumptions may lead to many conflicts.

*Making assumptions*

Figure 12.2
## How Frequency of Intercourse is Related to Satisfaction with Marital Sex

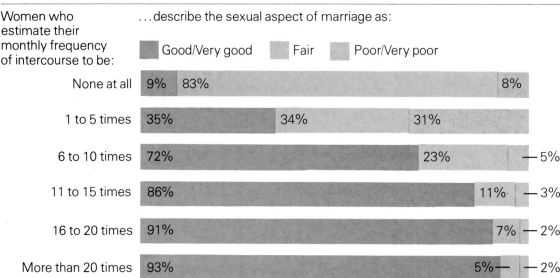

Women who estimate their monthly frequency of intercourse to be: ...describe the sexual aspect of marriage as:

Good/Very good    Fair    Poor/Very poor

| | Good/Very good | Fair | Poor/Very poor |
|---|---|---|---|
| None at all | 9% | 83% | 8% |
| 1 to 5 times | 35% | 34% | 31% |
| 6 to 10 times | 72% | 23% | 5% |
| 11 to 15 times | 86% | 11% | 3% |
| 16 to 20 times | 91% | 7% | 2% |
| More than 20 times | 93% | 5% | 2% |

The more frequently intercourse occurs each month, the more likely women are to say that sex is "good" or "very good." When it occurs 16 or more times a month, 9 out of 10 women say they have a good sexual relationship.

Source: Levin, R.J. & Levin, A. Sexual pleasure: the surprising preferences of 100,000 women. *Redbook Magazine*, 1975 (September), 145, 5.

There is a rich literature on what makes a sexually satisfying marital relationship. We suggested earlier, for instance, that when the frequency of sexual intercourse is greater than the frequency of marital arguments, the levels of marital happiness are higher. Levin and Levin (1975), working with the enormous resources of *Redbook Magazine,* analyzed a detailed survey of over 100,000 women who answered sex questionnaires that were published in one issue. Figure 12.2 shows that, from their analyses of the respondents, the more frequently intercourse occurs each month, the more likely a woman is to say that her sex life is "good" or "very good." They also found that among married women sexual satisfaction decreases slowly over the years, as shown in figure 12.3, from approximately 82 percent who feel very satisfied the first year to 67 percent after the tenth year of marriage. Not surprisingly, their data suggest too that frequency of orgasm increases marital sex satisfaction, although, "approximately 3 out of every 10 women who never experience orgasm have also rated the sexual aspect of their marriages as good. There were some other interesting results too. As shown in figure 12.4, communication between spouses was shown to be positively related to sexual satisfaction: "the less frequently wives can discuss their sexual feelings and desires with their husbands, the less likely are they to report the sexual aspect of marriage as 'good' or 'very good' " Levin and Levin (1975, p. 5). Finally, as we might expect, there was a high correlation between general marital satisfaction and sexual satisfaction, indicating clearly that the latter is a significant part of the former.

Extramarital relationships

Extramarital sexual relationships are a fact of life for many couples, and we should consider their effects on marriage. Extramarital relations are generally frowned on, however, although the social perceptions of an "errant" spouse depend largely on whether it is a casual fling or an affair also characterized by love and affection (Hartnett, Mahoney, and Bernstein 1977). A double standard exists too, where "cheating" by a wife is

Figure 12.3
**How Communication in Marriage is Related to Satisfaction with Sex**

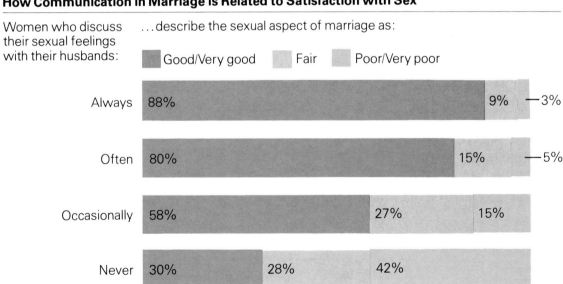

Women who discuss their sexual feelings with their husbands:

...describe the sexual aspect of marriage as:

■ Good/Very good    Fair    Poor/Very poor

| | Good/Very good | Fair | Poor/Very poor |
|---|---|---|---|
| Always | 88% | 9% | 3% |
| Often | 80% | 15% | 5% |
| Occasionally | 58% | 27% | 15% |
| Never | 30% | 28% | 42% |

The less frequently wives can discuss their sexual feelings and desires with their husbands, the less likely are they to report the sexual aspect of marriage as "good" or "very good" and the more likely are they to describe it as "poor" or "very poor."

Source: Levin, R.J. & Levin A. Sexual pleasure: The surprising preferences of 100,000 women. *Redbook Magazine*, 1975 (September), 145, 5.

Figure 12.4
**How Sexual Satisfaction Varies over the Years of Marriage**

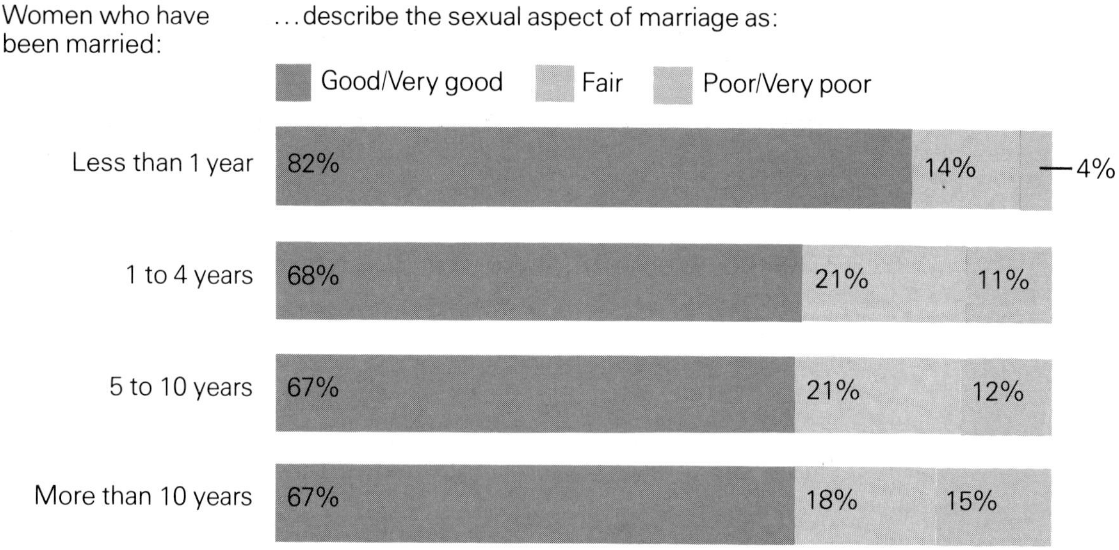

Women who have been married:   ...describe the sexual aspect of marriage as:

Good/Very good    Fair    Poor/Very poor

Less than 1 year    82%    14%    —4%

1 to 4 years    68%    21%    11%

5 to 10 years    67%    21%    12%

More than 10 years    67%    18%    15%

It seems hardly surprising that the overwhelming majority of women who have been married less than a year rate sex as "good" or "very good." But, astonishingly, almost 7 out of every 10 women continue to describe sex as "good" or "very good" regardless of how many years they have been married.

Source: Levin, R.J. & Levin, A. Sexual pleasure: the surprising preferences of 100,000 women. *Redbook Magazine*, 1975 (September), 145, 5.

perceived as worse than "cheating" by a husband. Interestingly, although it may be considered nonnormative, the majority of married people, with men tipping the balance heavily, have had sexual relations outside the marriage during the period of the marriage (Ross 1978). This situation will be explored when we look at marital dissolution.

The phenomenon of *swinging* falls somewhere in between marital fidelity and extramarital relationships. Swinging is defined as "the pursuit of sexual activities with extramarital partners by both spouses at the same time and usually in the same place" (Walshok 1971). In New York City, a small club called "Plato's Retreat" opened in 1974 for the purpose of introducing paired couples to other paired couples who want to swing. Within three years the club was so successful that over 50 similar clubs opened in the city, and most of them are still in business today.

The emergence of a form such as swinging is interesting because it is neither marital nor extramarital. How does this form affect the marriage relationship?

In what is probably the best research study on swinging, Henshel (1973) investigated which spouse first becomes aware of swinging, which one tends to initiate it, and who makes the final decision to swing. She found that the husband alone "made 59% of *all* the initial decisions, 28% were joint decisions, while only 12% were made by the women" (p. 78). This could lead us to conclude that while swinging is often cited by couples as a part of their marital sexual adjustment, it is actually more of a coercion of the wife by the husband. Many women, it was found in this and subsequent research, merely went along with their husbands' wishes in order to please them.

## When Adjustment Fails

Sometimes it becomes necessary for the spouses to seek outside professional help. This may happen because of an unmanageable adjustment problem, a set of role conflicts, or a general range of conflict and inadaptability that has come to permeate the marital relationship. In any case, at the point when outside help is needed our society offers outlets. In one subculture, it may be customary to consult with the clergyman; in another, the entire extended family may be called in to help; in a third, a physician, psychiatrist, or psychologist may be the appropriate person for the task. The partners in a troubled marriage invariably recognize that

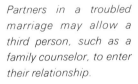

*Partners in a troubled marriage may allow a third person, such as a family counselor, to enter their relationship.*

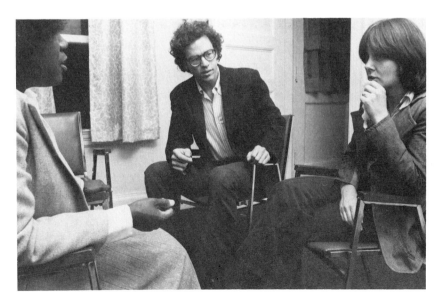

their respective roles are threatened and may be willing to allow a third person into their intimate dyad.

## Marriage and Family Counseling

Although the term *family counseling* or *family therapy* includes a range of related practices, such as marriage counseling, sexual counseling, child therapy, parent-child counseling, and counseling more than one family member in a joint session, we will focus our discussion on specific efforts to help the marriage partners and their children work out conflicts between themselves and other family members.

Nathan Ackerman's (1958, p. 9) historical comment helps explain how family therapy as a system compensated for the weaknesses inherent in the individual therapy approaches.

> We have somehow kept ourselves so busy, so preoccupied with studying and treating the suffering of individuals, that we have, in effect, blinded ourselves to the significance of the concurrent struggles of the family for mental health, and to the way in which the ongoing content of family experience affects the emotional struggles of its adult members. I do not mean to imply that the treatment of the individual patient, the alleviation of the very real sufferings of a single human being, is unimportant or unnecessary. To the contrary. But I do question the effectiveness of any such treatment that does not take into consideration the sum total of this individual, which must of necessity include his environment, and his interactions with it.

Nathan Ackerman is the founder of family therapy in the United States.

In practice, family therapy involves the joint participation of several family members. It is used descriptively for all settings in which family members are working together, under the guidance of a professional, to solve individual or family problems. However, most social scientists also emphasize the conceptualization of personality or conflict theory from a *family systems point of view,* that is, by looking at the family as an organic, functional unit, as opposed to looking at the individual's problems separate from the family functioning (Feldman 1976).

Therapeutic family interventions may take place in a therapist's office, in a school, in a clinic, in the family's home, in an institution, or in some other setting. Such interventions may be provided by a psychiatrist, counselor, psychologist, teacher, social worker, paraprofessional, or any other concerned professional helper.

What brings the members of a family to therapy? One member may have already been in therapy and have encouraged the other members to begin. Sometimes in the course of therapy a person realizes that his or her problem is one that is shared by the entire family. Or, the entire family may have made the decision to begin therapy based on some recent family crisis. In any case, "family therapy begins at the first moment of the therapist's contact with the family" (Prosky 1974, p. 45). The therapist will usually, from the beginning, convey the feeling that he or she is there for the entire family, not to take sides with individual members against other members of the family. By showing themselves as concerned but neutral individuals, therapists establish the comfortable, open setting in which productive family interventions can take place.

## Some Family Therapy Goals

Although the specific goals of therapy differ from family to family depending on the nature of the conflicts, we can offer a few general statements about the typical goals of family intervention approaches as opposed to the goals of individual therapy.

1.  The family should be taught to communicate openly with each other. This goal includes the principle of "constructive emotional honesty" (Spotnitz 1976) and learning to read verbal and non-verbal cues of other family members.
2.  The socioemotional intactness of the family should be preserved wherever possible. Even in cases where physical or legal separation becomes necessary, such as a family member leaving for prison or the military, a divorce, or an illness that confines a family member to a distant place, there are opportunities to maintain contact and to allow that family member to remain a part of the family.
3.  The family should learn constructive new ways of solving its problems. The family members should learn to come to grips with their conflicts by observing the way the family therapist helps them to do so.
4.  Each family member has to be able to individuate him- or herself from the family as a total unit.

In the following pages we will look briefly at each of these goals: improving intrafamily communication, maintaining intactness, increasing problem-solving skills, and facilitating individuation.

### Effective Communication    In many family situations, one of the major difficulties is the inability of members to communicate effectively

with each other. Communication has been stifled by years of inactivity and misunderstandings within the family. Many aspects of family relationships have a tendency to get "stuck" in patterns, and family communication is no exception. As Bell (1975, p. 177) points out,

> Many of the ways in which parents learn to communicate in early days during a child's infancy are clung to as the children and the parents mature. So we find later, where we may now be dealing with older children and adolescents, that the family still communicates on the same level. We now see it primarily in the subverbal language—through . . . facial expressions, gestures, postures, movement—rather than through words. This is private communication within the family, derivative of a time when words were not available for communication. These nonverbal modes of speech were functional, and continue to be so as they accumulate added significance by repeated use within the family.

The job of the family therapist then is to open up the channels of communication. Bolte (1970) has suggested that the framework of therapeutic family interventions should be based around *communications theory,* which focuses on changing behaviors through more effective communication. This does not mean that out-and-out honesty, irrespective of its consequences, is always the best policy. It isn't. Spotnitz (1976) introduces the idea of *constructive emotional interchange,* in which you provide another person with the kinds of honest communication that are most helpful for them to understand and accept what you are saying. The therapist teaches family members to honestly express constructive feelings to other family members. For example, in one family the parents who were having problems told their children intimate details of their feelings about each other, with the justification that they were "levelling" with the children. The therapist had to teach them that while they needn't lie to the children, neither should they burden the children with the full force of their feelings. More constructively, they can communicate to the children that they are having problems, but not go into such great detail.

Honest
communication

## Socioemotional Intactness
When we view the family as a unit, anything that preserves that unity either on a social or an emotional level is a sign of *socioemotional intactness* and is therefore productive. Anything that tears the family apart is viewed as counterproductive. Earlier, we referred to the "family systems conception" of conflict resolution. This view says that most family problems and conflict situations are a result of failures in communication between family members, failures that are viewed as signs of the dissolution of the family's intactness.

The family as a unit

## Problem Solving in the Family

One of the key goals of all family intervention efforts is to teach the family how to solve its problems on its own. In fact, quite often the family conflict can be defined as an inability to find direct means of solving fairly simple problems. This has been emphasized time and again in different contexts. "In relation to diagnosis," Haley (1972) points out, "a sharp difference between the beginner and the experienced therapist is in the concern with using a diagnosis that defines a solvable problem" (p. 162). He goes on to point out how experienced family therapists use diagnosis as a way of helping the family learn to state the problems that they must solve.

The facilitator's role

It is not enough that the facilitator attempt to solve the immediate problems with the family, for this will do little good in the long run. Rather, he or she should determine what is blocking the family from solving its own problems. Families often find, as they explore what is preventing them from solving a specific problem, a general pattern of underlying resistance that, when resolved, can open up many new avenues for solving other problems. As Bell (1975, p. 142) points out,

> Sometimes parents will ask the therapist how to solve their problems. When they ask me, I say, in a simple way, "I could answer this question (assuming I could), but this is not my job. My job is not to provide information or give advice; my job is to help you arrive at your own answers for your own family. . . . The therapist's action is that which will help the family itself work out the problem. It may be through helping a child to express his anger, his desires, his needs, and his resistance to the dominance of a parent; or through helping the parent to expose the reasons for his point of view. . . . The course of problem solving is not always even. Digressions are common. Some problems outside the family may be introduced because they are pressing on the family and seem to have urgency.

It is not the primary job of the family therapist to solve the family's problems for them but to help them find appropriate ways of problem solving. These enable them to solve not only the immediate problem, but long-range problems as well.

### The Forester Family

The Forester family came to Dr. Singer for counseling after a year and a half of continual fighting between the parents and the children and between the children themselves. Richard, age 14, and Donna, age 12, couldn't get along together and teamed up only when they became involved in loud, nasty fights with their parents. Among themselves they fought about property and personal space: they shared a room, and there was constant bickering about who could use which drawer, about whose phonograph record was whose, about who could bring a friend to the room at a certain time. With the parents, they fought about rights and privileges. They found that they had to stick together because they both felt strongly that the parents were too strict with them. Richard complained that he was not being allowed any more liberties than Donna, who was two years his junior; Donna complained that she was not treated as an adult, as her friends were. The parents told Dr. Singer that Richard and Donna were "difficult children," and they expressed the feeling that there was little they or Dr. Singer would be able to do about them.

Dr. Singer was especially interested in finding the answers to two questions: (1) What was the relationship between the siblings' inability to get along with each other and their allied fights with the parents?; and (2) Were the parents being overly strict or did their children unfairly perceive them in that way?

Of course, simply asking the questions directly would only provoke another argument among them, and it was not the counselor's place to try to answer the questions on her own. She had to find a way for the family to answer the questions on its own.

After much work, in which channels of communication were opened, innuendos brought into the forefront, and some underlying conflicts clarified, three important points that the whole family could agree on emerged:

1. Richard and Donna had an inflexible attitude when it came to dealing with their parents: they expected the worst and they got it. When they approached the parents with a request, they did it in almost a challenging and brazen way, which they knew would encourage the parents to refuse their request.
2. Richard always gave Donna the feeling that *their* room was *his* room, a feeling she always resented. The parents subtly supported this, since during the first two years of her life they had actually called it "Richard's room."

3. Mr. and Mrs. Forester had some very firm beliefs about what their children could and could not do. Some of these beliefs did not tally with their friends' beliefs, and Richard and Donna were treated somewhat more harshly and firmly than most of the other children they were friends with.

As each of these points came to light, steps were taken to solve the problems. For example, it was soon discovered that Richard and Donna had deeply buried fears and anxieties about sharing a room and that neither had ever discussed it openly with each other or with their parents. This was one of the underlying causes of their fighting. It also came out that Mrs. Forester had had a miscarriage when Donna was three and that she had been told she could not have any more children. Perhaps she was trying to keep Richard and Donna as children and not let them grow up. This point was explored but not fully resolved. Mr. Forester's passive attitude in family conflicts did not make him a neutral party; rather, it contributed to the family's inability to resolve problems.

By examining forthrightly the ways in which they communicated or did not communicate, the members of this family learned ways to solve their own problems. The family therapist did not act as a mediator and judge but taught the family members to express, concretize, clarify, probe, and, in short, to use among themselves in the family the same techniques that help people understand each other outside the family.

Individuation   From within the context of the family unit, each family member develops his or her individual identity in the process of *individuation*. This identity is not a rejection of one's place in the family but an identity that refines and enriches the family identity. To be able to say, "I exist individually as a person with my own ideas, feelings, needs, insights, and a life of my own" is a cogent sign of emotional health and sound interpersonal functioning. The ability to individuate is in part a consequence of the relationship with the mother during the early years of life. Individuation may be seen as the socialized end product of the lengthy process of separating from the mother and forming one's own identity. Freid (1970, p. 452) relates this early phase of individuation to later, more sophisticated developmental signs:

Struggles to individuate

In the child, individuation . . . is assumed to start at the end of the second year of life. As the encompassing dependence on the mother that is the core of the symbiotic phase wanes, as the child begins to acquire the rudiments of body autonomy, as new ego skills are acquired, the now semiliberated child wants more often to do than to be done for. . . .

In higher measure than we usually acknowledge, the striving for individuation—for forming convictions that are truly self-made and for relying on inner strength to cope with perils and pleasures—continues throughout any vital life. Never is there an end to the process of achieving self-determination and self-expression.

Many difficulties arise from individual family members' struggles to individuate. Karpel (1975) has proposed a model for understanding the marital and family problems of adult couples based on the struggle of each person to individuate. Along the same lines, Robinson (1975) correctly points out that "family therapists have ample experience indicating that dysfunctional families are established by parents who have achieved low levels of separation from their own parents, and are poorly prepared to construct an independent marital relationship" (p. 1047). This is another example of how the failure to individuate becomes a multigenerational problem, handed down from parents to children, if the parents are not fully socialized for parenthood. When individuation has not been successfully completed early in life, it becomes the job of the family therapist to see that it takes place in the clinical setting.

## Some Practical Considerations

Plan of treatment

Because the family members may have different goals for or expectations about therapy, it is necessary at the outset that there be a clearly delineated plan of treatment and clearly formulated, although tentative, set of rules and guidelines. This delineation not only prevents counterproductive misunderstandings later on, but also allows each member of the family to express what he or she feels is his or her primary goal and rationale for participating in the therapy. Aponte (1974) suggests that the general direction of therapy has to be organized around the family's structure and the problems they bring with them into therapy. He views the therapeutic process as including three critical stages: (1) the family's agreement on the problem, (2) identification of the role each member plays in the problem, and (3) the family's pledge to cooperate in solving the problem. He emphasizes the need for this structural scheme, since several people have to work together to solve the problem, which may involve all of them.

## Contracting

Closely related to this structural approach is the use of *contracts*. These establish, either orally or in writing, the rules, regulations, guidelines, and goals of the treatment. The *behavioral contract* is the most commonly used. This type of contract sets out acceptable and unacceptable behaviors, and the parties to the contract agree to abide by it. Its purpose is to increase the frequency of desirable behaviors and decrease, or eliminate, the frequency of undesirable behaviors. Firestone and Moschetta (1975) suggest that behavioral contracts are a major tool in breaking down family members' resistances to change and that they encourage flexibility and the experimentation with new behaviors. The use of contracts has become so popular that a number of intervention approaches have developed around them.

Weathers and Liberman (1975), for example, have discussed an innovative use of the *family contracting exercise,* which is a therapeutic learning experience in which family members learn to negotiate with each other. The exercise consists of five steps: (1) identifying the family members' needs and desires, (2) setting the rewards, (3) empathizing with each other, (4) clarifying what is needed for helping other family members, and (5) bargaining and compromising. The purpose of the exercise is to help the family members learn to negotiate with each other so that they eventually provide for each other's needs. It is also, we should note, an exercise in role definition and clarification, as exchanges of power are negotiated. Weathers and Liberman suggest four guidelines for generating successful contracts. These guidelines are central to the entire procedure:

*Flexibility* (margin)

*Role definition* (margin)

1. The negotiation of a contract must be open and honest, free from explicit or subtle coercion.
2. The terms of a contract should be expressed in simple, explicit, clearly understood words.
3. For a contract to be effective it has to provide an opportunity for all participants to optimize their reinforcements or minimize their costs and losses in the areas of their lives covered by the contract. The contract must provide advantages to each party over the status quo.
4. The behaviors contracted for must be in the repertoire of the person agreeing to do them. It is very easy to make the mistake of asking too much from a person.

## Helpful Kinds of Interventions

Whether an intervention is effective or not is largely a product of its timing as well as its content. The same comment or interpretation or suggestion may be entirely inappropriate during one session and entirely appropriate the next. Foley and Dyer (1974) offer eight occasions when therapeutic interventions are most helpful. We will discuss each one briefly, keeping in mind that most can be used in the family setting, outside of therapy.

**Labeling**

1. When labeling takes place and a family member is classified according to the label, such as "the good child," "the dull child," or "the nice parent," the therapist can intervene to point out the inaccuracy of this classification, to show that people are too complex to be labeled.

2. When one family member speaks for another, the therapist may intervene to help the other member speak for him- or herself. "The therapist must constantly intervene and point out that each person is an individual with his own feelings and thoughts" (p. 378).

3. When the family denies that the problems stem from within and suggests instead "If it weren't for them," indicating that forces outside are causing all or most of their problems, the therapist will step in to show how the family is not meeting the challenge of dealing with these forces. "Obviously a family has to unload," Foley and Dyer (p. 376) point out, "has a need to ventilate. But when it has been given time to do this, the therapist must intervene and face it with the responsibility that *change is within its power and no one else's.*" (italics in original)

**Scapegoats**

4. Sometimes a single member of the family becomes the scapegoat for the family's problems. "If it weren't for you," the others, "we wouldn't have these difficulties." Again, it is the job of the family therapist to show how the total interaction among all the family members, rather than the actions of one member, are responsible for the problems the family is experiencing.

5. "Families believe that certain laws operate in their lives. . . . An intervention ought to be made whenever such an immutable law is articulated" (p. 378). These family myths—for example the belief that "whatever we do we are doomed to fail" or the principle "if you are honest, you're a sucker"—are often resistances that prevent the family from coming to grips with their real problems.

**"The mañana position"**

6. The therapist should intervene when the family adopts what Foley and Dyer call the "mañana [tomorrow] position," insisting that things will get better by themselves. "This hope," they point out, "is not one which flows from change in the interaction, but from hope based on fantasy rather than reality. The therapist must cut through the wish for improvement and insist that change will result from realistic steps which are accompanied by action" (pp. 378–79).

7. The therapist may help the family members learn the meanings of their nonverbal cues.

8. The therapist may intervene when ''discrepancies of feelings, words, or actions are noted'' (p. 379).

These eight criteria for growth-producing intervention, while not exhaustive, are extremely comprehensive and helpful to the family members. Each of them is a practical tool, in that when the appropriate intervention is used, it is likely to facilitate the family's growth and cohesiveness.

## Summary

1. There are many life changes that put stress on individuals and on their marriages. A quantitative scale of life change units (LCUs) has recently been developed to indicate the relative stress that these events place upon people.

2. Jealousy, especially irrational jealousy, can be a constant source of conflict between partners and can eventually lead to a total lack of trust and a severe breakdown in marital communication.

3. Marital partners often fight about money. Money can also represent power, love, or social status and may sometimes be a symbolic battleground in which marital battles are waged.

4. Another common ground for marital fighting is childrearing. This may involve specific decisions about whether to have children, when to have them, or what children should be allowed to do. The couple may fight about the very role of parent as either partner conceptualizes it.

5. Fighting about sex and sexual dissatisfaction in general are related to levels of marital discord.

6. Some other areas of marital conflicts include in-law problems and small domestic differences that are compounded by communication difficulties in trying to resolve them.

7. Marital satisfaction depends largely on the ability of the partners to define and enact mutually satisfying marital roles. This task is entwined with the ability to communicate role expectations and to offer constructive feedback.

8. As sexual needs and interests change in marriage as they are bound to over a period of many years, it is imperative that the partners be able to openly discuss these with each other.

9. When the couple's own efforts at marital adjustment fail, they may want to avail themselves of professional marriage and family counseling. This involves the cooperation and participation of both partners and often of other family members, especially children.

10. The goal of most marriage and family counseling is that the family members learn how to solve their own problems and that they fully understand what has been impeding them from doing so. There are four specific goals: improving intrafamily communication, maintaining family intactness, increasing problem-solving skills, and facilitating individuation.

11. Some practical aspects of family counseling include contracting and helpful forms of therapist intervention.

## Key Terms

The following terms were introduced and defined in this chapter. Definitions also appear in the glossary.

behavioral contract
communications theory
constructive emotional interchange
contract
family contracting exercise
family counseling
family systems point of view

individuation
jealousy
life change unit (LCU)
The Social Readjustment Rating Scale
socioemotional intactness
swinging

**Discussion
Questions**

1. If you are married, list some of the more difficult marital problems you have experienced during the course of your marriage. Try to figure out how you and your partner solved some of these problems successfully, and see what qualities enabled you to maintain marital stability. For any problems that are still not solved, see if you have been applying the same problem-solving skills that worked successfully for other problems.

2. Interview some of the married couples you know well to see what they fight about most. How do your results compare with what we have outlined in this chapter? In what ways do your findings significantly differ?

3. Using the premise that in order to maintain a functional marriage two people have to be able to adapt to compatible role situations, outline some of the common sources of marital conflict discussed in this chapter. How can each of these be resolved by successful adaptation; that is, what kinds of role learning and role clarification would minimize potential conflict?

4. From your reading of this chapter, construct a definition of family counseling, taking into account its goals and processes. Define the following terms: socioemotional intactness, individuation, and contracting.

5. Find out what marriage and family counseling resources are available in your regional area. What is the general fee and how many sessions do most couples require?

6. As a class experiment, have two students enact a problem-solving session for a typical marital problem. They may wish to use a nonmarital relationship problem that parallels a marriage problem. Illustrate how the problem arises because of poor communication and how communicating can help solve many problems.

7. How would you analyze the case of Dr. Singer and the Forester family in terms of the social psychological concepts discussed throughout this book? Specifically, gear your discussion to the following concepts: socialization in the family, sibling relationships, childrearing practices, gender-role differentiation and stereotyping, and reciprocal socialization effects.

## Suggested Readings

1. Robert O. Blood and Donald M. Wolfe. *Husbands and Wives: The Dynamics of Married Living.* Glencoe, Ill.: Free Press, 1960.

See number (1) in Chapter 7.

2. Harvey J. Locke. *Predicting Adjustment in Marriage: A Comparison of a Divorced and a Happily Married Group.* New York: Holt, 1951.

A report of one of the early studies of marital success through interviews with over 200 divorced and 200 happily married couples. It broke some methodological ground by combining the detailed interviews with a marital adjustment test.

3. John Scanzoni. *Sexual Bargaining: Power Politics in the American Marriage.* Englewood Cliffs, N.J.: Prentice-Hall, 1972.

A detailed social exchange analysis of power relations between men and women in American marriage, which is set within a cross-cultural perspective and uses national statistics on marriage and divorce.

4. Nelson N. Foote and Leonard S. Cottrell, Jr. *Identity and Interpersonal Competence.* Chicago: University of Chicago Press, 1955.

A very important early argument for the reorientation of research on the family in terms of the concept of interpersonal competence. This book is a thorough-going attempt to try to use social psychological theory to aid practitioners working with families.

5. Sherod Miller (Ed.). *Marriages and Families: Enrichment Through Communication.* Beverly Hills, Calif.: Sage Publications, 1975.

This book has important practical implications. It presents a model to enable couples to communicate more clearly, more constructively, and with better consequences. The emphasis is on how couples can, with some effort, grow together and develop a mutual understanding and respect.

6. Nathan W. Ackerman. *The Psychodynamics of Family Life.* New York: Basic Books, 1958.

A classic psychiatric work on the importance of examining the patient's total set of family relationships in the course of individual treatment. At the time, it broke new ground among psychoanalytically oriented therapists by highlighting the importance of the family as a social group and the relevance of its internal social processes to its individual members.

7. John Elderkin Bell. *Family Therapy.* New York: Jason Aronson, 1975.

This is a clearly written book that provides a solid overview of the field of family therapy. For those readers interested in learning about how the family functions, and the therapeutic implications, this work is a solid introduction to the subject. Many of the insights are useful to individuals who are considering the possibility of seeing a family therapist.

8. Jeff Bryson and Rebecca Bryson (Eds.). *Dual-Career Couples* (Special issues of *Psychology of Women Quarterly*). New York: Human Sciences Press, 1978.

A recent government survey indicated that about half the married women in the United States today are employed. This important book examines the effect on marriage and family relationships—and on society in general—of dual-career commitments.

## Chapter 13

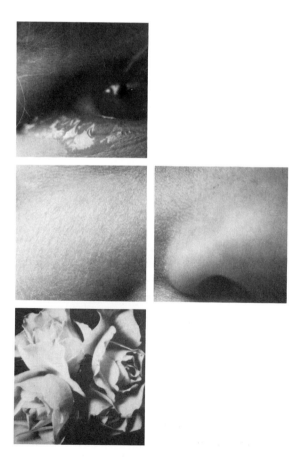

# Crises in the Family: Violence, Alcoholism, Divorce

**Family Violence**
Spouse Abuse
Child Abuse
**Alcoholism and the Family**
Alcoholics and Problem Drinkers
The Path to Alcoholism
Effects of Alcoholism on the Family
Adolescent Alcohol Abuse
Treatment of Alcoholism
**Separation and Divorce**
Divorce Rates
Causes of Divorce

## Chapter Aims

1. To explore in some detail spouse abuse and child abuse, focusing on their prevalence, their social psychological roots, and the social supports offered to abusers and victims.

2. To examine alcoholism and its effects on the functioning of the family.

3. To examine divorce in America, in terms of its frequency and in terms of the status it confers upon the divorced person.

4. To consider some of the factors that increase the risk of divorce.

## Overview

All families have problems and conflicts; however, in some cases these are severe. Spouse beats spouse, parent abuses or neglects a child, one of the family members is so dependent on alcohol that he or she can no longer function normally. Today there are groups that offer help and support to these families in crisis, and sometimes the disrupted family may become a working unit.

However, some internal crises and social factors may lead to the eventual breakup of the family, when the husband and wife no longer live together.

## Family Violence

As long as there have been families there has been family violence (Steinmetz 1978a). But it is only during the past decade that it has received a great deal of attention from the mass media and from social agencies, which, under federal and state funding, have begun to support wide-scale research and intervention efforts aimed at understanding and preventing family violence.

*Family violence* can be defined as the physical abuse of one family member by another. It can and does occur among any combination of family members. A recent article in the *New York Times* (July 2, 1979, p. 89) describes for example a new type of family violence: parents being battered by their adolescent offspring. Old people may be abused or killed by their children or grandchildren, just as grandchildren have been abused and killed by their grandparents. Siblings may do violence to each other, and there are many cases of children inflicting violence on their parents (Steinmetz 1978b). Forced incest and rape can occur between brother and sister or between parent and child. By far the most serious problems are violence by one spouse against the other or violence including sexual abuse by a parent against a child. The former is called *spouse abuse* or *wife abuse* because it typically occurs when the husband inflicts harm on the wife. The latter is called *child abuse.* Both are serious, often life-endangering, social problems.

Both spouse abuse and child abuse have two central points in common. First, they are both part of a pattern that Renvoize (1978) has called the "web of violence," to indicate that family violence spreads from member to member, from generation to generation, and that it invariably "traps every newborn member of long-ensnared families" (p. 31). The web of family violence, like a spider's web, traps its victims without killing them right away; and no matter how hard the victims try to escape, they may remain inextricably trapped for life.

The "web of violence"

Secondly, spouse abuse and child abuse are complex social problems that are more likely to afflict individuals with certain psychological predispositions. They are classic examples of how some types of personalities under certain social conditions and pressures will react in detrimental ways, while other personality types under the same social conditions will react quite differently. While it was once believed that these problems were predominantly limited to lower-class, uneducated families, more comprehensive and convincing data show that they are spread, although not evenly, across all social classes and all educational levels.

## Spouse Abuse

While there is no question that wifebeating is a widespread practice in the United States today, there are many unanswered questions about just how prevalent it is and what its underlying causes are. Some of the central questions we are still investigating, although we do have some tentative answers, are:

- Why are some women socialized to accept physical abuse from their husbands? Do they see their victimization as a part of the normative marital role of "wife"?
- What types of family backgrounds, social-class variables, and educational levels have been associated with wife abuse?
- What social supports or lack of support for the abused wife mitigates or worsens the problem of spouse abuse?
- Is husband abuse a real social problem, or is it a fiction of the mass media, which has attempted recently to portray victimized husbands along with victimized wives?

As we examine these questions, it is important to understand the appropriate background, so as to place all aspects of family violence in perspective.

### Socialization Factors
There is considerable evidence that the chronically abused wife has been socialized for that role. She does not necessarily cause her victimization, but to her it is a predictable part of the marital experience.

*Socialization of victims*

### Chris and Joe

"Sure, I think of leaving Joe sometimes," Chris explains, "especially after what he did to me last week. I mean spending a night in the hospital's just too much, even for me. But what do you think? It'd be any different with any man? *All men are like that*, especially after they've been drinking.

The key phrase, "all men are like that," shows that this woman's perception of the man's role includes the fact that he will abuse "his" woman when he's been drinking. If a woman has not been socialized to accept this pattern as normative, it would seem incredible when it happened, and such a situation would become intolerable.

It has been suggested that wifebeating is simply another manifestation of the view of women as property, literally "owned" by their husbands and subject to their husbands' whims and caprices. Interestingly, too often both abusive husbands and abused wives may view their relationships in this way.

There are many specific causes that precipitate abuse, none of which explains its deeper roots. Heavy drinking is probably the foremost reason. Some people under the influence of alcohol tend to be more violent than normal anyway; and if a man is angry with his wife, he may suddenly do what he would not do if he were sober. Some abusing husbands suffer from severe psychological problems and cannot control their violent impulses even when sober. They take out their frustrations and failures brought on by their jobs or by their interpersonal relationships on their wives, who are less physically powerful. Gelles (1977) has also suggested that wife abuse often precedes forced sexual compliance and that there are many more instances of marital rape than have generally been acknowledged.

### Backgrounds of Spouse Abusers and Victims

Women who are continually abused by their husbands tend to come from families where either or both of her parents physically abused her or where her father demonstrated frequent violence against her mother. Most of the men come from families where warmth and a sense of familial love was missing. A relatively large number of the husbands and wives come from stepparent families, where they were mistreated or neglected (Carroll 1977). Although spouse abuse occurs in all economic levels, it is more common among the lower classes and among the less educated (Wolfgang 1976). In short, it is argued that the backgrounds of spouse abusers and victims play a part in their present situations.

### Social Supports

The seriousness and extent of this problem is finally beginning to be recognized. Violence from spouse abuse results in one-fourth of all murders committed in the United States today (Meyers 1978). It is only in the past few years, primarily in response to the vocal demands of the feminist movement, that social agencies have developed

Society's response

systematic procedures for handling cases of wife abuse. For many years, police and judicial institutions had not taken a wife's charges of abuse seriously, and there was a general reluctance to prosecute abusing husbands. The situation was casually written off as a "domestic quarrel,"

*Women are beginning to receive social support and reinforcement to deal with intolerable and dangerous marital situations.*

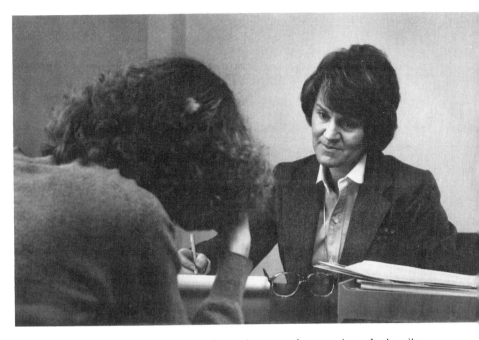

and the wife had little recourse. In fact, she was often made to feel guilty that she had somehow "provoked" the husband into beating her. "If things are so bad," she was told, "then leave him." It was not recognized that she could not leave her husband because, among other things, she might not have had the economic resources to live on her own. It became a vicious cycle.

Recently, a Domestic Violence Project, initiated by the National Organization of Women (NOW), was set up at Ann Arbor, Michigan, to serve as a clearinghouse on information about wife abuse for organizations that were contemplating programs (Higgins 1978). Also, there have been important legal changes in the past five years, governing not only abuse but marital rape as well (Meyers 1978). Women are finally beginning to get some of the social support and reinforcement necessary to deal with intolerable and dangerous marital situations.

## Child Abuse

Historical tolerance

As with spouse abuse, only in recent years has the widespread problem of child abuse been recognized for what it is: a serious social issue that produces psychological disturbances in the perpetrators and victims alike. Throughout history, there is shameful evidence that mistreatment and abuse of children has been tolerated in many cultures. Recorded incidents range from institutional infanticide, in which the society advocates the systematic murder of children for population control, to the intentional training of children into the criminal professions as in *Oliver Twist,* to the unprovoked torture and mistreatment of children. The horrors of the *comprachicos* is described by Ayn Rand (1971), who tells us how this seventeenth-century nomadic association bought children and purposely deformed them, making them into hunchbacks and cripples for the pleasures of the aristocracy and the amusement of the king.

Recognition of the extent of the problem has led to a flood of research attempting to understand the causes of child abuse. Sociologists, psychologists, and other behavioral scientists have put forth a number of theories to account for the existence of child abuse, which is usually at the hands of the child's parents.

## Background

The first comprehensive effort to view child abuse as a syndrome, commonly dubbed the *battered-child syndrome,* is credited to C. Henry Kempe, a pioneer in the field, who published a noted article on the problem in 1962 (Kempe et al. 1962), setting the stage for further study. Six years later, Helfer and Kempe (1968) edited a major work on the battered-child syndrome; and in the years since the publication of this book, hundreds of articles, many case histories, and scores of research studies have appeared in professional journals. The subject is clearly multidisciplinary, although there are sharp differences in emphasis between the psychologists and sociologists.

## What Is Child Abuse?

There is no clear-cut, universally accepted definition of child abuse. Generally, however, care is taken to distinguish between the physically abused, or "battered," child and the child who is psychologically or physically "neglected" but not physically assaulted by the parents. A number of operational definitions have been suggested for research purposes. *Child abuse* may be defined narrowly to include only physical assault (Lauer, Ten Broeck, and Grossman 1974) or more broadly to include severe neglect as well as assault (Burland, Andrews and Headsten 1973). The broader definition poses a certain problem inasmuch as the evidence against the abusive parent usually emphasizes the violent physical assault in which the parent loses control. However, this definition is probably more helpful, since it includes more children who are in danger.

Definitions

## Who Is The Child-Abusing Parent?

This question has been studied in some depth and a great deal is now known about parents who abuse their children. In many ways, they are not much different than spouse abusers. There are two perspectives to this issue: the psycho-pathological and the sociological. But certain facts are recognized by both. Child-abusing parents are often highly disturbed individuals who were severely abused themselves in childhood. Child abuse is viewed as a self-perpetuating disorder in which the abused child grows up to be an abusing parent. Moreover, the abusing parent is usually insecure, violent, and unable to control anger and has a tendency to project his or her own inadequacies on the child. There is also considerable evidence that in abusing families there is ''a high incidence of divorce, separation, and unstable marriages, as well as minor criminal offenses.'' Child-abusing parents also ''share common misunderstandings with regard to the nature of child-rearing, and look to the child for satisfaction of their own parental emotional needs'' (Spinetta and Rigler 1972).

A self-perpetuating disorder

Many studies reflect what is generally called the *psychopathological position.* This position explains child abuse as a result of an ''emotional sickness'' of the parents. While this is an important position, certainly in terms of clinical psychology, it pays too little attention to the matrix of social forces that bears on the family. Many of these social forces can lead to family disorganization and increased violence among its members—particularly economic pressures, prejudice and discrimination, difficult early socialization experiences of the parent, disagreements among parents about childrearing, etc. Some recent criticisms along these lines by sociologist Richard Gelles (1973, 1978) have received wide attention.

Gelles provides a sociological critique and reformulation of the portrait of child-abusing parents. Responding to this predominantly psycho-pathological model, he argues that the psychopathological theory is inconsistent and that the literature on child abuse is not based on hard-core empirical research that meets the rigorous standards of social science. Instead, Gelles suggests what he calls a sociocultural analysis of the situation. His model combines the processes of socialization with psycho-pathological insights to provide a synthesis. ''Concentrating on social factors rather than individual pathology,'' explains Rappaport (1979), describing the reports of research conducted by Gelles and his colleagues, ''the study shows violence toward children to be highest among parents who are: under 30 years of age, living in the Midwest (and to a lesser extent the West), living in large cities, members of minority races (excluding blacks) or religions, high school graduates only, earning less than $6,000 a year, blue-collar workers, and under considerable stress'' (p. 4). We see that what is emphasized here is not individual psychological disturbance, important as that may be in particular cases, but a sociological portrait—a set of social conditions that apparently creates the personal and familial strains that lead to child abuse and other forms of family violence.

Sociocultural analysis

Roberta Kalmar (1977), in a recent book she edited on child abuse,

*Child abuse seems to be a self-perpetuating disorder in which the abused child grows up to be an abusing parent.*

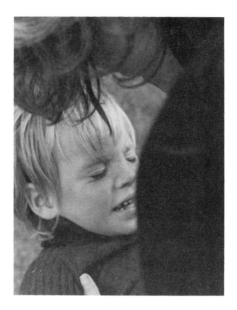

also emphasizes the role of society in the problems of child abuse. Writing as a practicing social worker, Kalmar (p. iv) points out:

> While the parents of abused children may be held directly responsible for their acts, society too must bear part of the blame for child abuse. This is so in part because ours is a society which is prone to violence and exploiting the powerless and because ours is a society which does not adequately meet the needs of minorities, the unemployed, the emotionally ill or the mentally retarded. The continued manifestations of child abuse is also related to our Constitutional structure which mandates greater emphasis on parental rights than on children's rights. In reality there appears to be an inherent conflict between parental rights and the best interests of the child.

Whatever the specific causes, it is widely agreed that the abusing parent is a product of social and psychological strains that lead to such behavior.

Social Supports   What kind of help is available to the abused child and to the parents? The answer to this varies greatly from state to state and from county to county within states. In recent years, most states have enacted specific laws for the reporting of child abuse. Many schools, social agencies, and hospitals have issued guidelines for physicians, nurses, teachers, and public administrators who observe instances or suspect the existence of child abuse, including severe neglect—although the ex-

Reporting child abuse

tremely neglectful parent may fail to send the child to any agency, including school! Equally interesting is the fact that an increasing number of voluntary self-help groups, similar to Alcoholics Anonymous, have begun to spring up all over the country for parents who realize they have a problem.

Nagi (1975) conducted a national survey to evaluate the services available. One troubling finding of this survey is that about one-third of the estimated cases are never reported to the appropriate agencies. This lack may in part be the fault of the school or agency personnel who are reluctant to report cases for fear of social or legal repercussions. As Sanders et al. (1975) point out, "the biggest barrier to aiding the abused child is the unwillingness of those who notice the child's distress to report the abuse" (p. 336). And no matter how well-intentioned the system is, this remains a difficult barrier that only a change in social attitudes and individual conscience can overcome.

## Alcoholism and the Family

One of the major problems associated with family disruption and marital dissolution in our contemporary American society is alcoholism. Alcoholism, in fact, is the largest single factor cited in the cause of marital failure. It is not clear which causes which—does marital strain cause one to drink heavily or does heavy drinking cause marital strain? Probably each feeds the other.

A cross-cultural phenomenon

There are an estimated 10 to 12 million alcoholics or serious problem drinkers in the United States today, "approximately one-third [of whom] are women" (Eddy and Ford 1979). Alcoholism straddles all social classes, all ethnic groups, most religions, and all regions of the country. A large number of alcoholics are parents, heads of nuclear families, financial providers, or primary caretakers of their children. If either parent is an alcoholic, a problem drinker, or is prone to any form of drug dependence or abuse, there is an indication that the family-as-unit is in serious trouble. If both parents are alcoholics, the family is in even greater difficulty. In this section we will look at the effect of an alcoholic parent on the family and briefly consider the problem of teen-age alcoholism, which has been the subject of much scrutiny during the past decade.

## Alcoholics and Problem Drinkers

Addiction

An *alcoholic* is a person with a physical and psychological dependency on alcohol. Alcoholism is an addictive disorder. The alcoholic is, for all intents and purposes, unable to function normally and tends to focus his or her life energy and goals on consuming enough alcohol to feel psychologically numb and physically relieved from the terrible withdrawal symptoms, the DTs, caused by not having sufficient alcohol in the system. While many alcoholics may be able to function reasonably well at least part of the time, emotionally the alcoholic is much like an infant, who, when not fed, cries and cries without the ability to do much about the hunger. Then, like the infant, when the true alcoholic is fed, that is, intoxicated, he or she goes to sleep or blacks out, to awaken only when the body craves more alcohol. Socially, the alcoholic has withdrawn from most situations, and is unable to interact with others under expected role conditions.

*Problem drinking,* which is more common, is one step before alcoholism. Typically, problem drinkers exhibit normal role behaviors most of the time but need alcohol as a regular part of their routines. While they are not suffering yet from alcoholism per se, they may experience many of the alcoholic effects. Eddy (1979) points out that they drink to escape from an inner anxiety, from which they know no other effective form of escape.

Usually, those people closest to the problem drinker, with the most opportunity to directly observe his or her private behaviors, will be more aware of the problem than those with whom the problem drinker has less consistent contact. Therefore, many people who socialize with a problem drinker may not be aware that the person has a problem because in the social setting drinking is an expected behavior. But in these situations ironically the need to drink becomes especially pronounced. The popular saying, "If you need a drink to be social then you're not a social drinker," best explains the problem drinker's needs in terms of his or her anxiety in interacting with others.

While both the problem drinker and the full-fledged alcoholic are disruptive influences on their families, the alcoholic is worse by far. For while the problem drinker may experience a serious loss of functioning, he or she is able for much of the time to keep the family together. Unfortunately, problem drinking is usually a step on the way to alcoholism.

## The Path to Alcoholism

"Social drinking"

Alcoholism does not happen overnight, but develops over a period of many years, usually in a fairly predictable progression. Of course, to become an alcoholic, one first has to be a problem drinker. But the large majority of drinkers never become alcoholics or problem drinkers. The signs that one is becoming an alcoholic stand out from casual social drinking, and others can see these signs if they are open to them.

Stages of alcoholism

Many psychiatrists and mental health researchers have attempted to clearly define the path to alcohol dependency. Jellinek (1971) delineates four stages of alcoholism, which are widely accepted. During the first stage, which is called the *prealcoholic phase,* the person becomes a heavy social drinker and finds that drinking relieves tension and reduces levels of anxiety. This continues to the point where the person can no longer tolerate even the normal tensions of living and has to use alcohol almost daily.

## Gus

"When Gus and I got married we both used to drink a lot because it was a part of our business. It was strictly social drinking, I'm sure. We'd drink at lunch with the client, then we'd have a cocktail with the other salespeople after work, and then maybe a nightcap when we were home. It didn't seem like much, and I never gave it any thought with regard to myself. I only started to worry when I began to notice that Gus was tense, highstrung, and sensitive if he weren't drinking. In the mornings, it was almost as if he were counting the minutes waiting for that first drink of the day. I can't honestly say he was drinking that much more: it was the *way* he was drinking that worried me."

During the next stage, the *prodromal phase,* people begin to exhibit many of the behaviors we associate with true alcoholics: sneaking a drink so that others don't "hassle" them about drinking too much; thinking about alcohol almost obsessively; always being sure to have a bottle "handy," sometimes even going as far as keeping a small flask in the suit pocket or pocketbook; avoiding the company of people who don't drink and especially those who attempt to tell them that they have a drinking problem; adamant self-denial about their dependency on alcohol. Also during this prodomal phase, these are often amnesiac episodes, in which they forget days or hours of their lives.

## Carlota's Mother

"Mom used to drink as far back as I can remember," Carlota explains, "even though I only saw her really drunk a few times. But I remember she used to sleep a lot during the day. I'd come home from school and the house would be really filthy and she'd be sleeping on the couch in the living room. Once when I said to her, 'You shouldn't be drinking so much, mom,' she hauled off and slapped me across the face. Hard. Then she began to cry and sob, begging me to forgive her. But two minutes later, guess what?: she was pouring herself a vodka on the rocks and chugging it down like there was no tomorrow.

Physical dependency

The third phase is what Jellinek calls the *crucial phase,* and it is here that the person loses complete control and becomes physically dependent upon alcohol. It is here too that the alcohol itself serves as a triggering mechanism for more alcohol, and the vicious cycle of alcohol dependency becomes painfully evident. It is also at this particular phase that Alcoholics Anonymous' message is truest: ONE DRINK IS TOO MANY AND ALL THE DRINKS IN THE WORLD ARE NOT ENOUGH.

## Leo

"I was doing all right for a while, I really was," says Leo, describing what happened. "I'd been on the wagon for about five months, and the wife and I were working out our problems. We were living together again. We were even going for psychotherapy. But then my brother came into town—you know, I hadn't seen him in years—and we began to BS about old times. I was feeling great, better than I'd felt in years, and we went out for a beer. I figured a beer—what's a beer?—it's not going to hurt me. Besides, I wasn't depressed: I was feeling great. But as that beer started going down my gullet, I swear I heard myself calling out to the bartender, 'A double bourbon straight up,' and before I even realized what I was saying it was in front of me, whiffing up my nose. I was boozing again within the hour—like I was never on the wagon at all."

Finally, there is what Jellinek calls the *chronic phase,* in which the individual's life beomes dominated by drinking. It is here that normal interpersonal relations cease and the quality of life becomes one drunken binge after another. It is also at this point that the family tends to experience the greatest degree of hopelessness and the greatest stress.

## Linda and Marge's Mother

"We knew our mother was an alcoholic, but we kept hoping things would change," Linda and Marge recalled sadly. "She kept *promising* and we kept believing her. We wanted to believe her because we love her. I realize now that our mistake was in believing it was a promise she *could* keep. She couldn't: by that point, she was beyond the stage of being able to help herself."

We see that these stages of alcoholic deterioration, even if they take years, gradually wreck havoc on family unity and place unbearable strains on the marital relationship.

## Effects of Alcoholism on the Family

It is not difficult to imagine the profound effects one alcoholic family member has on family functioning and stability. Depending upon which family member it is and the strength of the other members, these effects can cause severe problems for all other family members. The most serious problems are caused when one or both of the parents are alcoholics.

Effects on marriage

Within the context of the marital relationship, the bottle can replace the spouse as the basic source of solace and relief. In the classic film *Days of Wine and Roses,* alcohol played a major role in tearing apart a marriage. There the couple both became alcoholics, and when either one would try to reform, the other would fight against it. They sunk into despair and hopelessness together. When both partners are alcoholics, each one reinforces the other's behavior for fear of being isolated if the other were to go on the wagon.

Family conflict

Alcoholism signals to the family that at least one of its members is experiencing some serious difficulties which are not only affecting that member but the overall quality of the family's life. Steinglass, Weiner, and Mendelson (1971), in their analysis of drinking behavior in the family, point out two possible roles it may serve within the organization of the family system. It may signal a sign of stress inside the system, expressing to all members of the family through one member's drinking that a problem exists. This may serve as a releaser of intrafamily tension and force the family to seek outside help, which it would not otherwise seek. Family therapists are well aware that problem drinking is often the superficial symptom of role tension or conflict that brings a troubled family into treatment. For example, gender-related role conflicts within the marital relationship may be expressed through drinking. As Kirkpatrick (1977, p. 91) points out, the conflicts differ for men and women, showing some consistent patterns:

Many women's emotional problems and disturbances are all tied up in the male-female relationship. . . . All women in our culture feel a modicum of guilt for not being ''perfect,'' for not fitting into the unrealistic mold that American society has cast for them. For alcoholic women, this guilt is almost unbearable at times. . . . *Women alcoholics have this strong feeling of having failed as a wife, as a mother, as a sister or daughter, or as a woman.* . . .

On the other hand, the male alcoholic feels much remorse for having hurt his family . . . his wife and children. He rarely feels guilt and he never feels the same as women do. There is a vast and distinct difference in this particular area between male and female alcoholics (italics ours).

On the other hand, according to the Steinglass model, heavy drinking may be an integral part of the family system. For example it may be a part of the clarification of role differentiation or power distribution in the family. In this sense, it is a central part of the family's social functioning. The perennially drunken father who abuses his family when drunk is using his alcoholism as the raison d'être of his physical force. Or, the mother who disables herself through drinking may not want to face what she thinks is her role, using alcohol as the excuse.

The social stigma

There are many practical problems to deal with when a family member is an alcoholic. There may be a social stigma, whereby all the family members feel ''contaminated'' by the antisocial behavior of one. Children of alcoholic parents feel ashamed of their parents' behavior. There is also a much higher incidence of family violence in alcoholic families. Financial problems are common, especially where the family breadwinner becomes unable to adequately provide because of the alcohol addiction. Sexual relationships between the spouses invariably suffer as does the ability to communicate with other family members. In short, one alcoholic family member can short-circuit the entire family network.

## Adolescent Alcohol Abuse

A particularly poignant problem in recent years has been the increasing dependence upon alcohol by young people. Beginning about 1974, alcohol began to emerge as the single most abused drug among the adolescent population. No one knows exactly why, but it may represent an ironic adolescent rebellion against the prevailing adult acceptance of marijuana use.

*One alcoholic family member can short-circuit the entire family network; communication can suffer as a result.*

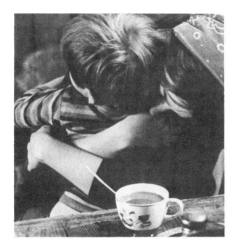

## Marion and Her Friends

Marion, a fifteen-year-old, and her friends go over to Peter's house after school and drink wine. Peter's parents both work and leave a well-stocked liquor cabinet unattended. Bob, one of the "tough guys" at the school drinks whiskey and puts down the other kids because they only drink wine or beer. Peter's older brother Edward comes by with his friends and smokes grass downstairs in the basement. Marion's friends put this down. It's the behavior of college kids, whom they don't admire.

One interesting study revealed parallels between antisocial patterns in abusers of alcohol and abusers of drugs. Globetti (1972) investigated problem high school drinkers in two small towns where alcohol was prohibited. He found that the alcohol abuser, like the drug abuser, tended to have generally antisocial and mildly criminal characteristics, although this result may not be valid for communities where there are no restrictions on the sale and use of alcohol. More importantly, another study (Block & Goodman, 1978) pointed to the patterning of drug usage. They showed that adolescents who used alcohol were also more likely to smoke, to use illegal drugs, and to use over the counter medicines and to do so more frequently than adolescents who were nonusers.

Patterns and symptoms

The symptoms of alcohol abuse among teen-agers include family conflicts and school-related conflicts. Adolescents with drinking problems are likely to have high absentee rates from school, may appear intoxicated in class, and invariably fall behind in their school work. They may fight frequently with their parents, even if the parents themselves are alcoholics.

Why do adolescents increasingly turn to alcohol? A person undergoing such stresses as are inherent in adolescence is more likely than a mature person to rely on getting high for escape, for fantasy, and for peer group approval and recognition. Jessor and Jessor (1975) have suggested that adolescent drinking behavior is related either to the degree of rapid transition to new adult-oriented roles, such as having sexual relations, or to problem proneness in personality. The escape value of alcohol lies in its potential for allowing one to forget one's problems and to seek refuge temporarily from the real world? And who needs this escape more than the conflict-torn, changing adolescent. A fantasy world is set up, a world where the individual is freed of all responsibilities, where nothing is important, and where there is no way to get hurt by others.

*Escapism*

## Treatment of Alcoholism

It is generally agreed that the successful treatment of alcoholism in the family depends on two things: the motivation of the alcoholic member to change and the support given that member by the family. Because it is usually a battle with many setbacks, a great deal of family unity is needed to offer the degree of encouragement necessary for cure. The prognosis is not always good. Dinaburg, Glick, and Feigenbaum (1977) point out that although marital or family therapy can be helpful in preventing the development of alcoholism of a family member it is of little value once a member is an alcoholic. They recommend that it be used in conjunction with an effective self-help group such as Alcoholics Anonymous and along with other supportive therapy, such as sex therapy for example.

*Prognosis and treatment*

In recent years there has been an enormous increase in alcoholic support groups and therapy groups, especially for women alcoholics. While AA, Alcoholics Anonymous, is still widely regarded as the best source of help available, some women believe the program is geared more toward the male alcoholic, and female-oriented organizations such as Women for Sobriety have been springing up throughout the country with the special needs of women in mind (Kirkpatrick 1977).

## Separation and Divorce

Sometimes crises lead to family dissolution when the spouses separate or divorce each other. Most societies provide a prescribed method for terminating a marital relationship when it becomes impossible for the partners to maintain what they or the culture deem a functional marital relationship. The act of dissolving a marriage is called *divorce*. The criteria are called the *grounds for divorce.*

Methods of divorce

Acceptable reasons for divorce vary from culture to culture, as do the rites of divorce. In Jewish and Moslem law, for example, the man need not give any reason for wanting to divorce his wife. He may do so at his will, as long as he follows the detailed procedures for making it known that he is divorced. According to orthodox Moslem law, the husband simply repeats three times in public that he wants a divorce and they are divorced. The wife has no say in the matter. In Hindostan, the husband can dissolve the marriage unilaterally by calling his wife "Mother" (Mace and Mace, 1959, p. 245). Among the Nayar, a matrilineal society, on the other hand, the woman can "divorce" her "husband" simply by placing his belongings out on the front veranda. These are rites that make divorce relatively easy, but one-sided. The Catholic Church, at the other extreme, prohibits divorce for any reason. Under extreme cases a marriage can be annulled by Church ritual—meaning in effect that the marriage never actually took place.

Just as marriage is surrounded by customs that enable the newly married couple to present themselves socially as a pair, divorce requires a certain type of social presentation. Any kind of paired relationship is subject to dissolution, but divorce is a special case with a public side to it. "While breakups of less established pairs go unrecorded and often unrecognized," Levinger (1976) points out, "marital breakups have a public status"; that is, when you are divorced you are not simply "not married" (p. 21). Divorce confers a special social status on the individual. Levinger continues, "there are few data about the dissolution of friendships or acquaintanceships, but there is a large literature on marital separation" (p. 43). The available data on divorce indicate strongly that it is culturally controlled, in terms of attitude and rate. For example, Catholics have a low rate of divorce, in part because of the prohibitions of their religion.

Methods of divorce

Research in the field

Research on marital dissolution and divorce has generally concentrated on four areas: (1) rates of divorce by variables such as age when married, social class, and legal provisions; (2) specific reasons within the marriage and pressures from without that precipitate divorce; (3) the actual process of dissolving the marriage; and, (4) readjustment after marital dissolution. We will refer to the first three areas in this section and to the last one in the following chapter.

## Divorce Rates

What is the frequency of divorce? Who gets divorced? These are the basic questions that social scientists and statisticians try to answer as they examine the data on divorce and analyze its demographic characteristics. The questions are complicated by the way we present our statistics. Should we measure the "rate" of divorce as a percentage of the population, as a percentage of the population over a certain age or between certain ages, or as a percentage of the number of existing marriages in a given year? The way one computes the figures drastically affects what one infers from them.

"If you get married the chances are 50/50 that it will end in divorce," some people say. How true is this, and how can you determine if a specific marriage is one of the ones more or less likely to end in divorce. For instance, how do variables such as age when married, social class, educational level, and whether this is the first or a later marriage affect the statistical outlook for a specific marriage? "Divorce rates do not by themselves measure levels of marital disruption in society," Stetson and Wright (1975) correctly point out, "but they are important as the *official* certification of marriage failure" (p. 537). In short then, although we can't rely on statistics alone, they do give us some clues that we can follow to conclusions.

Here are three generally accepted facts about divorce rates:

Factors to consider

1. Within a society, the rate of divorce is likely to vary over the years, increasing or decreasing at certain periods in history.
2. In our society, there are some significant variations in the divorce rate, according to ethnicity, age at marriage, whether it is a first or a later marriage, religious affiliation, and socioeconomic level.
3. Among cultures there are likely to be differences in divorce rates.

As we can see in table 13.1, which shows the rates of divorce and marriage from the turn of the century to the present time, the number of divorces in the United States has increased dramatically, although it has not been a continuous increase. In the period of 1945–1947, for example, the divorce rate suddenly shot up, along with the marriage rate. This jump was clearly related to the end of World War II, when our veterans came home from the war and either married their "sweethearts" who had been waiting for them, or divorced their wives who had not. This is an example of how profound social strains affect the divorce rate as well as the marriage rate.

The calculation of the divorce rate, we should emphasize, is not a simple matter. In fact, as we can see from the following excerpt (from *New York Review of Books,* May 3, 1979, p. 26), there are several different ways to derive such data, each giving a different "fact," which is really only one of several ways of interpreting the data:

Table 13.1

**Marriages, Divorces, and Rates in the U.S.**

| Year | Marriages[1] No. | Rate | Divorces[2] No. | Rate | Year | Marriages[1] No. | Rate | Divorces[2] No. | Rate |
|------|------|------|------|------|------|------|------|------|------|
| 1890.... | 570,000 | 9.0 | 33,461 | 0.5 | 1940.... | 1,595,879 | 12.1 | 264,000 | 2.0 |
| 1895.... | 620,000 | 8.9 | 40,387 | 0.6 | 1945.... | 1,612,992 | 12.2 | 485,000 | [3]3.5 |
| 1900.... | 709,000 | 9.3 | 55,751 | 0.7 | 1950.... | 1,667,231 | 11.1 | 385,144 | 2.6 |
| 1905.... | 842,000 | 10.0 | 67,976 | 0.8 | 1955.... | 1,531,000 | 9.3 | 377,000 | 2.3 |
| 1910.... | 948,166 | 10.3 | 83,045 | 0.9 | 1960.... | 1,523,000 | 8.5 | 393,000 | 2.2 |
| 1915.... | 1,007,595 | 10.0 | 104,298 | 1.0 | 1965.... | 1,800,000 | 9.3 | 479,000 | 2.5 |
| 1920.... | 1,274,476 | 12.0 | 170,505 | 1.6 | 1970.... | 2,158,802 | 10.6 | 708,000 | 3.5 |
| 1925.... | 1,188,334 | 10.3 | 175,449 | 1.5 | 1975.... | 2,152,662 | 10.1 | 1,036,000 | 4.9 |
| 1930.... | 1,126,856 | 9.2 | 195,961 | 1.6 | 1976.... | 2,154,807 | 10.0 | 1,083,000 | 5.0 |
| 1935.... | 1,327,000 | 10.4 | 218,000 | 1.7 | 1977(p) | 2,176,000 | 10.1 | 1,090,000 | 5.0 |

Data refer only to events occurring within the United States, including Alaska and Hawaii beginning with 1960. Rates per 1,000 population.
(1) Includes estimates and marriage licenses for some states for all years. (2) Includes reported annulments. (3) Divorce rates for 1945 based on population including armed forces overseas. (p) provisional.

Source: National Center for Health Statistics, Public Health Service

THREE WAYS TO COMPUTE THE "DIVORCE RATE"

If present patterns continue, 40 percent of all women in their late twenties currently getting married will end up being divorced. As follows:

Among every 100 first marriages, 38 will result in divorce. Among these 38 divorced women, 29 will remarry. And 13 of those 29 will get divorced again.

Methods for calculating

So the original 100 women will have 51 divorces (38 plus 13) out of their 129 marriages (100 plus 29). And 51 out of 129 makes a rate of 40 percent.

(The divorce rate for first marriages is 38 per 100, as noted. For second marriages, it is 45 per 100.)

Another way to compute the divorce "rate" is by comparing the annual ratio of marriages to divorces. In 1976 there were 50 divorces for every 100 marriages in the country as a whole. Oregon and California led the list with 83 and 89 per 100. South Carolina and South Dakota were at the bottom with 21 and 22 per 100.

A third method simply records the number of divorces per 1,000 people in the population. In 1915, the national rate was one per 1,000. By 1966, it was 2.5 per 1,000. The latest figure, for 1977, is 5.1 per 1,000.

Table 13.1 is an example of the third way mentioned (divorces per 1,000 people in the population), and Table 13.2 is an example of the second method (ratio of marriages and divorces). Each method offers a different kind of picture of current trends. The media have tended in the past two decades to compute divorce rates in a way that is most dramatic and newsworthy; namely, by implying that there is a divorce epidemic in contemporary society. For example, using the second method of comparing the ratio of couples getting married to those obtaining divorces, it would appear that California's 89 divorces for every 100 marriages undoubtedly proves the decline of the institution of marriage in California. But this figure fails to tell us what percentage of the married couples in California are remaining married and not opting for divorce. This, of course, would be nowhere near 89 percent.

Table 13.2

**Divorces as a Percentage of Marriages**

| Year | Divorces as % of marriages |
|------|----------------------------|
| 1900 | 7.8% |
| 1910 | 8.8% |
| 1920 | 13.4% |
| 1930 | 17.4% |
| 1940 | 16.5% |
| 1950 | 23.1% |
| 1960 | 25.8% |
| 1965 | 26.6% |
| 1970 | 32.8% |
| 1975 | 48.1% |
| 1976 | 50.3% |

SOURCE: National Center for Health Statistics, Public Health Service

There is a fourth way to look at divorce data which, in our view, is at least as useful as the other three in assessing changes in the frequency of marriage and divorce, although it is less sensational and hence less likely than some of the others to capture the attention of the media. This method, described by Clayton (1975, p. 72) is to compare the number of divorces per 1,000 *existing marriages*. This figure would more accurately reflect the percentage of married couples opting to stay married against the percentage opting for divorce. Different methods of computation can yield vastly different conclusions about divorce and marriage.

The stringency of a state's divorce laws also has been shown to affect the divorce rate. The more permissive the divorce laws, the higher the rate of divorce (Stetson & Wright, 1975), although this of course cannot in itself be an explanation of why people divorce. Permissive divorce laws

Figure 13.1
**The Marriage Odds**

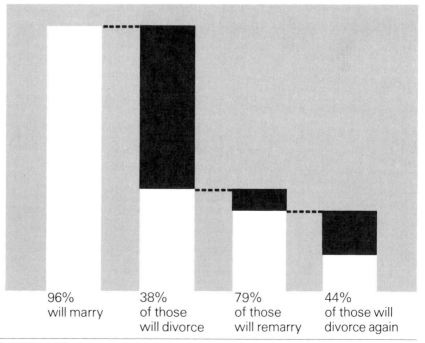

96%
will marry

38%
of those
will divorce

79%
of those
will remarry

44%
of those will
divorce again

Source: *Newsweek*, May 15, 1978, p. 67

Table 13.3

**Grounds for Divorce**

| State | Breakdown of marriage / incompatibility | Cruelty | Desertion | Non-support | Alcohol &/or drug addiction | Felony | Impotency | Insanity[1] | Living separate and apart | Residence time | Other grounds |
|---|---|---|---|---|---|---|---|---|---|---|---|
| Alabama | X | X | X | X | X | X | X | X | | 1 yr. | X |
| Alaska | X | X | X | . . . | X | X | X | X | | 1 yr. | X |
| Arizona | X | . . . | | | | | | | | 90 days | |
| Arkansas | . . . | X | X | X | X | X | X | X | 3 yrs. | 3 mos. | X |
| California | X | . . . | | | | | | X | | 6 mos. | |
| Colorado | X | | | | | | | | | 90 days | |
| Connecticut | X | X | X | X | X | X | . . . | X | 18 mos. | 1 yr. | X |
| Delaware | X[4] | | | | | | | | 18 mos. | 3 mos. | |
| Dist. of Columbia | . . . | . . . | X | . . . | | X | X | . . . | 6 mos.-1 yr. | 6 mos. | X |
| Florida | X | . . . | | | | | | X | | 6 mos. | |
| Georgia | X | X | X | . . . | X | X | X | X | | 6 mos. | X |
| Hawaii | X | . . . | | | | | | | 2 yrs. | 6 mos. | X |
| Idaho | X | X | X | X | X | X | . . . | X | 5 yrs. | 6 wks. | |
| Illinois | . . . | X | X | . . . | X | X | X | . . . | | 3 mos. | |
| Indiana | X | . . . | | | | X | X | X | | 6 mos. | |
| Iowa | X | . . . | | | | | | | | 1 yr. | |
| Kansas | X | X | X | . . . | X | X | X | X | | 60 days | X |
| Kentucky | X | | | | | | | | | 180 days | |
| Louisiana | . . . | . . . | | | | X | . . . | | 2 yrs. | 1 yr. | X |
| Maine | X | X | X | X | X | . . . | X | . . . | 3 yrs. | 6 mos. | |
| Maryland | . . . | . . . | X | | | X | X | X | 1-3 yrs. | 1 yr. | X |
| Massachusetts | X | X | X | X | X | X | X | . . . | 6 mos.-1 yr. | 2 yrs. | |
| Michigan | X | . . . | | | | | | | | 6 mos. | |
| Minnesota | X | . . . | | | | | | | 6 mos. | 6 mos. | X |
| Mississippi | X | X | X | . . . | X | X | X | X | | 6 mos. | X |
| Missouri | X | . . . | | | | | | | 1-2 yrs. | 3 mos. | |

Adultery is either grounds for divorce or evidence of irreconcilable differences and a breakdown of the marriage in all states. The plaintiff can invariably remarry in the same state where he or she procured a decree of divorce or annulment. Not so the defendant, who is barred in certain states for some offenses. After a period of time has elapsed even the offender can apply for permission. Grounds not recognized for divorce may be recognized for separation or annulment. Local laws should be consulted.

Table 13.3
**Grounds for Divorce**

| State | Breakdown of marriage/ incompatibility | Cruelty | Desertion | Non-support | Alcohol &/or drug addiction | Felony | Impotency | Insanity[1] | Living separate and apart | Residence time | Other grounds |
|---|---|---|---|---|---|---|---|---|---|---|---|
| Montana | X | | | | | | | | | 3 mos. | |
| Nebraska | X | | | | | | | | | 1 yr. | |
| Nevada | X | | | | | | | X | 1 yr. | 6 wks. | |
| New Hampshire | X | X | X | X | X | X | X | | | 1 yr. | X |
| New Jersey | | X | X | | X | X | | X | 6 mos. | 1 yr. | X |
| New Mexico | X | X | X | | | | | | | 6 mos. | |
| New York | | X | X | | | X | | | 1 yr. | 1 yr. | X |
| North Carolina | | | | | | | X | X | 1 yr. | 6 mos. | X |
| North Dakota | X | X | X | X | X | X | X | X | | 1 yr. | X |
| Ohio | X | X | X | | X | X | X | | 2 yrs. | 6 mos. | X |
| Oklahoma | X | X | X | X | X | X | X | X | | 6 mos. | X |
| Oregon | X | | | | | | | | | 6 mos. | |
| Pennsylvania | | X | X | | | X | X | X | 3 yrs. | 1 yr. | X |
| Rhode Island | X | X | X | X | X | X | X | | 3 yrs. | 1 yr. | |
| South Carolina | | X | X | | X | | | | 3 yrs. | 1 yr. | |
| South Dakota | | X | X | X | X | X | | | | actual | |
| Tennessee | X | X | X | X | X | X | X | | | 6 mos. | X |
| Texas | X | X | X | | | | X | | X | 3 yrs. | 1 yr. |
| Utah | | X | X | X | X | X | X | X | | actual | X |
| Vermont | | X | X | X | | X | | X | 6 mos. | 6 mos. | |
| Virginia | | X | X | | | | | | 1 yr. | 6 mos. | X |
| Washington | X | | | | | | | | 2 yrs. | actual | |
| West Virginia | | X | X | | | X | X | | X | 2 yrs. | 2 yrs.-S |
| Wisconsin | X | | | | | | | | 1 yr. | 6 mos. | X |
| Wyoming | X | | | | | | | X | 2 yrs. | 60 days | |

(1) Cal. has a procedure whereby if the couple has been married less than 2 years, have no children, no real estate, little personal property, and few debts they can get a divorce without an attorney and without appearing in court.

Source: Adapted from William F. Mariano, Council on Marriage Relations, Inc., 110 E. 42d St., New York, NY 10017 (as of Oct. 1, 1978).

permit people to get out of unhappy marriages, thereby increasing the divorce rate, but don't explain why people are unhappy in their marriages. If we look at the grounds for divorce by state (Table 13.3) we see there is great variation, from ''no-fault'' divorce to very severe reasons only.

Beyond general trends, it is difficult to predict what specific factors lead to a high divorce rate. As shown in figure 13.1, *Newsweek* (May 15, 1978, p. 67), using U.S. census data, reported that statistically 96 percent of the adults in the United States marry and 38 percent of these people get divorced. We also know that 79 percent of those who divorce then remarry and that 44 percent of these marriages end in divorce. We also know that a number of social factors have been associated with the incidence of divorce. For example, second marriages have a higher divorce rate than first marriages. People who marry in their teens have the highest divorce rate. The divorce rate is lower for college-educated people than for less educated and higher for the poor than for the upper-middle class. Blacks, we know, have a significantly higher divorce rate than whites of comparable income levels. And, blacks who do divorce have more children, so that in 1978 approximately half the black children under 18 were living with only one of their natural parents. Also, even among blacks with a college education there is a considerably higher divorce rate than among whites with a college education. Several reasons for this difference have been suggested, ranging from the increased pressures brought upon blacks as minority groups to the residual effects of historical racism and slavery. But at the present time it is still not clear what the reasons actually are.

## Causes of Divorce

We saw that the incidence of divorce varies according to certain social factors, such as race, socioeconomic level, and educational attainment. Now we are going to look at some factors within the marriage that increase the risk of divorce. Research has identified a number of concrete factors, aside from general marital instability, that affect the likelihood of divorce.

Grounds for divorce

In trying to understand the reasons couples choose divorce over reconciliation, we must recognize that the explicit legal grounds for divorce tell us little about what really breaks apart a marriage. In North Carolina, for example, the only legal grounds for divorce are impotency and insanity, and yet we can assume that the vast majority of failed marriages are dissolved for other reasons, despite what official documents state. The legal grounds for divorce reflect only a society's attitude toward marital dissolution, not the realistic problems of marriage in that society.

Contemporary divorce laws in the United States give basically equal rights to husbands and wives, at least insofar as grounds for divorce are concerned. The search for the real reasons for divorce, then, must go beyond the legal records and into the minds and hearts of the spouses. In an important study, George Levinger (1966) examined the counseling

Table 13.4

**Marital Complaints among 600 Couples Applying for Divorce, Classified by Sex and by Social Position of Respondents**

| | Proportion of complaints by respondent groups | | | | | |
| | | Husbands | Social position of | | | |
| | Wives | | Wives | | Husbands | |
| Complaint | Total[a] | Total[a] | Middle[b] | Lower[c] | Middle[b] | Lower[c] |
|---|---|---|---|---|---|---|
| Physical abuse | .368[d] | .033 | .228 | .401[e] | .029 | .035 |
| Verbal abuse | .238[d] | .075 | .200 | .245 | .048 | .082 |
| Financial problems | .368[d] | .087 | .219 | .402[e] | .124 | .079 |
| Drinking | .265[d] | .050 | .143 | .294[e] | .048 | .051 |
| Neglect of home or children | .390[e] | .262 | .457 | .374 | .200 | .276 |
| Mental cruelty | .403[e] | .297 | .372 | .408 | .267 | .306 |
| In-law trouble | .067 | .162[e] | .038 | .074 | .200 | .153 |
| Excessive demands | .025 | .040 | .057[f] | .018 | .057 | .035 |
| Infidelity | .240 | .200 | .324[f] | .223 | .114 | .198[f] |
| Sexual incompatibility | .138 | .200[e] | .124 | .141 | .267 | .188 |
| Lack of love | .228[e] | .135 | .324[e] | .206 | .200[f] | .120 |

[a] N = 600; all husbands or wives.
[b] N = 105; "Middle" refers to Class I–III on Hollingshead's Index of Social Position.[3]
[c] N = 490; "Lower" refers to Class IV–V on the Hollingshead Index. Note that 5 cases could not be categorized for social position, by dint of insufficient information.
[d] p<.001, indicating a significant difference in favor of the lettered number in the pair, by t test (two-tailed).
[e] p <.01.
[f] p <.05.

Source: Levinger, G. Sources of marital dissatisfaction among applicants for divorce. *American Journal of Orthopsychiatry,* 1966, 36 (5), 803–807.

records of 600 couples seeking divorce in the Cleveland area. While the stated grounds for divorce in Ohio were limited, these in-depth records of legally mandated counseling sessions enabled Levinger to ascertain a broader spectrum of the causes of divorce.

Table 13.4 presents Levinger's data. Wives had about twice as many complaints as did husbands, complaining frequently about physical and verbal abuse, their husbands' drinking, about neglect of family, and financial problems. Only in two areas did the husbands have more complaints than their wives: in-law difficulties and sexual incompatibility.

Levinger also made some social class comparisons which revealed some interesting differences in the patterns of dissatisfaction and complaints across socioeconomic lines (pp. 129–130):

> Lower-status wives were considerably more likely than middle-status wives to complain about financial problems, physical abuse, and drinking. Middle-class wives were significantly more prone to complain about lack of love, infidelity, and excessive demands. Middle-class husbands paralleled the wives in their significantly greater concern with lack of love; on the other hand, they were significantly *less* likely than lower-class husbands to complain of the wife's infidelity.

From these differences, he concludes that "in general, the evidence indicates that spouses in the middle-class marriages were more concerned with psychological and emotional interaction, while the lower-class partners saw as most salient in their lives financial problems and the unsubtle physical actions of their partner" (p. 130).

Noting these differences, Levinger arrives at an explanation which may be applicable in helping us understand marital satisfaction or dissatisfaction in general. Using Maslow's hierarchy of basic needs (see figure 4.1), he points out that in lower-status marriages, the spouses may be so involved in fulfilling subsistence and safety needs that they have little interest in the higher level needs of mature love and interpersonal respect. This suggests that marital difficulties which lead to divorce are directly related to the socioeconomic level of the spouses and to the level of needs which are or are not being met. This model may also help us understand why premarital pregnancy and early motherhood have been associated with a higher divorce rate.

Fulfillment of needs

## Premarital Pregnancy

There is a considerable body of evidence now that there is a causal association between premarital pregnancy and subsequent marital dissolution. Couples who marry when the woman is pregnant are more likely to divorce each other later than are other couples.

Several reasons have been suggested for this phenomenon, most of which emphasize either or both partners' lack of preparation for their respective marital roles. This is sometimes known as *accelerated role transition,* meaning that a person has to assume a new role before he or she is capable of fully understanding or enacting it.

Furstenberg (1976), who has investigated this phenomenon longitudinally, using a sample of 203 adolescent mothers, found specifically that "disruption in the courtship process and limited economic resources are the most important factors contributing to marital dissolution" (p. 63) in the case of couples who marry when the wife-to-be is pregnant. He found that the unplanned pregnancy prevented the newly married couple from building up the financial resources that are often so important at the beginning of a marriage. Because the expectant wife's income-earning potential is decreased, the couple becomes dependent entirely on the husband's salary, which more times than not is insufficient to meet the couple's needs. This dependency, in turn, places a strain on the husband, which further prevents him from being able to support a family and to be supportive of his wife.

## Mel and Crystal

"I think things started to go wrong the day Crystal told me she was pregnant," Mel, her ex-husband explains. "I was finishing my second term at the computer school and if I just had another year I could've landed a great job as a programmer and then we would have gotten married like we planned. But she couldn't work for long, and I couldn't keep up my grades going nights and working days, so I dropped out and took the job I have now, which pays 'beans.' That's all we ever fought about: money-money-money. And that used to make me feel really bad as a father too—like I was letting my kid down."

Disruption of courtship

Just as important to the subsequent dissolution of marriage is the sudden interruption of the courtship process, which we know is a necessary preparation for marital roles (see chapters 4 and 6). The disruption of courtship prevented the two partners from easing into their new roles: instead, they were suddenly thrust into roles for which they were unprepared socially, emotionally, and economically. Furstenberg (1976, p. 83) goes on to say,

> Persons who are "out of phase," that is, premature in their movement to a new role, may be both reluctant to relinquish familiar positions and poorly equipped to assume new ones. Even

if they are adequately prepared, others on whom they depend for support may not be. Ill-timed transitions may remove them from customary sources of social support while denying them the necessary resources to function effectively in their new positions. These reasons help explain why the occurrence of a premarital pregnancy augues so poorly for a couple's prospects of marital success.

### Early Marriage and Early Motherhood

Two other factors that have been shown to affect marital dissolution rates and that are closely related to the above are early marriage and early motherhood. The younger the partners are at the time they marry, the greater the likelihood that their marriage will end in divorce (Schoen 1975).

Early motherhood aggravates early marriage as a factor in divorce. We know that the earlier in a marriage a child is born, the greater the likelihood of marital separation (Bacon 1974). As figure 13.2 shows, early motherhood is positively correlated with a high divorce rate. The very reasons suggested above for premarital pregnancy as a cause of divorce are generally applicable here too. As Bacon points out, "early motherhood, a form of accelerated role transition, is closely associated with high incidence of marital dissolution, poverty, and truncated education" (p. 333). It takes a period of enacting marital roles before one can feel comfortable and can perform well in a parenting role.

*Marital success and age*

There is, then, a direct statistical causal relationship between the potential for marital success and the age at the time of marriage and at first parenthood. In fact, using demographic and statistical data, Lasswell (1974, p. 242) concluded that

> when all of the evidence is in, it appears that women should wait until they are 25 to marry and that they should have their two children at age 28 and age 30. This gives them ample time before they are 35 [when childbearing risks are greater] and it also gives three years after marriage to get the marriage on solid ground emotionally and financially. Men should marry at age 28 and father those two children at age 30 and 32. This allows for what still seems to be a popular notion in our society that it is desirable, for whatever reasons . . . for the husband to be older."

Of course, even if this model were followed exactly it would only give a couple a statistical edge, not a practical one. For the more important factors leading to divorce are not found in statistics but in the quality of the marital relationship itself.

Other Factors  We mentioned earlier the differences in black-white divorce rates. There is also some preliminary evidence that under the so-called *no-fault divorce* laws, which are becoming more commonplace, the divorce rate among blacks jumps even higher, while the rate among whites remains constant (Mazur-Hart and Berman 1977). Also, interracial marriages have a very high rate of dissolution, higher than any other group except teen-age, out-of-wedlock pregnancies (Barron 1972). These rates vary geographically and over time and are apparently highly responsive to the social pressures brought to bear upon the marital partners. Thus social background differences between the spouses, inherent in most intergroup marriages, as well as external social disapproval of a non-normative situation, conspire to create more difficulties—in addition to those found in all marriages. These difficulties produce a greater strain than many interracial couples can bear.

Figure 13.2
**Early Motherhood and Social Pathologies**

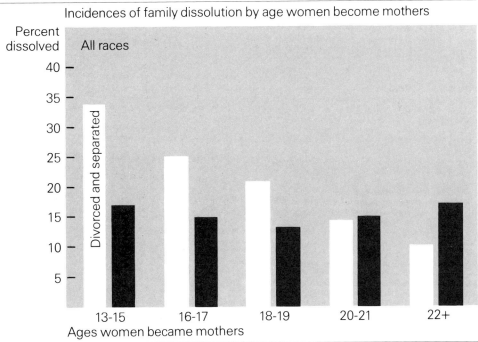

Incidences of family dissolution by age women become mothers

Source: Bacon (1974, p. 336)

## Summary

1. Family violence is the physical abuse of one family member by another. It occurs between any combination of family members. However, the most common problems are violence by one spouse against the other or violence including sexual abuse by a parent against a child. The former is called spouse abuse and the latter child abuse.

2. Spouse abuse and child abuse have two central points in common. First, they are both part of a pattern that has been called the "web of violence," to indicate that family violence spreads from member to member and from generation to generation. Secondly, both are complex social problems that afflict individuals with certain psychological predispositions.

3. There are two perspectives to understanding the roots of child abuse: the psychopathological and the sociological. However, certain facts are recognized by both. Child-abusing parents are often highly disturbed individuals who themselves were severely abused in childhood. Child abuse is a self-perpetuating disorder in which the abused child grows up to be an abusing parent. Moreover, the abusing parent is usually insecure, violent, and unable to control anger, with a tendency to project his or her own inadequacies on the child. The abusing parent is a product of social and psychological strains leading to abusive behavior.

4. A person may become an alcoholic in stages as the dependency on alcohol increases to the point at which his or her life is dominated by drinking.

5. Alcoholism causes severe problems for the family. There may not be enough money or anyone to take care of the children or an adequate sexual relationship between the spouses when one partner drinks. What there is is suffering for every member of the family.

6. Most societies provide a prescribed method for terminating a marital relationship. The act of dissolving a marriage is called divorce. The criteria are called the grounds for divorce. Acceptable reasons for divorce vary from culture to culture.

7. Just as marriage is surrounded by customs that enable the newly married couple to present themselves socially as a pair, divorce requires a certain type of social presentation. Any kind of paired relationship is subject to dissolution, but divorce presents a special case with a public side to it.

8. There are many problems in accurately indicating what the divorce rate really is. The way one computes the figures drastically affects what one infers.

9. Some factors within the marriage that increase the probability of divorce are early marriage and early motherhood. There is also a considerable body of evidence now that there is a causal association between premarital pregnancy and subsequent marital dissolution. Marriages that take place because the bride is pregnant are more likely to end in divorce than are other marriages.

10. It is difficult to predict what specific factors lead to a high divorce probability although the incidence of divorce does vary according to certain social factors such as race, socioeconomic level, and educational attainment.

## Key Terms

The following terms were introduced and defined in this chapter. Definitions also appear in the glossary.

| | |
|---|---|
| accelerated role transition | family violence |
| alcoholic | grounds for divorce |
| battered-child syndrome | prealcoholic phase |
| child abuse | problem drinking |
| chronic phase | prodromal phase |
| crucial phase | psychopathological position |
| divorce | spouse abuse |

**Discussion
Questions**

1. What, if any, violence did you experience or witness in your nuclear family of orientation? Survey your classmates to determine their experiences, either in their own families or in families they knew? What, if any, generalizations can you make about violence in the family?

2. Find out the resources in your community that are available to spouses and children who are victims of family abuse. Assess their adequacy or inadequacy with respect to the prevalence of the family violence problem in your area.

3. From your reading of this chapter, what are some of the common problems underlying all forms of family disruption and dissolution, including violence, alcoholism, and divorce? What do these problems tell us about the structure of the contemporary American family?

4. Investigate the various self-help and support groups for alcoholics in your area. What differences do you find in their approaches? At which of Jellinek's four stages of alcoholism would you try to have a friend of yours seek the help of AA?

5. What are some of the difficulties in accurately and usefully computing the divorce rate? Specifically, what do we mean by *rate* and how can this figure be manipulated to change even as the actual number of divorces would remain constant?

6. From your reading of this chapter, what would you cite as some of the main causes of divorce? Also, what specific social psychological factors at the time of marriage contribute to a poor prognosis for a long and successful marital relationship?

**Suggested
Readings**

1. Paul Bohannan (Ed.). *Divorce and After.* Garden City, New York: Doubleday, 1970.

A short collection of articles analyzing the social and emotional problems both during and after divorce in this and other countries.

2. Richard J. Gelles. "Child Abuse as Psychopathology: A Sociological Critique and Reformulation," *American Journal of Orthopsychiatry,* No. 43 (1973), pp. 611–621.

In this article Gelles sets forth his views on the necessity of taking into account important sociological and contextual factors in the analysis of the causes and remediation of child abuse.

3. D. G. Gil. *Violence Against Children.* Cambridge, Mass.: Harvard University Press, 1970.

A comprehensive report drawing largely on two nationwide surveys, one in 1965 of the knowledge, opinions, and attitudes about the physical abuse of children in the U.S., and the other an epidemiological survey of those children whose physical abuse had been reported to official channels in 1967 and 1968. Gil also reviews the available literature and develops a conceptual framework for his broad-scale, activist-oriented recommendations which includes supporting programs to eliminate poverty, providing a national health service, providing family life education, and counseling for adolescents and adults preparing for marriage and even after marriage.

4. Elizabeth Kubler-Ross. *On Death and Dying.* New York: Bantam, 1973.

An analysis of grief as a definable process by means of which patients deal with the reality of their impending death. This particular book puts the discussion of death and the problems of the dying into the consciousness of society as a whole.

5. Helena Z. Lopata. *Widowhood in an American City.* Cambridge, Mass.: Schenkman, 1973.

The report of a thoughtful and well executed piece of research on the problems of widowhood among a sampling of both black and white women in Chicago over the age of 50, primarily from a role theory perspective.

6. Max Rheinstein. *Marriage Stability, Divorce, and the Law.* Chicago: University of Chicago Press, 1972.

An important, though difficult book by an extremely competent professor of comparative law on the history and contemporary workings of family law in the U.S., Japan, Sweden, Italy, and the Soviet Union. Rheinstein views the major problem in the family as that of marital breakup, with divorce being merely the consequence, and calls for remedial action in terms of counseling and family life education.

7. Suzanne Steinmetz and Murray A. Strauss (Eds.). *Violence in the Family.* New York: Dodd, Mead, 1974.

A 1970 Conference of the National Council on Family Relations on "Violence in the Family" revealed a paucity—and scattering—of research and theoretical analyses of this important topic. Steinmetz and Strauss have done the field a service by pulling together a good deal of the relevant literature and publishing some of the more important pieces in this particular volume.

8. Robert S. Weiss. *Marital Separation.* New York: Basic Books, 1975.

A sensitive analysis of the difficulties of marital dissolution in easily readable form.

# Chapter 14

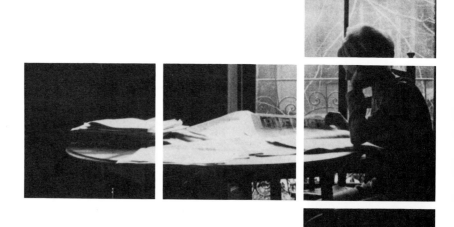

# Reestablishing Equilibrium: Readjustment and Remarriage

**A Complex New Life**
**Postdivorce Adjustment**
**Children of Divorce**
Custody
**Readjustment after a Death**
**The Reconstituted Family**

## Chapter Aims

1. To look at the patterns of reestablishing family equilibrium following family dissolution by death or divorce

2. To examine the social psychological processes of readjustment, for the formerly married and for the children of divorce or death.

3. To consider new trends in child custody.

4. To examine readjustment in a reconstituted family, which is a new family created from two family units dissolved either by death or divorce.

## Overview

Whether a divorce occurs or one of the spouses dies, the resulting dissolution of the family is traumatic. There is an adjustment period that may involve physical changes, such as moving or learning to live with less money, as well as emotional upheaval and a different status among one's friends.

When formerly married people marry other people, they form new families, with new conflicts and patterns of adjustment. The chances of success for these new families vary greatly and harmony between the new spouses is a critical factor.

## A Complex New Life

In a modest brownstone in Boston's Back Bay area, Louise, age twelve, Jill, age nine, and Brad, age six, live with their mother, Emily, and her second husband, Grant. With them live two of Grant's children from his former marriage: Alex, age fifteen, and Damian, who is nine. Not more than a couple of miles away live Emily's former husband, Peter, with his wife, Corrine, along with Valerie, who is Peter and Emily's sixteen-year-old daughter. Corrine is pregnant now, so there will soon be a new member of the household. Also not far away live Alex and Damian's little brother, Eric, with their mother, who is Grant's ex-wife. If this *sounds* confusing imagine how confusing it is when any of the family members named above are trying to explain their relationships to one another to a person from outside the family network.

### The Greenes

Jeannette divorced Lars and married Bob who'd been divorced from Judy who married Rex. Meanwhile, Lars proceeded to marry Ruth who'd been divorced from Sal who then married Anne.

Sound like something from "Mary Hartman, Mary Hartman?" Actually, it's the "family" of Jeannette Lofas Greene, a West Sider who became part of all this by divorcing Lars Lofas in 1968 and marrying Bob Greene in 1972. Also involved are 26 kids residing in a total of five new households.

Early on, the Greenes had to overcome problems familiar to many wed-agains: for instance, dealing with the kids (his four daughters and her son). They've also endured remarriage's financial strain. Investment banker Bob says his divorce was a zero investment—financially speaking, of course. He departed on terms that were highly favorable to his first wife—and enormously money-sapping to his second marriage.

An unexpected problem has been personal dealings within the new extended "family"—all the "exs" (husbands and wives) and "steps" (fathers, mothers, sons, and daughters). One wife, for instance, says she would like to be friendlier with her spouse's ex-wife than he would like her to be. Still, he has to remain on good terms with his "ex" to see his daughters. Meanwhile, a son is depressed because he doesn't like his dad's new stepdaughter. And on it goes . . .

Jeannette has become so intrigued with remarrieds' problems that she has founded the Step Foundation (333 West End Ave., N.Y.C.) to, among other functions, publicize available professional help.

She also counsels many problem-beset remarrieds, drawing complex charts of their new "families" in an effort to explain why they're all not getting along.

Still, a good sense of humor helps one handle the confusion caused by everyone's continually getting divorced and remarried.

Recently, for instance, one of Jeannette's stepdaughters gave birth. When the baby is old enough to understand it all, Jeannette will show him a chart of his extended family.

"By then," she says, "it will be like trying to explain, piece by piece, how a B-1 bomber is assembled."

Source: Michael Pousner, *New York Daily News*, Sept. 1, 1977, p. 57.

Still, as confusing as it may be, this type of social arrangement is becoming more and more common each year. Three things account for it: the increase in the marriage-divorce-remarriage pattern, the trend toward giving fathers as well as mothers custody of children, and the practice of people with children remarrying other people with children and joining the two families together in a single household.

When the family dissolves, reestablishing equilibrium is a complex pattern, including either the process of adjustment to former family dissolution by remaining outside a marital relationship or adjustment through remarriage. Families dissolved by separation or divorce and those dissolved by death face common problems in some areas but have some different readjustment patterns. Let us begin by considering the effects of divorce and separation on the spouses and the children.

## Postdivorce Adjustment

Regardless of the circumstances, divorce is always a traumatic, emotionally difficult situation. A new residence has to be established, financial plans that may have been working well for years have to be revamped, the wife may have to return to work if she has been home raising the children, and the husband may find his spending capacity severely cut, as his income is divided into supporting two separate households.

One of the more complex decisions that has to be made following di-

Living arrangements

vorce is the choice of living arrangments. Does the husband or wife return to the family in which they were raised? Do they live alone? Do they move in with single or married friends? Bernard (1975) has examined some of the changes in living arrangements of divorced men and women during the early to mid-1970s, when the trends that continue to this day began to appear.

First, as we can see in table 14.1, more divorced women than men were living as heads of households and heads of families following a divorce. Fewer divorced women than men were living in families as nonheads, a condition which is commonly referred to as "going home to mother." In short, after a divorce, it is more likely that the woman, rather than the man, will function as a head of a family. This probably reflected the common practice of granting the wife, rather than the husband, custody of the children. Therefore, the wife became head of a one-parent household, while the husband might have gone to live alone or returned to his parents' home.

Additionally, Bernard has shown (1975, pp. 586–587) that the most important determinant of how divorced men and women reestablish themselves is the presence or absence of children:

> The greater the probability that if there are young children they will be with the mother means that: (1) more women than men will be heads of households; (2) fewer will live alone; (3) fewer will live in families as nonhead; and (4) fewer will live in households of unrelated individuals, usually not hospitable to children.

Socially, both ex-spouses have to learn to be single again: an especially tricky adjustment if a person has been out of the dating scene for a long time.

Health trauma

Sudden changes in health may follow marital dissolution as a reaction to the enormous stress caused by the divorce process. Chester (1973) found that 85 percent of a group of divorced women experienced some kind of postdivorce health trauma, including the following most common symptoms:

- serious weight change
- sleep difficulties
- exhaustion and weepiness
- difficulties concentrating
- self-neglect
- increased use of tobacco and alcohol

It is interesting to note that at present less attention seems to be directed toward the post-divorce feelings of men than of women. Even

Table 14.1

**Differences Between Divorced Men and Women in Living Arrangements, 1970, 1974***

| | 1970 | | 1974 | |
|---|---|---|---|---|
| | More men than women[§] | More women than men[§] | More men than women[§] | More women than men[§] |
| In families | | 27.8 | | 26.2 |
| As head | | 33.2 | | 38.2 |
| As nonhead | 5.4 | | 12.0 | |
| Not in families | 27.6 | | 26.0 | |
| Living alone | 16.6 | | 14.4 | |
| Living with non-relatives | 11.0 | | 11.6 | |
| Head of household | | 14.0 | | 20.2 |
| Family | | 33.2 | | 38.2 |
| Nonfamily | 2.5 | | 3.6 | |
| Alone | 16.6 | | 14.4 | |
| Not head of household | 14.0 | | 20.2 | |
| Family | 5.4 | | 12.0 | |
| Nonfamily | 8.5 | | 8.2 | |

[§]Differences in percentage points.

Source: Bernard, J. Note on changing family lifestyles, 1970–1974. *Journal of Marriage and the Family*, 1975, 37, (3), 582–593.

though almost half a century ago, Waller (1930) examined the emotional consequences of divorce for both men and women, much that has been written on divorce in the 1970s focuses on a woman's post-divorce adjustment. In part, this is a consequence of the impact of the women's movement, which has been active in calling public attention to the social disparities between men and women.

The Postdivorce Reaction    There is a tendency to form a set of attitudes and behaviors that have sometimes been referred to as the *post-divorce reaction*. Especially for a person who has either felt trapped in an unhappy marriage or heavily burdened by the arduous and emotionally wearing process of trying to work out complex marital problems, there may be mixed feelings of elation and depression following the divorce. The elation is based on being free of the burden: the situation is finally over with. The depression is a residual feeling of having failed at something that at one time was viewed as important.

**Role transformation**

At the same time that the individual is experiencing these ambivalent feelings and this complex role transformation, an adjustment to a new social status—that of divorced person—is required. Suddenly and without any preparation, the formerly married person is perceived differently by others, and this person is acutely aware of the new reactions.

## Sandra

"After my divorce," Sandra tells us, "I really found out who my friends were. I was quite shocked at how many couples that Stanley and I had been friendly with just dropped me like that. I don't know if Stanley remained friends with them or not. I also noticed that a lot of the women we had known as part of a couple saw me as a threat now because I was single. And you know, a lot of the married men that we had been friends with did 'come on' to me. You may think I'm naive, but I couldn't believe it at first. After all, I was still friendly with their wives."

In an important and sensitive work entitled *Divorced in America* (1974), Joseph Epstein analyzes in considerable depth the complex processes of readjustment required after divorce. There are the serious financial problems of maintaining two households where before there was one, questions over the division of joint property, alliances of friends, associates, and family, and of course the question of custody if children are involved. But perhaps most perplexing, Epstein goes on, is the question of role transformation—how to become accustomed to the new role of divorced person. Despite its high incidence, and despite the fact that divorce no longer stigmatizes as it once did, Epstein argues, "how a divorced person ought to view himself, or how others ought to view themselves in relation to him is not much clearer now than it ever was" (1974, p. 209). He gives some examples of uncertainties of social conduct newly divorced people face: What should be the attitude toward the ex-spouse? How does one behave toward the new spouse (and stepparent) if the "ex" remarries? What about former in-laws?

In a similar vein, in a classic paper on the subject of readjustment after divorce, Waller (1930) makes the important point that even "if one escapes the deep trauma of the experience of divorce itself, he is not yet free, but must encounter . . . being treated as people think that a divorce should be treated. If not the divorce, then perhaps his status as a divorced person wounds him" (p. 103). Often, a lack of additional social support increases the difficulty of interpreting how one feels following divorce, and adds in its own way to the possibility of chronic physical complaints, malaise, severe depression, and even a possible mental breakdown. It has been noted, for example, that there is a higher frequency of depression and breakdown among divorced people than among those who remain married or who never marry (Briscoe and Smith, 1973).

Kin relations can also be complicating factors, especially if there is real attachment to the family of the ex-spouse. The friendliness or antipathy of the postdivorce relationship with the ex-spouse if there is contin-

*The depression that follows divorce may be a residual feeling of having failed at something that once was important.*

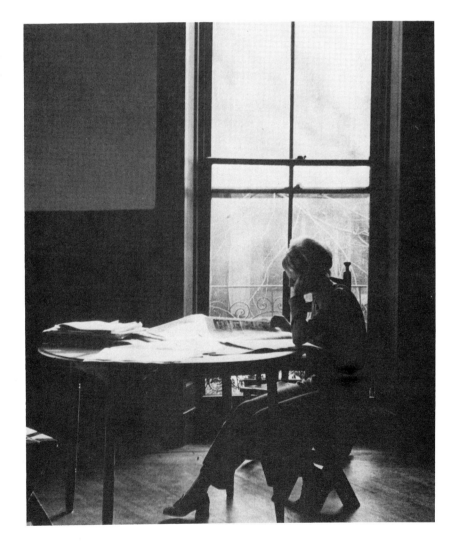

uing contact can make the adjustment easier or more difficult. If one of the ex-partners has found a new partner and the other has not, there may be envy or anger, which could slow down the adjustment.

**Transitional groups**

In recent years, specialized transitional groups, such as postdivorce groups or divorce-adjustment seminars, have been appearing throughout the country, ostensibly to help individuals adjust to the postdivorce period (Fisher 1977). But they also provide the important service of helping formerly married people who are now single meet others who may be looking for companionship.

## Children of Divorce

About 60 percent of the couples obtaining a divorce have children at home, most of these below high school age. For the children, the adjustments following parental divorce are even more complicated and difficult than they are for the parents. They are made so by a number of factors: the children's probable dependency on both parents, their dual loyalties and mixed feelings, the divided time they spend with each parent, and the reactions of their peers.

Where at one time "it may have been conventional wisdom that couples, no matter how unhappy with one another, should stay together for the sake of the children," Weiss (1975) points out that nowadays, "couples appear to believe that a stressful two-parent home provides a less satisfactory setting for a child's development than a tranquil one-parent home" (p. 167). With this change in attitude, a greater number of parents with dependent children are willing to separate and divorce.

Even the most conscientious of parents will have difficulty helping the child through the postdivorce trauma. The parent with whom the child lives for the majority of time is, after all, not only emotionally involved in the situation and working out his or her own adjustment, but may well be viewed by the child as the one responsible for the divorce or at least half-responsible. Since so many of these children are of school age, some schools are taking an increasing role in providing group and individual counseling support for children of divorce in much the same way as adult postdivorce adjustment groups are springing up for the ex-spouses (Green 1978). In a way, what this is telling us is that divorce is becoming recognized as a fact of life in the United States and social institutions are changing to accommodate to it.

Lora Heims Tessman, who has done extensive research on the social and psychological processes of child adjustment following divorce has published an important book, entitled *Children of Parting Parents* (1978). She describes some of the complex stages and situations children may go through during the period of readjustment. We have summarized three of the main types of reactions:

**The child's reactions**

1. *Identification With the Lost Parent*—the child imagines he or she is the lost parent (the parent not living at home) and behaves as that parent did in the home—or imagines a fantasy relationship with the absent parent. We see this when, for example, a boy will suddenly take on his absent father's mannerisms, even to the extent of doing imitations of the father. Or, a child may tell friends that the missing father is on a secret government mission and will be back in a few months.

2. *Quest for the Wanted Absent Person*—the ''quest'' may be psychological or expressed through such behaviors as restlessness, creativity, hyperactivity, or antisocial behavior. This can be considered a part of the adjustment process because the child is still working through the disquieting feelings of abandonment.

3. *Grieving*—the child goes through a reaction as if the parent had died, but without the support that would be present from the living parent if the other had died. This reaction becomes especially strong when the child's expected contact with the missing parent is frustrated, for example, if the parent fails to show up on visiting day.

## Custody

In years past, unless the mother could be shown beyond a reasonable doubt to be unfit to care for a child, the custody of the child of divorce was routinely awarded to the mother. Women were viewed as more fit as parents, with ''natural instincts'' for taking care of their children. And the role of the ex-husband following divorce was to earn enough money to support his ex-wife and child in the style to which they had become accustomed.

This common practice was known in law as the *tender years doctrine.* It said in effect that children are better off with their mothers than with their fathers. It resulted in a consistent policy of maternal custody, supported by many specialists in the child-care disciplines, such as psychologists, pediatricians, educators, and sociologists. They argued that paternal custody or dual custody was dangerous to the welfare of the child (Woody 1978). Especially influential was the book *Beyond the Best Interest of the Child* by Joseph Goldstein, Anna Freud, and Albert Solnit, published in 1973 and cited as evidence in many court cases.

But as studies began to indicate that there is nothing natural about mothering and that many fathers could be good ''mothers,'' there came to be some leeway in this doctrinaire position. Several important books, such as *The Disposable Parent* (Haddad and Roman 1978), cogently challenged the ''tender years doctrine.''

Just as important to the question of custody was a simultaneous social phenomenon and its affect on the family. As women began to enter the work place en masse, many divorcing couples were living on two incomes, not one. Thus, the argument about the father being the sole financial support lost ground as well. As a result, and in view of the expanding social role of women, a new concept, *joint custody*, came into prominence.

*Watts v. Watts*

In 1973 in New York's Family Court, the old doctrine was discarded altogether in a landmark case (*Watts* v. *Watts*), where Judge Sybil Hart Kooper found the ''tender years doctrine'' was based largely on social stereotypes and not supported adequately by the bulk of research (Pick 1978). Several other important cases followed, the most notable being the ''Salk case,'' in which Dr. Lee Salk won custody of his child, even though his wife was not found to be wanting as a mother. For the first time, a man was being awarded custody of his child, not by elimination, but because he merited the award on the facts of the case.

*The belief that the mother is best qualified to receive custody is now being questioned and more fathers are winning custody of their children.*

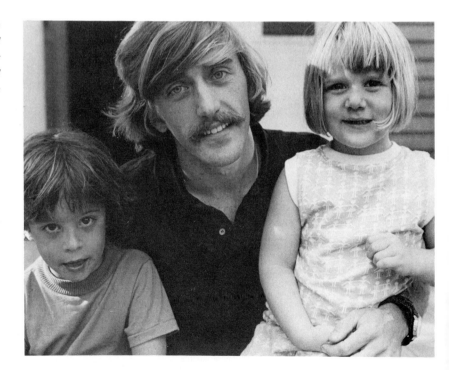

The awarding of paternal custody or joint custody has required some serious rethinking of the entire question of custody. It has also influenced much of the divorce process. Where once mothers took it for granted that they would be awarded custody, they may now have to fight for it, and so custody becomes a part of the total divorce battle in which the child is a pawn. In recent years the custody struggle has led to an increase in children's problems, especially as they are caught in the middle of a division of loyalties between their battling parents (Musetto 1978).

**Adam**

"When I look at Adam, I really feel I've failed as a mother," Mrs. Kramer says sincerely. "I can only say in defense that I did it for his own good. When my 'ex' got joint rights, I was as shocked as my lawyer. I knew I had to fight it for Adam's own benefit, for a stable home for him. He didn't like to see me and his father going at each other, and sometimes it was vicious. But that was the way it had to be. Someday, Adam will realize that I fought this way because I love him, not to hurt him. But he got hurt in the process, and now he's angry at me."

## Readjustment after a Death

A large number of marriages terminate with the death of a spouse. For the surviving spouse this is probably the most significant life crisis. In the case of a family with children, suddenly left motherless or fatherless, there are profound social as well as personal implications. Dissolution by death requires considerable psychological adjustment by each individual family member and usually attracts a broad range of social support from kin relations to intimate friends and from business associates to social institutions.

Dissolution by death

When a spouse or parent dies either unexpectedly or after a long illness and the surviving family members are unable to reorganize themselves under these difficult and painful circumstances, there is a *grief crisis:* a turbulent period of major psychosocial readjustment.

Funerals and formal periods of mourning are designed to help readjustment. The surviving spouse and other family members may want to talk about their memories of the deceased, possibly expressing such feelings as "I was never as good [to the deceased] as I should have been." Or they may want to talk about how the deceased enjoyed life and deserved to live longer or pine about how unjust and unfair the world is, tak-

*Funerals and formal periods of mourning help in the readjustment of survivors to the loss of a loved one.*

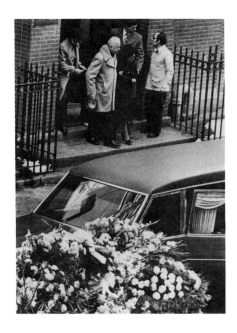

ing away such a good person. The surviving spouse often recalls with painful clarity long-past incidents involving his or her interactions with the deceased and may long to express feelings about these incidents that have been forgotten for some time.

"The duration of a grief reaction," Lindeman (1944) points out in his classic paper on the subject, "seems to depend on the success with which a person does the *grief work;* namely, emancipation from the bondage to the deceased, readjustment to the environment in which the deceased is missing, and the formation of new relationships" (p. 143). Mourning rituals are designed to speed up this process. Until the grief work is completed and the grief worked through, the survivor is, in Lindeman's words, "in bondage" to the deceased.

*On Death and Dying*

The most significant recent work on grief crisis and on dealing with death as a reality of life has been done by Elizabeth Kubler-Ross. Her book *On Death and Dying* (1973) paved the way for much of the subsequent research on this subject. Her theory is especially important because it represents the first serious effort to deal with the grief crisis experienced by the dying person while in the process of dying, rather than by the survivors after the death has occurred. This period of dying, as we can well imagine, places an enormous strain upon the family members, who know they are going to lose someone they love and can do nothing about it. Under certain circumstances, the strain can pull a family apart at the very moment they should be solidifying their bonds.

Kubler-Ross (1969) emphasizes the need to keep communication open between the dying person and the family and suggests that the grief crisis can be worked through before the person dies, not only after. She delineates a five-stage process through which a person adjusts to the idea of death. The first stage involves *denial,* where the person refuses to believe he or she is dying. Then there is *anger*—''Why is this happening to me?'' followed by *bargaining, depression,* and finally, with the appropriate supportive family interventions, a stage of *acceptance.* Her book is well worth reading for any person who is going through this painful experience.

### Factors in Working through Grief
There are a number of significant factors that play a part in how well or how poorly a grief crisis can be resolved. First, the suddenness of the death is of great practical importance. Even though it is said that we can never fully prepare for a loved one's death, there is a qualitative difference between our loved one suddenly dropping dead and a loved one lingering on for a period of time, wasting away with illness.

Untimely death

Weisman (1973) differentiates between three kinds of untimely death: premature, unexpected, and calamitous, and suggests that they cause different types of reactions. *Premature* refers to the death of a young person, a child. *Unexpected* refers to the sudden death of a normal and healthy person. ''The emotional impact upon survivors,'' he points out, ''is gauged and sharpened by how [the deceased] happens to be at the time of death.'' It is not uncommon to hear, ''He was such a vital, alive person . . . I can't believe he's dead.'' Finally, *calamitous death* ''is not only unpredicted, but violent, destructive, demeaning, and even degrading (p.371). This last category would include murder and suicide.

The important point is that every grief situation requires a different process of readjustment and family reorganization, and this always requires strong social supports. The family members' responses to each form differ, but Weisman correctly points out, ''there are no ready made, cookbook recipes for coping with untimely death.''

## The Reconstituted Family

The majority of people who divorce with children or whose spouse dies while they have growing children, eventually remarry. There are probably a number of reasons that so many people whose first marriage ends in divorce choose to marry a second time. People who were divorced once may feel that they now know how to make a marriage work this time. People who were divorced once may be members of socioeconomic and religious groups that are more likely to view divorce as a possibility. Likewise, people who lose a spouse may, as a part of getting over the grief period, find someone else to love and to marry. This is especially important where children are involved, since many people feel it is better for the children to be a part of a two-parent family. This pattern has become so widespread that now it is estimated there are about eight million families in the United States with at least one child and a stepparent. These hybrid families are called *reconstituted families*.

Remarriage

Whether or not a remarriage will work, and whether the newly formed family will be successful as a unit depends on many different factors. "The most important predictor of a remarriage's success," according to Weiss (1975), "appears to be its acceptability to other individuals in the lives of the prospective spouses. A remarriage that not only has the approval of the two spouses' children, but also the support of their kin and friends, appears especially likely to be successful" (p. 304). This, as we will see below, has been borne out by further research which emphasizes the importance of a number of external social factors as predictors of success or failure in second marriages.

The reconstituted family has more than its share of problems. The questions of dual loyalties, of the development of appropriate new roles and the understanding of family statuses are complicated enormously by the experiences the children and spouses had in the previous family setting. Understandably, there is a high divorce rate among families reconstituted after divorce. Cherlin (1978, p. 640) has suggested that this is so because remarriage after divorce is not institutionalized enough yet to enjoy the effective (and necessary!) social controls that first marriages have. What this means, in effect, is that we do not have as many rules and expectations regarding remarriage as we do the first marriage:

> Persons who are remarried after a divorce and have children from
> previous marriages face problems unlike those encountered in
> first marriages. The institution of the family provides no standard
> solutions to many of these problems, with the result that the
> unity of families of remarriages after divorce often becomes pre-
> carious. The incomplete institutionalization of remarriage shows
> us, by way of contrast, that family unity in first marriages is still
> supported by effective institutional controls.

Compared with first marriages, remarriages involve more complex decisions on matters which earlier seemed to be just routine. Should there be a honeymoon? What remnants of the former marriage do the spouses retain (such as the wife's formerly married name by which she may be known professionally) What name do the children use? How are former in-laws accepted by the new spouse? Are the children to be legally adopted by the new spouse?

However, people whose spouses die and who then remarry tend to have more successful remarriages and to get along better with their stepchildren than people whose first marriages were dissolved by divorce (Duberman 1975). It is possible, although not proven, that one reason for this success is the social support that is offered after the death of a spouse but withheld after divorce. Another explanation for this has been suggested by Leitner and Stecher (1974), who point out that "crises can lead to self-exploration and this may lead to clearer personal meaning and identity [in life]" (p. 29). They go on to suggest (p. 32) that crisis states give the individual a motivation for change and growth:

> When forces of life push our daily existence to some edge whereupon we find ourselves in the midst of crisis, then we have a chance to emerge as changed beings. Growth implies change and change may imply growth. Emerging from a crisis can be a movement toward a new being-state, one that we may not have been capable of before the crisis. . . . Crises call for *risking.* People in crisis, under intense pressure, become introspective— they can look at themselves more deeply and honestly than in times of tranquility. (italics in original)

In her landmark study of the reconstituted family, sociologist Lucile Duberman (1975), herself a member of a reconstituted family, investigated in depth remarried couples and their children, focusing on the

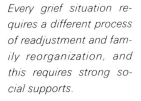

*Every grief situation requires a different process of readjustment and family reorganization, and this requires strong social supports.*

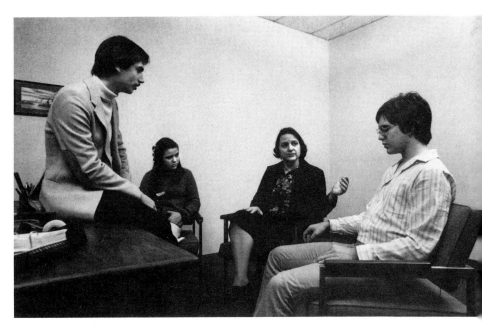

stepchild-stepparent-stepsibling interactions. This is a fascinating book, well worth reading, and we summarize here only a few of the key points from her research.

1. For most remarried people, the greatest single problem and the cause of the most arguments with their spouses is childrearing beliefs. Middle-class remarried husbands viewed money as the second most bothersome problem that caused marital discord. Table 14.2 displays some of the problems remarried couples encounter.

2. The younger the remarried couple, the greater is the "integration" of their reconstituted family. There is more integration if the previous marriage dissolved because of the death of a spouse and if the parents in the reconstituted family have a child together.

3. Husband-wife relationships were rated as excellent in 54 percent of the sample and "poor to good" in 46 percent, with about 70 percent of the couples perceiving their relationship as "improving." The main sources of argument were childrearing and money.

4. The better the relationship between husband and wife, the more integrated is the family.

5. Stepfathers, especially those who had never been married

Table 14.2

**Major Problems Encountered by Remarrieds**

| Problem | Husbands percent | Wives percent |
|---|---|---|
| Child-rearing | 35 | 35 |
| Money | 20 | 16 |
| Sex relations | 11 | 6 |
| Religion | 10 | 6 |
| Political differences | 9 | 11 |
| Outsiders | 9 | 14 |
| Recreation | 6 | 11 |
| Total | 100 | 100 |

Adapted from: L. Duberman, *The reconstituted family: A study of remarried couples and their children* (Chicago: Nelson-Hall, 1975).

before, generally had better relationships with their stepchildren than did stepmothers, regardless of the sex of the stepchild.

6. Stepsibling relationships varied. ''When both sets of children lived in the same house, the relations between them were more likely to be 'Excellent' than if they lived in different houses. Furthermore, when the remarried couple had a child together, their children were likely to have more harmonious relations'' (p. 75). Table 14.3 displays how well remarried couples think their reconstituted families are getting along.

7. While most remarried people are fairly indifferent to their ex-spouses, there was a higher incidence of ex-spousal conflicts and anger for men than for women. This was probably because the men were responsible for alimony, and sometimes fought with their ex-wives about money.

When we consider the implications of these findings, it becomes clear that a reconstituted family can only work as well as the remarried spouses are able to get along together. Where there is harmony between the parents, there is more likely to be harmony among the children. Moreover, to increase the chance for a successful reconstituted family, the remarried parents might consider having their own child, since it has been shown that this offers a greater sense of integration, more family stability, and better relations with the children of the former marriage(s).

Table 14.3

**Parental Estimation of the Direction of Change in the Relationships Between Stepsiblings**

| Direction | Percent of families | |
| | percent | number |
| --- | --- | --- |
| Worse | 16 | ( 7) |
| Same | 42 | (19) |
| Better | 42 | (19) |
| Total | (100) | (45) |

Source: Duberman (1975).

## Summary

1.  Divorce is a traumatic, emotionally difficult situation. A new residence has to be established, financial plans that may have been working well for years have to be revamped, the wife may have to return to work if she has been home raising the children, and the husband may find his spending capacity severely cut, as his income is divided into supporting two separate households. Socially, both ex-spouses have to learn to be single again.

2.  There is a tendency to form a set of attitudes and behaviors that have sometimes been referred to as the ''postdivorce reaction.'' Especially for a person who has felt trapped in an unhappy marriage or terribly burdened by the arduous process of trying to work out complex marital problems, there may be mixed feelings of elation and depression following the divorce. At the same time that the individual is experiencing these ambivalent feelings and a complex role transformation, an adjustment to a new social status—that of divorced person—is required.

3.  About 60 percent of the couples obtaining a divorce have children at home, most of these below high school age. For the children, the adjustments following parental divorce are even more complicated and difficult than they are for the parents. They are made so by a number of factors: the children's probable dependency on both parents, their dual loyalties and mixed feelings, the divided time they spend with each parent, and the reactions of their peers.

4.  In years past, unless the mother could be shown beyond a reasonable doubt to be unfit to care for a child, the custody of the child of divorce was routinely awarded to her. But as studies began to indicate that there is nothing natural about mothering and that many fathers could be good caretakers, this practice began to change.

5.  A large number of marriages end with the death of a spouse, at which point there may be a grief crisis when the family goes through a period of turbulent readjustment.

6.  The reactions of the survivors are influenced by whether the death followed a long illness or was untimely. In any case, the family members have the tasks of working out their grief and readjusting and reorganizing the family.

7. The majority of people who divorce or whose spouses die and who have children eventually remarry. This pattern has become so widespread that it is estimated now there are about eight million families in the United States with at least one child and a stepparent. These hybrid families are called reconstituted families.

8. In her landmark study of the reconstituted family, sociologist Lucile Duberman investigated remarried couples and their children in depth, focusing on the stepchild-stepparent-stepsibling interactions. The chances for success in reconstituted families are greater when the remarried spouses get along well together, when the previous marriage ended with the death of the spouse, and when the remarried parents have a child together.

## Key Terms

The following terms were introduced and defined in this chapter. Definitions also appear in the glossary

acceptance
anger
bargaining
calamitous death
denial
depression
grief crisis

grief work
joint custody
postdivorce reaction
premature death
reconstituted families
tender years doctrine
unexpected death

**Discussion Questions**

1. Interview one or two people, preferably at least one man and one woman, who have been through a divorce. What do they cite as the major difficulties of postdivorce adjustment, and what personal characteristics and social supports were most helpful in enabling them to adapt to their "new lives?" If you know any children of divorce, attempt to find out what types of difficulties they experienced and what factors affected, positively or negatively, their adjustment process.

2. Assume you have been asked to present a brief in support of joint or paternal custody. What findings from throughout this book could be cited in support of your argument? Particularly, attempt to relate some of the information you learned in chapters 3 and 10 that would be relevant to this issue.

3. After reading this chapter, what do you see as the common points of readjustment following a grief crisis and a divorce? List the four major kinds of life-changes and changes in emotional perspective that help an individual with each of these.

4. Focus on a reconstituted family with whom you are familiar. Which of the Duberman findings would you say are most consistent with your own observations of this family? With which would you disagree?

## Suggested Readings

1. Jesse Bernard. *Remarriage*. New York: Dryden, 1956.

   Prepared basically as a supplementary textbook for courses in ''marriage and the family,'' this book also includes a good deal of Bernard's own research on this question. It did much to raise the consciousness of family sociologists to the increasing numbers of persons involved in remarriage and the attendant problems they faced.

2. Lucile Duberman. *The Reconstituted Family*. Chicago: Nelson-Hall, 1975.

   This important work, a detailed study of remarried couples and their children, points out answers to some of the basic questions affecting second marriages, including discussions of step-parent/step-children relationships, step-sibling relationships, family integration, the husband-wife relationship, etc.

3. Joseph Epstein. *Divorced in America*. New York: Penguin Books, 1974.

   A well written book by a literary scholar about divorce among middle-class Americans that blends reporting with his own personal experiences of divorce.

4. William J. Goode. *After Divorce*. New York: Free Press, 1956 (Reissued as *Women in Divorce*, 1965).

   A thorough-going sociological study of the factors that lead to divorce and the consequences of marital dissolution. Specifically, Goode analyzes the institutionalization of adjustment after divorce, the effects of divorce on the children, dating and economic activities that occur after divorce, remarriage, and a number of other important issues.

5. Morton Hunt. *The World of the Formerly Married*. New York: McGraw-Hill, 1966.

   A description and analysis of the heretofore largely invisible world of the formerly married by a perceptive and thoughtful writer. Hunt combines in-depth interviews, survey questionnaires, and personal observation with a review of a good deal of the existing social science literature on divorce to focus on the issue at hand. In part, this book made the problems of the formerly married more visible and lead in some cases to the development of voluntary organizations to assist individuals finding themselves in this circumstance.

# Epilogue: The Future of Marriage and the Family

We have attempted, throughout this book, to point out some of the major trends which characterize changes in marriage and family life in the United States today. In this section, we will try to synthesize some of this information and indicate which of the present trends are likely to continue as well as some possible new directions in the 1980s in marriage and family life.

Rather than present this information as a series of formal propositions, since it would be presumptuous to try to predict the future with any semblance of authority, we have tackled this task in a question and answer format. The questions are those most asked by students in our courses, or by others who have an interest in this subject matter. The answers are drawn from the material presented throughout this book, or, where cited, from other relevant contemporary sources. We will attempt to focus as much as possible on basic interpretations of the the available data. Consider each question and our answers. Then, write down predictions and plans for *your* future in each of these areas. It may be quite interesting years hence to look back and see how you fared in predicting your future.

## Is the nuclear family still a viable institution?

Evidence seems to indicate that indeed it is. Not only is there considerable support to suggest its universality, as we indicated in Chapter 2, but in the past two decades it has been put to some severe tests—and has survived! This is probably the best indication of its strength as a viable institution.

For example, during the turbulent 1960s and 70s the proliferation of communes, the increasing frequency of nonmarital cohabition, the considerably greater mobility of young people—all these social trends seemed at the time to pose a threat to the stability of the nuclear family. Yet, the most recent census data indicate that people are still getting married and having children. Even though divorce is becoming more common, individuals tend to remarry and establish second families. Moreover, attitude surveys and public opinion polls, as well as these census data show clearly "the persistence of commitments to family life" by most Americans (Bane 1978). So, we conclude that the nuclear family is going to be around for a long time, and although we may see many other tests where it will have to prove itself, it should survive as an institution.

### How will the form and structure of the family change?

The fact that the nuclear family will survive does not mean that its form will remain the same as it has been during the past half century, nor that its contemporary structure will endure. Presently, in fact, only 17% of American families consist of the traditional model of a fulltime working father and a "homemaking" mother taking care of the children, while 28% of the families consist of both mother and father as contributing wage-earners, with one or more children at home (Freidan 1979, p. 92). For example, over the past 50 years there have been notable changes in family size and in the incidence of extended vs. modified extended families. Westoff (1978) points out several changes that are presently affecting the form and structure of families. People are getting married later, often after some years of childless cohabitation. Women are having their first children later in life and are bearing, on the average, fewer children. A larger number of children are being raised in single family settings. Fertility is on the decline and will probably fall below replacement level shortly: that is, we will have a negative population growth. Such changes will undoubtedly continue.

### Will there be changes in the roles of different family members?

Clearly, the most pronounced changes in this area involve the changing role of women in our society. As the social and personal expectations of women have risen over the past decade, along with higher levels of education and economic attainment, the option of becoming a housewife and mother is now one of several available to girls who enter womanhood. Some choose a career followed by marriage and motherhood; others choose not to marry at all. In any case, because the contemporary American woman recognizes that domestic life is but one option of many, she regards it differently than would the woman who historically felt that this was her only choice. However, we will not know the full impact of evolving the feminist consciousness on marriage, childrearing, and family life for several years (Hymowitz and Weissman 1978).

The sexual roles of the spouses are also undergoing changes in the family. The wife's traditional position as a sexual subordinate, whose job it was to please her husband, has come under intense challenge. Women, both married and single, have shown a willingness to speak out for their sexual satisfaction, which has influenced men's attitudes about sex. Since the husband is no longer viewed as the primary sexual force in a marriage—the one to be satisfied—he has a role that includes pleasing the wife.

### Will the relationship between family roles and work roles be any different?

Since family roles have traditionally been tied up with work roles (and work opportunities), we can expect the changes in the latter to affect the former. This has been shown to be particularly true when we look at the marital functioning of dual-career couples, both with and without children. The research is not entirely clear at this time, but we do know that during the past decade the number of such couples has tripled. Many studies have indicated that these couples can function at least as well, and in certain areas (such as flexibility in problem solving) possibly better than traditional couples (Huser and Grant 1978). Certainly the available data seem to indicate that in the 1980s "the dual-career family is an emergent family form in our society that offers new satisfaction [and] also presents new types of problems for families" (Hopkins and White 1978). Just how these problems will be resolved will be a test of the strength and viability of this new form.

### What are the present trends with regard to family size and how is this expected to affect family stability and marital happiness?

Important technological, social, and attitudinal changes in the United States have made it easier and more acceptable for a woman to remain childless. Effective female contraception is available, abortions are widely and legally performed, and an increasing number of women are now encouraged to pursue a career in lieu of bearing children. Does this mean that more and more women are remaining childless? According to Poston and Gotard (1977), there is indeed an increasing number of young women who are remaining voluntarily childless and this is probably "linked to broader societal changes regarding fertility control, contraceptive technology, female work preferences and patterns, and sexual and family norms" (p. 212).

There is considerable speculation about how this change will affect the institution of marriage which is, to a large extent, designed for the rearing of children. While many people believe that childless marriages tend to be unhappy (an old stereotype, perhaps perpetuated to encourage couples to have children), there is some evidence to the contrary. For example, Renne (1976) investigated the overall physical health and dimensions of marital satisfaction for married couples with children and without children. She found that "parenthood may be detrimental to both health and marital satisfaction." Specifically, she points out

> that parenthood detracts from the physical and psychological health of husbands and wives, particularly among younger couples. Rates of joint marital satisfaction also were lower for active parents than for former parents and childless couples, regardless of the duration of the marriage and the wife's age and employment status. (p. 183)

These results would certainly have to be replicated to be truly meaningful but they do raise some serious questions about the effect that childrearing has on a marriage.

### Will reproduction continue to be an important part of the form of family life that we know?

From the beginning of history, reproduction has been an important part of family life, although its importance relative to other functions has changed from time to time. Nowadays, child-free marriage is a more likely option than at any other time in history for three reasons: better, more effective, and comfortable methods of contraception; more career and educational opportunities for women who, years ago, would have had little choice but to bear children soon after marriage; and, finally, the considerable expense of finding a suitable place to live for a family (as opposed to a couple). This does not mean that married couples will not have children, but rather that they now have a choice. For many couples, the bearing of children will be a more carefully thought-out act than it has been in the past.

### How will the increasing divorce rate affect the future of the family?

If present trends continue, and the divorce rate rises annually while the marriage rate remains relatively stable, within the decade we will be seeing a common pattern of sequential marriage as the norm, rather than the exception. What this means is that there may be at any given time as many people married a second time as there are couples in first marriages. Moreover, many of these couples will have children from a previous marriage.

The fact that there are so many children involved in these remarriage situations leads to a second type of situation; namely, that there will be an increasing number of reconstituted families, with children and their step-parents and step-siblings living in a common residence. Because, as we pointed out earlier, many of the decisions that are easy to make in first marriages become more complex in second marriages, it seems likely that new rules, regulations, and conventions will evolve for the reconstituted family. In short, it is likely that there will evolve the kinds of social definitions and supports for remarriages and reconstituted families that are available for first marriages and primary families.

### How will the preparation for marriage and family life change?

Several trends in recent years indicate some changes in the way people prepare for marriage and family life, and in the way entering into marriage is approached in general. First, there seems to be an increasing emphasis on institutionally supported preparation for marriage and parenthood. Schools and civic and religious organizations provide guidance, and reading material that helps young people assess their future prospects is more readily available. Colleges offer courses which emphasize effective communication and understanding of what marital roles entail. Many of these courses are practical and problem-solving oriented, offering information on such areas of potential conflict as premarital sex, birth control, extramarital affairs, financial management, wife's earnings, and alcohol problems in the family (Knox and Knox 1974). This kind of preparation, along with courses on parenting offered in high schools and colleges, should provide young people entering into marriage more information than was available to their parents, information which can be put into practice in family life.

Second, for various reasons, such as the pervasive cynicism of the late 1960s, the fact that people entering into marriage know more and more people who are getting divorced, and because we no longer view the first marriage as inevitably permanent, young people especially are willing to work on their marriages to make them succeed. This includes the growing phenomenon of couples' groups, growth groups, self-help books, and private marriage therapy. Many more people today recognize that marriage is something that has to be continually worked on, not some natural path to lifelong happiness after taking the vows.

Each of us could certainly generate an equal number of interesting questions about the future of the family, but we tried to limit ourselves to what we discussed before and to what is most frequently asked by our students. It might be interesting as an exercise to see what questions and what answers you could come up with.

In short, then, it seems to us that the twin institutions of marriage and the family are still strong and viable—at least for the foreseeable future. They will be somewhat different institutions from what they have been in the past, marked by more equality, greater flexibility in role relationships, and more opportunities for reevaluation and change. This transition has been and will continue to be painful to many—as is often true in cases of rapid social change. However, marriage and the family have proved to be resilient institutions in the past, and they will undoubtedly continue to adapt to the changing social circumstances of the present and to the demands of the immediate future. We conclude by agreeing with Mary Jo Banes (1978), that American family life is "here to stay."

# References

**Abernathy, V.**
1976. Prevention of unwanted pregnancy among teenagers. *Primary Care,* 3 (3), 399–406.

**Abramowitz, R.**
1977. Parenthood in America. *Journal of Clinical Child Psychology,* 5 (3), 43–46.

**Ackerman, N. W.**
1958. *The psychodynamics of family life.* New York: Basic Books.

**Adams, B.**
1968. *Kinship in an urban setting.* Chicago: Markham.

**Anthony, E. J. & Chiland, C.**
1978. *The child in his family.* Vol. 5, "Children and their parents in a changing world." New York: John Wiley & Sons.

**Aponte, H. J.**
1974. Organizing treatment around the family's problems and their structural bases. *Psychiatric Quarterly,* 48 (2), 209–222.

**Aranoff, J. & Crano, W.D.**
1975. A reexamination of the cross-cultural principles of task segregation and sex role differentiation in the family. *American Sociological Review,* 40 (1), 12–20.

**Araoz, D. L.**
1977. Marital problems and the exceptional child. *International Journal of Family Counseling,* 5 (1), 64–69.

**Ashworth, A. E. & Walker, W. M.**
1972. Social structure and homosexuality. *British Journal of Sociology,* 23 (2), 146–158.

**Aubrey, R. T.**
1975. *Experimenting with living: Pros and cons.* Columbus: Charles E. Merrill.

**Bacon, L.**
1974. Early motherhood, accelerated role transition, and social pathologies. *Social Forces,* 52 (8), 333–340.

**Bagley, C.**
1969. Incest behavior and incest taboo. *Social Problems,* 16 (4), 505–518.

**Baker, S. L. et al.**
1967. *Impact of father absence on personality factors of boys.* Paper presented at American Orthopsychiatric Association meeting. Washington, D. C. March.

**Bane, M. J.**
1978. *American families in the twentieth century.* New York: Basic Books.

**Bandura, A.**
1969. *Principles of behavior modification.* New York: Holt, Rinehart & Winston.

# References

**Baranowski, M. D.**
1978. Perception of adolescents' attempted influence on parental behaviors. *Dissertation Abstracts International,* 38 (10–A), 6342.

**Barron, M. L.**
1972. *The blending American: patterns of intermarriage.* Chicago: Quadrangle.

**Baum, P.**
1973. *Another way of life: The story of communal living.* New York: Putnam.

**Baumrind, D.**
1971. Current patterns of parental authority. *Developmental Psychology Monographs,* 4 (1, Pt. 2).

**Becker, H. S.**
1963. *Outsiders: Studies in the sociology of deviance.* New York: The Free Press.

**Bell, J. E.**
1975. *Family therapy.* New York: Jason Aronson.

**Bell, R. R. & Chaskes, J. B.**
1970. Premarital sexual experience among coeds, 1958 and 1968. *Journal of Marriage and the Family,* 81–84.

**Belser, J. L.**
1977. Empathy as a two-component process. *Dissertation Abstracts International,* 38 (2–B), 887–888.

**Berg, D. H.**
1975. Sexual subculture and contemporary heterosexual interaction patterns among adolescents. *Adolescence,* 10 (40), 543–547.

**Berscheid, E. & Walster, E.**
1974. Physical attractiveness. In L. Berkowitz (Ed.), *Advances in experimental social psychology* (Vol. 7). New York: Academic Press.

**Bettelheim, B.**
1969 *The children of the dream.* New York: Macmillan.

**Bettinger, C.**
1978. Maternal-infant bonding. *New Age,* 4 (4), 16–18.

**Biller, H. B.**
1971. Father absence and the personality development of the male child. *Developmental Psychology,* 2, 181–201.

**Bird, C.**
1979. *The two-paycheck marriage.* New York: Rawson Wade.

**Black, K. N.**
1974. Working mother: What effect is she having? *Forecast of Home Economics,* 19, 50–52.

**Block, J. R. & Goodman, N.**
1978. Illicit drug use and consumption of alcohol, tobacco, and over-the-counter medicines among adolescents. *International Journal of the Addictus,* 13 (6), 951–964.

**Blood, R. O. & Wolfe, D. M.**
1960. *Husbands and wives.* New York: Macmillan.

**Bolte, G. L.**
1970. A communication approach to marriage counseling. *The Family Coordinator,* Jan., 32–40.

# References

**Bradley, R. W.**
1968. Birth order and school-related behavior: A heuristic review. *Psychological Bulletin,* 70 (1), 445–57.

**Braen, B. B. & Forbush, J. B.**
1975. School-age parenthood: A national overview. *Journal of School Health,* 65 (5), 256–260.

**Bragg, B. W. & Allen, V. L.**
1970. Ordinal position and conformity. *Sociometry,* 33, 371–381.

**Bossard, J. & Boll, E. G.**
1966. *The sociology of child development* (4th ed.). New York: Harper.

**Bowlby**
1958. The nature of the child's tie to his mother. *International Journal of Psychoanalysis,* 39, 350–373.

**Bowlby**
1960. Separation anxiety. *International Journal of Psychoanalysis,* 41, 69–113.

**Bowlby**
1969. *Attachment and loss.* (Vol. I). New York: Basic Books.

**Bradburn, N. M.**
1969. *The structure of psychological well-being.* Chicago: Aldine.

**Brazelton, T. B.**
1978. Early parent-infant reciprocity. In J. K. Gardner (Ed.), *Readings in developmental psychology.* Boston: Little, Brown, pp. 71–78.

**Brehm, J. et al.**
1974. Psychological arousal and interpersonal attraction. Unpublished paper cited in P. M. Middlebrook, *Social psychology and modern life.* Glencoe, Il. Scott, Foresman, p. 437.

**Brim, O. G. Jr.**
1978. Family structure and sex role learning by children: A further analysis of Helen Koch's data. *Sociometry,* 21 (1), 1–16.

**Briscoe, W. C. & Smith, J. B.**
1973. Depression and marital turmoil. *Archives of General Psychiatry,* 29 (9), 811–817.

**Brody, E. B. & Brody, N.**
1976. *Intelligence: Nature, determinents, and consequences.* New York: Academic Press.

**Brody, G. H., Lahey, B. B. & Combs, M. L.**
1978. Effects of intermittent modeling on observational learning. *Journal of Applied Behavioral Analysis,* 11 (1), 87–90.

**Bronfenbrenner, U.**
1961. Some familial antecedents of responsibility and leadership. In L. Petrullo & B. M. Bass (Eds.), *Adolescents in leadership and interpersonal behavior.* New York: Holt.

**Bronowski, J.**
1973. *The ascent of man.* Boston: Little, Brown.

**Brook, D.**
1976. *Naturebirth: You, your body, and your baby.* New York: Pantheon.

**Browning, D. H. & Boatman, B.**
1977. Incest: Children at risk. *American Journal of Psychiatry,* 134 (1), 69–72.

# References

**Burgess, E. W. & Cottrell, L. S., Jr.**
1939. *Predicting success or failure in marriage.*
Englewood Cliffs, N.J.: Prentice-Hall.

**Burgess, E. W. & Wallin, P.**
1953. *Engagement and marriage.* Philadelphia:
J. P. Lippincott.

**Burland, J. A., Andrews, R. G. & Headsten, S. J.**
1973. Child abuse: One tree in the forest. *Child
Welfare,* 52 (9), 585–592.

**Burlingham, D.**
1972. *Psychoanalytic studies of the sighted and
the blind.* New York: International Universities
Press.

**Carroll, J. C.**
1977. The intergenerational transmission of family
violence: The long-term effects of aggressive
behavior. *Aggressive Behavior,* 3 (3), 289–299.

**Caudill, W. A. & Schooler, C.**
1973. Child behavior and child rearing in Japan and
the United States: An interim report. *The Journal
of Nervous and Mental Diseases,* 157, 323–327.

**Chafetz, J. S. et al.**
1974. A study of homosexual women. *Social
Work,* 19 (6), 714–723.

**Cherlin, A.**
1978. Remarriage as an incomplete institution.
*American Journal of Sociology,* 84 (3), 634–650.

**Cherlin, A.**
1978. Teen-age pregnancy: Carter sees half the
problem. *The Nation,* 226 (23), 727–730.

**Chester, R.**
1973. Health and marital breakdown: Some
implications for doctors. *Psychosomatic Research,*
17 (6), 317–321.

**Chester R.**
1977. The one-parent family: Deviant or variant. In
R. Chester & J. Peel (Eds.), *Equalities and
inequalities in family life.* New York: Academic
Press.

**Chiland, C.**
1976. Social adaptation of the child in the latency
period. *Canadian Psychiatric Association Journal,*
21 (4), 192–196.

**Chilman, C. S.**
1974. Some psychosocial aspects of female
sexuality. *The Family Coordinator,* 23 (2), 123–131.

**Clanton, G. & Smith, L. G. (Eds.).**
1977. *Jealousy.* Englewood Cliffs, N.J.:
Prentice-Hall.

**Clark, R. & Spengler, J.**
1978. Population aging in the 21st Century. *U.S.
Dept. of Health, Education and Welfare,* 8,
279–280.

**Clarke-Stewart, K. A.**
1978. Popular primers for parents. *American
Psychologist,* 33, 359–369.

**Clayton, R. R.**
1975. *The family, marriage and social change.*
Lexington, Mass.: D. C. Heath.

**Cleveland, M.**
1976. Sex in marriage: At 40 and beyond. *The
Family Coordinator,* 25, 237–240.

**Cogswell, B. E. & Sussman, M. B.**
1972. Changing family and marriage forms:

# References

Complications for human service systems. *The Family Coordinator,* 21 (4), 505–516.

**Cole, S.**
1979. *The sociological orientation.* 2nd Ed., Chicago: Rand McNally.

**Collard, R. R.**
1968. Social and play responses of first-born and later-born infants in an unfamiliar situation. *Child Development,* 39 (1), 325–334. (Reprinted in and quoted from J. F. Rosenblith, W. Allinsmith & J. P. Williams (Eds.), *Readings in child development.* Boston: Allyn & Bacon, 1973.)

**Collins, J. K.**
1974. Adolescent dating intimacy: Norms and peer expectations. *Journal of Youth & Adolescence,* 3 (4), 317–328.

**Constantine, L. & Constantine, J.**
1973. *Group marriage: A study of contemporary multilateral marriages.* New York: Macmillan.

**Coombs, L.**
1978. How many children do couples really want? *Family Planning Perspectives,* 10 (5), 303–308.

**Corsini, R. J. (Ed.).**
1977. *Current personality theories.* Itasca, Il.: F. E. Peacock.

**Cornelius, S. W. & Denney, N. W.**
1975. Dependency in day-care and home-care children. *Developmental Psychology,* 11 (5), 75–82.

**Cotugno, H. E.**
1975. Parent and peer influence on adolescent decision-making. Doctoral Dissertation, Rutgers University, 1974. Dissertation Abstracts International, April, 75–8386.

**Cox, F. D.**
1974. *Youth, marriage and the seductive society.* 2nd Ed. Dubuque, Iowa: Wm. C. Brown.

**Cronkite, R. C.**
1977. The determinants of spouses' normative preferences for family roles. *Journal of Marriage and the Family,* 39 (3), 575–585.

**Crosby, J.**
1976. A marriage wake: Myths that die hard. In F. D. Cox (Ed.), *American marriage: A changing scene.* 2nd Ed., Dubuque, Iowa: Wm. C. Brown Co., pp. 85–96.

**Curtis, F. L. S.**
1974. Observations of unwed pregnant adolescents. *American Journal of Nursing,* 74 (1), 100–102.

**Denzin, N. K.**
1977. *Childhood socialization.* San Francisco: Jossey-Bass.

**Devereux, E. C. et al.**
1974. Socialization practices of parents, teachers, and peers in Israel: The Kibbutz vs. the city. *Child Development,* 45, 269–281.

**Dion, K. K., Bersheid, F. & Walster, E.**
1972. What is beautiful is good. *Journal of Personality and Social Psychology,* 24, 285–290.

**Dion, K. L. & Dion, K. K.**
1977. Love, liking and trust in heterosexual relationships. *Personality and Social Psychology Bulletin,* 2 (2), 187–190.

**DiRenzo, G. J.**
1977. Socialization, personality, and social systems. *Annual Review of Sociology,* 3, 261, 295.

# References

**Downs, P. E.**
1977. Intra-family decision making in family planning. *Journal of Business Research,* 5 (1), 63–74.

**Doyle, A. B.**
1975. Infant development in day care. *Developmental Psychology,* 11 (5), 655–656.

**Dranoff, S. M.**
1974. Masturbation and the male adolescent. *Adolescence,* 9, 169–179.

**Driscoll, R., Davis, K. E., & Lipetz, M. E.**
1972. Parental interference and romantic love: The Romeo & Juliet effect. *Journal of Personality and Social Psychology,* 24, 1–10.

**Duberman, L.**
1975. *The reconstituted family: A study of remarried couples and their children.* Chicago: Nelson-Hall.

**Dunbar, J., Brown, M. & Vuorinen, S.**
1973. Attitudes toward homosexuality among Brazilian and Canadian college students. *Journal of Social Psychology,* 90, 173–183.

**Durkheim, E.**
1893. *On the division of social labor* (George Simpson, Tr.). New York: Free Press (1966).

**Eddy, C.**
1979. The effects of alcohol on anxiety in problem and nonproblem drinkers. In C. Eddy & J. Ford (Eds.), *Women and Alcohol.* Dubuque, Iowa: Kendall/Hunt.

**Eddy, C. & Ford, J. (Eds.)**
1979. *Women and alcohol.* Dubuque, Iowa: Kendall/Hunt.

**Edwards, D. D. & Edwards, J. S.**
1977. Marriage: Direct and continuous measurement. *Bulletin of Psychonomic Society,* 10 (3), 187–188.

**Endler, N. S. & Marino, C. J.**
1972. The effects of source and type of prior experience on subsequent conforming behaviors. *Journal of Social Psychology,* 88, 21–29.

**Essman, C. S.**
1977. Sibling relations as socialization for parenthood. *The Family Coordinator,* 26 (3), 259–262.

**Falk, G.**
1975. Mate selection in America. *International Behavioral Scientist,* 7 (1), 68–80.

**Fast, J.**
1977. *The body language of sex, power and aggression.* New York: Jove [Harcourt Brace Jovanovich].

**Fawcett, J. T.**
1974. Psychological research and population policy: A preview. *Journal of Social Issues,* 30 (4), 31–37.

**Fein, S. B. & Nuehring, E. M.**
1975. Perspectives on the genderintegrated gay community: Its formal structure and social functions. *Homosexual Counseling Journal,* 2 (4), 150–163.

**Feldman, L. B.**
1976. Processes of change in family therapy. *Journal of Family Counseling,* 4, 14–20.

**Finkel, M. L. & Finkel, D. J.**
1975. Sexual and contraceptive knowledge,

# References

attitudes and behavior of male adolescents. *Family Planning Perspectives,* 7 (6), 256–260.

**Firestone, E. & Moschetta, P.**
1975. Behavioral contracting in family therapy. *Family Counseling,* 3, 27–31.

**Fisher, B. F.**
1977. Identifying and meeting needs of formerly-married people through a divorce adjustment seminar. *Dissertation Abstracts International,* 37 (11–19,) 7–36.

**Fisher, W. A. & Byrne, D.**
1978. Sex differences in response to erotica? Love versus lust. *Journal of Personality and Social Psychology,* 36 (2), 117–125.

**Foley, V. D. & Dyer, W. W.**
1974. "Timing" in family therapy: The "when," "how," and "why" of intervention. *The Family Coordinator,* 23 (4), 373–382.

**Ford, C. S.**
1966. Self-stimulation. In M. F. DeMartino (Ed.), *Sexual behavior and personality characteristics.* New York: Grove Press.

**Fried, E.**
1975. *On love and sexuality.* New York: Grove Press.

**Furstenberg, F. F., Jr.**
1976. Premarital pregnancy and marital instability. *Journal of Social Issues,* 32 (1), 63–83.

**Gadpaille, W. J.**
1975. *The cycles of sex.* New York: Charles Scribner & Sons.

**Gagnon, J. H. & Simon, W. (Eds.).**
1967. *Sexual deviance.* New York: Harper & Row.

**Garfinkle, M., Massey, R., & Mendel E.**
1976. Adlerian guidelines for counseling. In G. S. Belkin (Ed.), *Counseling: Directions in theory and practice.* Dubuque, Iowa: Kendall/Hunt, pp. 145–150.

**Garris, L., Steckler, A. & McIntire, J. R.**
1976. The relationship between oral contraceptives and adolescent sexual behavior. *The Journal of Sex Research,* 12, 2, 135–146.

**Gelles, R. J.**
1973. Child abuse as psychopathology: A sociological critique and reformulation. *American Journal of Orthopsychiatry,* 43, 611–621.

**Gelles, R. J.**
1977. Power, sex and violence: The case of marital rape. *The Family Coordinator,* 26 (4), 339–347.

**Gelles, R. J.**
1978. Violence toward children in the United States. *American Journal of Orthopsychiatry,* 48 (4), 580–592.

**Giuffra, M. J.**
1975. Demystifying adolescent behavior. *American Journal of Nursing,* 10, 1725–1727.

**Globetti, G.**
1972. Problem and non-problem drinking among high-school students in abstinence communities. *International Journal of Addictions,* 7 (3), 511–523.

**Godenne, G. D.**
1974. Sex and today's youth. *Adolescence,* 9 (33), 67–72.

**Goffman, E.**
1974. *Stigma: Notes on the management of spoiled identity.* New York: Jason Aronson.

## References

(Originally published Englewood Cliffs, N.J.: Prentice-Hall, 1963).

**Goode, W. J.**
1959. The theoretical importance of love. *American Sociological Review,* 24 (1), 38–47.

**Goode, W. J.**
1976. Family patterns and human rights. In F. D. Cox (Ed.), *American marriage: A changing scene.* 2nd Ed. Dubuque, Iowa: Wm. C. Brown, pp. 159–167.

**Goodman, N.**
1969. Adolescent norms and behavior: Organization and conformity. *Merrill-Palmer Quarterly,* 15, 199–211.

**Goodman, N. & Marx, G. T.**
1978. *Society today* (3rd ed.). New York: CRM/Random House.

**Goodman, N. & Ofshe, R.**
1968. Empathy, communication efficiency and marital status. *Journal of Marriage and the Family,* 30 (4), 597–603.

**Goodsell, W.**
1915. A history of the family as a social and economic institution. Norwood, Pa.: Norwood Editions.

**Gough, K.**
1971. The origin of the family. *Journal of Marriage and the Family,* 33 (4), 760–771.

**Green, B. J.**
1978. Helping children of divorce: A multimodal approach. *Elementary School Guidance and Counseling,* 13 (1), 31–45.

**Guthrie, H. A. et al.**
1977. Behavior and malnutrition. *Journal of Cross-Cultural Psychology,* 8 (2), 170–179.

**Hainline, L. & Feig, E.**
1978. The correlates of childhood father absence in college-aged women. *Child Development,* 49 (1), 37–42.

**Haley, J.**
1972. Beginning and experienced family therapists. A Ferber, M. Mendelsohn & A. Napier (Eds.), *The Book of Family Therapy.* New York: Aronson, pp. 155–167.

**Hamilton, M. L.**
1977. *Father's influence on children.* Chicago: Nelson-Hall.

**Hansen, S. L.**
1977. Dating choices of high school students. *The Family Coordinator,* 26 (2), 133–138.

**Hartnett, J., Mahoney, J. & Bernstein, A.**
1977. The errant spouse: A study in person perception. *Perceptual and Motor Skills,* 45 (3, Pt. I), 747–750.

**Hawkins, J. L., Weisberg, C. & Ray, D. L.**
1977. Marital communication style and social class. *Journal of Marriage and Family,* 39 (3), 479–492.

**Heiman, J. R.**
1975. The physiology of erotica: Women's sexual arousal. *Psychology Today,* 8, 91–96.

# References

**Helfer, R. E. & Kempe, C. H. (Eds.)**
1968. *The battered child.* Chicago: University of Chicago Press.

**Henshel, A. M.**
1973. Swinging: A study of decision making in marriage. *American Journal of Sociology,* 78, 885-891.

**Hertz, D. G.**
1977. Psychological implications of adolescent pregnancy. *Psychosomatics,* 18 (1), 13-16.

**Herzog, E. & Sudia, C. E.**
1973. Children in fatherless families. In B. H. Caldwell & H. N. Riciuti (Eds.), *Review of child development research.* Chicago: University of Chicago Press, pp. 141-232.

**Hetherington, E. M.**
1972. Effects of father absence on personality development in adolescent daughters. *Developmental Psychology,* 7, 313-326.

**Higgins, J. J.**
1978. Social services for abused wives. *Social Casework,* 59 (5), 266-271.

**Hines, R. L.**
1976. Socialization for marital roles among select young adult marriages: A multivariate analysis of media influence in relation to parents and peers. *Dissertation Abstracts International,* 37 (5-A), 3212-3213.

**Hoffman, L. W.**
1961. Mother's enjoyment of work and effects on the children. *Child Development,* 32 (1), 187-197.

**Hoffman, M. L.**
1970. Consciousness, personality, and socialization techniques. *Human Development,* 13, 90-126.

**Hoffman, M. L.**
1971. Father absence and conscience development. *Developmental Psychology,* 4, 400-406.

**Hollingshead, A. B.**
1950. Cultural factors in the selection of marriage mates. *American Sociological Review,* 15 (5), 619-627.

**Holmes, T. H. & Rahe, R. H.**
1967. The social readjustment rating scale. *Journal of Psychosomatic Research,* 2, 213.

**Hoon, E. H., Hoon, P. W. & Wincze, J. P.**
1976. An inventory for the measurement of female sexual arousability: The SAI. *Archives of Sexual Behavior,* 5 (4), 294-95.

**Hopkins, J. R.**
1977. Sexual behavior in adolescence. *Journal of Social Issues,* 33 (2), 67-85.

**Hopkins, J. & White, P.**
1978. The dual-career couple: Constraints and supports. *The Family Coordinator,* 27 (3), 253-259.

**Hoult, T. F.**
1974. Dictionary of modern sociology. Totawa, N.J. Littlefield, Adams.

**Howard, J.**
1978. *Families.* New York: Simon & Schuster.

**Hughes, H. M.**
1971. *Life in families.* Boston: Holbrook Press.

# References

**Huser, W. R. & Grant, C. W.**
1978. A study of husbands and wives from dual-career and traditional-career families. *Psychology of Women Quarterly,* 3 (1), 78–89.

**Hymowitz, C. & Weissman, M.**
1978. *A history of women in America.* New York: Bantam.

**Isaacs, A. D. & Post, F. (Eds.).**
1978. *Studies in geriatric psychiatry.* New York: Wiley.

**Jacques, J. M. & Chason, K. J.**
1978. Cohabitation: A test of reference group theory among black and white college students. *Journal of Comparative Family Studies,* 9 (2), 147–165.

**Jay, J. & Birney, R. C.**
1973. Research findings on the kibbutz adolescent: A response to Bettelheim. *American Journal of Orthopsychiatry,* 43 (3), 347–354.

**Jellinek, E. M.**
1971. Phases of alcohol addiction. In G. D. Shean (Ed.), *Studies in abnormal behavior.* Chicago: Rand McNally.

**Jessor, R. & Jessor, S. L.**
1977. *Problem behavior and psychological development: A longitudinal study of youth.* New York: Academic Press, 1977.

**Jones, C. R.**
1974. *Homosexuality and counseling.* Philadelphia: Fortress.

**Jones, W. H., Hansson, R. O. & Phillips. A. L.**
1978. Physical attractiveness and judgments of psychopathology. *Journal of Social Psychology,* 105, 79–84.

**Kaats, G. R. & Davis, K. E.**
1970. The dynamics of sexual behavior of college students. *Journal of Marriage and the Family,* 32, 390–399.

**Kalmar, R. (Ed.).**
1977. *Abortion: The emotional implications.* Dubuque, Iowa: Kendall/Hunt.

**Kanter, R. M.**
1972. "Getting it all together": Some group issues in communes. *American Journal of Orthopsychiatry,* 42 (4), 632–643.

**Kanter, R. M.**
1973. Communes: Creating and managing the collective life. New York: Harper & Row.

**Karpel, M.**
1975. Individuation: From fusion to dialogue. *Family Process,* 65–82.

**Kempe, C. H. et al.**
1962. The battered-child syndrome. *Journal of American Medical Association,* 181, 17–24.

**Kemper, T. D.**
1978. *A social interactional theory of emotions.* New York: Wiley.

**Kimmel, D. C.**
1976. Adult development: Challenges for counseling. *Personnel and Guidance Journal,* 55, 103–105.

**King, E. W.**
1973. *Educating young children: A sociological interpretation.* Dubuque, Iowa: Wm. C. Brown.

**King, K., Balswick, J. O. & Robinson, I. E.**
1977. The continuing premarital sexual revolution

# References

among college females. *Journal of Marriage and the Family,* 39 (3), 455–459.

**Kinkade, K.**
1974. Power and the Utopian assumption. *Journal of Applied Behavioral Science,* 10 (3), 402–414.

**Kirkpatrick, J.**
1977. Turnabout: *Help for a new life.* New York: Doubleday.

**Klatskin, E., Jackson, E. & Wilkin, C.**
1956. The influence of degree of flexibility in maternal care practices on early childhood behavior. *American Journal of Orthopsychiatry,* 26, 79–93.

**Kleinke, C. L.**
1977. Assignment of responsibility for marital conflict to husbands and wives: Sex stereotypes or a double standard? *Psychological Reports,* 41 (1), 219–222.

**Kleinke, C. L., Meeker, F. B. & La Fong, C.**
1974. Effects of gaze, touch, and use of name on evaluation of engaged couples. *Journal of Research in Personality,* 7 (4), 368–373.

**Knox, D. & Knox, F.**
1974. Preparation for marriage: Beyond the classroom. *Journal of Family Counseling* 2, 16–22.

**Kogan, N.**
1961. Attitudes toward old people: The development of a scale and an examination of the correlates. *Journal of Abnormal & Social Psychology,* 62, 44–54.

**Kogan, N. & Shelton, F. C.**
1962. Images of "old people" and "people in general" in an older sample. *Journal of Genetic Psychology,* 100, 3–21.

**Kogan, N. & Shelton, F. C.**
1962a. Beliefs about "old people": A comparative study of older and younger samples. *Journal of Genetic Psychology,* 100, 93–111.

**Kohn, M.**
1969. *Classes and conformity: A study in values.* Homewood, Ill.: Dorsey.

**Komarovsky, M.**
1964. *Blue-collar marriage.* New York: Random House.

**Komarovsky, M.**
1973. Cultural contradictions and sex-roles: The masculine case. *American Journal of Sociology,* 78 (4), 873–884.

**Komarovsky, M.**
1974. Sociologists look at the family. In H. M. Hughes (Ed.), *Life in families.* 2nd Printing, Boston: Holbrook Press.

**Konopka, G.**
1966. *The adolescent girl in conflict.* Englewood Cliffs: Prentice-Hall.

**Korner, A. F.**
1975. Mother-child interaction. In W. C. Sze (Ed.), *Hunan life cycle.* New York: Jason Aronson, pp. 85–91.

**Kotelchuck, M.**
1973. *The nature of the infant's tie to his father.* Paper presented at the meeting of the Society for Research in Child Development, Philadelphia, March 29.

**Krich, A. & Blum, S.**
1974. Marriage and the mystique of romance. In C. E. Williams & J. F. Crosby (Eds.), *Choice and*

challenge: Contemporary readings in marriage. Dubuque, Iowa: Wm. C. Brown, pp. 55–62.

**Kubler-Ross, E.**
1969. *On death and dying.* New York: Bantam.

**Laden, C. J. & Crooks, M.**
1976. Some factors influencing the decision of mature women to enroll for continuing education. *Canadian Counselor,* 10, 29–36.

**Lamb, M. E.**
1977. The development of mother-infant and father-infant attachments in the second year of life. *Developmental Psychology,* 13 (6), 637–648.

**Laswell, M. E.**
1974. Is there a best age to marry? An interpretation. *The Family Coordinator,* 23 (3), 237–242.

**Lauer, B., Ten Broek, E. & Grossman, M.**
1974. Battered-child syndrome review of 130 patients with controls. *Pediatrics,* 54 (1), 67–70.

**Lauarakas, P.**
1975. Female preferences for male physiques. *Journal of Research in Personality,* 9 (4), 324–334.

**Leboyer, F.**
1975. *Birth without violence.* New York: Random House.

**Leitner, L. A. & Stecher, T.**
1974. Crisis intervention for growth: Philosophical dimensions and strategies. *Psychology,* 11, 29–32.

**Levin, R. J. & Levin, A.**
1975. Sexual pleasure: The surprising preferences of 100,000 women. *Redbook Magazine,* 145, 5.

**Levinger, G.**
1977. Re-viewing the close relationship. In G. Levinger & H. L. Rausch (Eds.), *Close relationships: Perspectives on the meaning of intimacy.* Amherst, Mass.: University of Massachusetts Press.

**Levinger, G.**
1976. A social psychological perspective on marital dissolution. *Journal of Social Issues,* 32 (1), 21–43.

**Levinson, D. J.**
1978. *The Seasons of a man's life.* New York: Random House.

**Levinson et al.**
1977. Periods in the adult development of men: Ages 18 to 45. In N. K. Schlossberg & A. D. Entine (Eds.), *Counseling adults.* Monterey, CA: Brooks/Cole, pp. 47–59.

**Levitt, E. P. & Klassen, A. D.**
1974. Public attitudes toward homosexuality: Part of the 1970 national survey by the Institute for Sex Research. *Journal of Homosexuality,* 1 (1), 29–43.

**Libby, R. W., Gray, L. & White, M.**
1978. A test and reformulation of reference groups and role correlates of premarital sexual permissiveness theory. *Journal of Marriage and Family,* 40 (1), 79–101.

**Lindeman, E.**
1944. Symptomatology and management of acute grief. *American Journal of Psychiatry,* 101, 141–148.

**Lindert, P. H.**
1978. *Fertility and scarcity in America.* Princeton, N.J.: Princeton University Press.

# References

**Linton, R.**
1963. *The study of man.* New York: Appleton, Century, Crofts.

**Litwak, E.**
1960. Occupational mobility and extended family cohesion. *American Sociological Review,* 25 (1), 9–21.

**Litwak, E.**
1960a. Geographic mobility and extended family cohesion. *American Sociological Review,* 25 (3), 385–394.

**Lyell, R. G.**
1973. Adolescent and adult self-esteem as related to cultural values. *Adolescence,* 8 (29), 85–92.

**Lynn, D.**
1974. *The father: His role in child development.* Monterey, CA: Brooks/Cole.

**Lynn, J. (Ed.)**
1976. *Day Care and Child Development Reports.* 5 (8).

**MacDonald, A. P., Jr.**
1976. Homophobia: Its roots and meaning. *Homosexual Counseling Journal,* 3 (1), 23–33.

**Macklin, E. D.**
1978. Nonmarital heterosexual cohabitation. *Marriage & Family Review,* 1 (2), 1–11.

**Mahoney, J.**
1976. Age and values: The generation non-gap. *Psychological Reports,* 39, 62.

**Malinowski, B.**
1964. Avenues to marriage among the Trobrianders. In R. L. Coser (Ed.), *The family: Its structure and functions.* New York: St. Martin's Press, pp. 93–104.

**Manis, J. G. & Meltzer, B. N. (Eds.).**
1967. *Symbolic interaction: A reader in social psychology.* Boston: Allyn & Bacon.

**Markowski, E. M., Croake, J. W. & Keller, J. F.**
1978. Sexual history and present sexual behavior of cohabiting and married couples. *Journal of Sexual Research,* 14 (1), 27–39.

**Marver, J. D. & Larson, M. A.**
1978. Public policy toward child care in America: A historical perspective. In P. K. Robins & S. Weiner (Eds.), *Child care and public policy.* Lexington, MA: Lexington Books.

**Maschoff, T. A., Fanshier, W. E. & Hansen, D. J.**
1976. Vasectomy: Its effects on marital stability. *Journal of Sex Research,* 12 (4), 295–314.

**Mazur-Hart, S. F. & Berman, J. J.**
1977. Changing from fault to no-fault divorce: An interrupted time series analysis. *Journal of Applied Social Psychology,* 7 (4), 300–312.

**McBride, M. C. & Enders, K. L.**
1977. Sexual attitudes and sexual behavior among college students. *Journal of College Student Personnel,* 18 (3), 183–187.

**McCauley, C. & Swann, C. P.**
1978. Male-female differences in sexual fantasy. *Journal of Research in Personality,* 12 (1), 78–86.

**McCary, J. L.**
1967. *Human sexuality.* New York: Van Nostrand Reinhold.

# References

**McGowan, C. A.**
1977. Celibacy, sexuality, and meaning in life: A comparative study of religious Catholic lay women. *Dissertation Abstracts International,* 38 (2-A), 634–635.

**McGurk, H. & Lewis, M.**
1972. Achievement motivation and ordinal position of birth. *Developmental Psychology,* 7 (3), 364–367.

**McLoughlin, W. G.**
1976. Evangelical childrearing in the age of Jackson: Francis Wayland's view of when and how to subdue the willfulness of children. *Journal of Social History,* 8, 21–43.

**Mechling, J.**
1976. Advice to historians on advice to mothers. *Journal of Social History,* 9, 44–63.

**Mencher, J. P.**
1965. The Nayars of South Malabar. In M. F. Nimkoff (Ed.), *Comparative family systems.* Boston: Houghton Mifflin, 163–191.

**Meyers, L.**
1978. Battered wives, dead husbands. *Student Lawyer,* 6 (7), 46–51.

**Miller, S., Corrales, R. & Wackman, D. B.**
1975. Recent progress in understanding and facilitating marital communication. *The Family Coordinator,* 24 (2), 143–152.

**Milligan, L. W.**
1972. Wives, women and wife role behavior. *International Journal of Comparative Sociology,* 13 (1), 36–47.

**Mitchell, J. J.**
1972. Some psychological dimensions of adolescent sexuality. *Adolescence,* 7, 447–458.

**Mitchell, J. J.**
1974. Moral dilemmas of early adolescence. *The School Counselor,* 22, 16–22.

**Mitchell, J. J.**
1975. Moral growth during adolescence. *Adolescence,* 10 (38), 221–226.

**Monahan, T. P.**
1976. The occupational class of couples entering into interracial marriage. *Journal of Comparative Family Studies,* 7 (2), 175–192.

**Money, J.**
1977. Interview with Dr. John Money. In *Gallery Magazine,* September.

**Montagu, A.**
1965. *Life before birth.* New York: New American Library.

**Moscowitz, D. S., Schwarz, J. C. & Corsini, D. A.**
1977. Initiating day-care at three years of age. *Child Development,* 48, 1271–1276.

**Murdock, G. P.**
1949. *Social structures.* New York: Macmillan.

**Murdock, G. P.**
1937. Comparative data on division of labor by sex. *Social Forces,* 15 (2), 551–553.

**Murdock, G. P.**
1957. World ethnographic sample. *American Anthropologist,* 59 (4), 664–687.

# References

**Murdock, G. P. & Whiting, J. W.**
1951. Cultural determination of parental attitudes: The relationship between the social structure, particularly family structure, and parental behavior. In M. Senn (Ed.), *Problems of infancy and childhood*. New York: Josiah Macy, Jr. Foundation.

**Murstein, B. I.**
1973. A theory of marital choice applied to interracial marriage. In I. R. Stuart & L. E. Abt (Eds.), *Interracial marriage: Expectations and realities*. New York: Grossman.

**Murstein, B. I.**
1976. *Who will marry whom? Theories and research in marital choice*. New York: Springer.

**Musetto, A. P.**
1978. Evaluating families with custody or visitation problems. *Journal of Marriage and Family Counseling*, 4 (4), 59-65.

**Nagi, S. Z.**
1975. Child abuse and neglect programs: A national overview. *Children Today*, 4 (3), 13-17.

**Nass, D. R. & Nass, S.**
1976. Counseling the fatherless child. In G. S. Belkin (Ed.), *Counseling: Directions in theory and practice*. Dubuque, Iowa: Kendall/Hunt.

**Nass, S. & Weidhorn, M.**
1978. Turn your life around. Englewood Cliffs, N.J.: Prentice-Hall.

**Neubauer, P. (Ed.).**
1965. *Children in collectives: Child-rearing aims and practices in the kibbutz*. Springfield, Il.: Charles C. Thomas.

**Neugarten, B. L.**
1977. Adaptation and the life cycle. In N. K. Schlossberg & A. D. Entine (Eds.), *Counseling adults*. Monterey, CA: Brooks/Cole, pp. 34-46.

**Newsweek Magazine.**
1979. Legal battle of the sexes. April 30, pp. 68-75.

**Nye, F. I.**
1976. *Role structure and analysis of the family*. Beverly Hills: Sage.

**Nye, F. I. & Berardo, F. M.**
1966. *Emerging conceptual frameworks in family analysis*. New York: Macmillan.

**Nye, F. I. & McLaughlin, S.**
1976. Role competence and marital satisfaction. In F. I. Nye, et al. *Role structure and analysis of the family*. Beverly Hills, CA: Sage Publications.

**Nye, F. I. et al.**
1976. *Role structure and analysis of the family*. Beverly Hills, CA: Sage Publications.

**Okada, L. M. & Gillespie, D. G.**
1977. The impact of family planning programs on unplanned pregnancies. *Family Planning Perspectives*, 9 (4), 173-176.

**Oshman, H. P. & Manosevitz, M.**
1976. Father absence: Effects of stepfathers upon psychosocial development in males. *Developmental Psychology*, 12 (5), 479-480.

**Osofsky, H. J.**
1971. Adolescent sexual behavior: Current status and anticipated trends for the future. *Clinical Obstetrics and Gynecology*, 14 (2), 393-406.

# References

**Otterbein, C. S. & Otterbein, K. F.**
1974. Believers and beaters: A case study of supernatural beliefs and child rearing in the Bahama Islands. *American Anthropologist,* 75, 1670–1679.

**Papalia, D. E. & Olds, S. W.**
1979. *Human development.* New York: McGraw-Hill.

**Parsons, T.**
1943. The kinship system of the contemporary United States. *American Anthropologist,* 45 (1), 23–38.

**Parsons, T.**
1954. The incest taboo in relation to social structure and the socialization of the child. *British Journal of Sociology,* 5, 101–117.

**Payne, B. & Whittington, F.**
1976. Older women: An examination of popular stereotypes and research evidence. *Social Problems,* 23 (4), 488–504.

**Peplau, L. A., Rubin, Z. & Hill, C. T.**
1977. Sexual intimacy in dating relationships. *Journal of Social Issues,* 33 (2), 86–109.

**Petroni, F. A.**
1973. Interracial dating—the price is high. In I. R. Stuart & L. E. Abt (Eds.), *Interracial marriage: expectations and realities.* New York: Grossman.

**Phipps, W. E.**
1977. Masturbation: Vice or virtue? *Journal of Religion and Health,* 16 (3), 183–195.

**Pick, G.**
1978. Father knows best: The new trend in child custory. *Student Lawyer,* 6 (9), 38–43.

**Piehl, J.**
1977. Integration of information in the courts: Influence of physical attractiveness on amount of punishment for traffic offenders. *Psychological Reports,* 41 (2), 551–556.

**Pitts, J. R.**
1964. The structural-functional approach. In H. T. Christensen (Ed.), *Handbook of marriage and the family.* Chicago: Rand McNally, 88–90.

**Place, D. M.**
1975. The dating experience for adolescent girls. *Adolescence,* 10, (38), 157–274.

**Pomeroy, W. B.**
1973. Playboy panel: New sexual life styles. *Playboy,* September, p. 86.

**Porterfield, E.**
1978. *Black and white mixed marriages: An ethnographic study.* Chicago: Nelson-Hall.

**Poston, D. L. & Gotard, E.**
1977. Trends in childlessness in the United States, 1910–1975. *Social Biology,* 24 (3), 212–224.

**Prescott, E.**
1978. Is day care as good as a good home? *Young Children,* January, 13–19.

**Prosky, P. O.**
1974. Family therapy: An orientation. *Clinical Social Work,* 2 (1), 45–56.

**Queen, S. A. & Habenstein, R. W.**
1974. *The family in various cultures.* 4th Ed. Philadelphia: J. B. Lippincott.

**Radin, N. & Epstein, A.**
1975. *Observed paternal behavior and the*

# References

intellectual functioning of preschool boys and girls.
Paper presented at a Meeting of the Society for
Research in Child Development, Denver.

**Rae, Grant, Q.**
1976. New family structures and the latency child.
*Canadian Psychiatric Association Journal,* 21 (4),
197–198.

**Rahe, R. H.**
1972. Subjects' recent life changes and their
nearfuture illness susceptibility. *Advances in
Psychosomatic Medicine,* 8, 2–19.

**Rainwater, L.**
1960. *And the poor get children: Sex,
contraception and family planning in the working
class.* Chicago: Quadrangle.

**Rainwater, L.**
1965. *Family design: Marital sexuality, family size
and contraception.* Chicago: Aldine.

**Ramey, J. W.**
1972. Emerging patterns of innovative behavior in
marriage. *The Family Coordinator,* 21 (4), 435–455.

**Rand, A.**
1971. *The new left: The anti-industrial revolution.*
New York: Signet, pp. 187–238.

**Rappaport, P.**
1979. Mixed views: A national conference on child
abuse. *APA* [American Psychological Association]
*Monitor,* January, 10 (1), pp. 4–5.

**Rebelsky, F.**
1975. *Life: The continuing process.* New York:
Knopf.

**Reichelt, P. A. & Werley, H. H.**
1975. Contraception, abortion, and venereal
disease: Teenagers' knowledge and the effect of
education. *Family Planning Perspectives,* 7 (2),
83–88.

**Reiss, I.**
1960. *Premarital sexual standards in America.*
New York: Macmillan.

**Reiss, I.**
1967. *The social context of premarital sexual
permissiveness.* New York: Holt, Rinehart and
Winston.

**Reiss, I.**
1971. *The family system in America.* New York:
Holt.

**Renne, K. S.**
1976. Childlessness, health and marital
satisfaction. *Social Biology,* 23 (3), 183–197.

**Renvoize, H.**
1978. *Web of violence: A study of family violence.*
London: Routledge & Kegan Paul.

**Ridley, C. L. Peterman, D. J. & Avery, A. W.**
1978. Cohabitation: Does it make for a better
marriage? *Family Coordinator,* 27 (2), 129–136.

**Rimmer, R.**
1966. *The Harrad experiment.* Los Angeles:
Sherbourne Press (New York: Bantam Books,
1973).

**Robertshaw, P. & Curtin, C. A.**
1977. Legal definition of the family: An historical
and sociological explanation. *The Sociological
Review,* 25 (2), 280–308.

# References

**Robinson, L. R.**
1975. Basic concepts in family therapy: A differential comparison with individual treatment. *American Journal of Psychiatry,* 132 (10), 1045–1048.

**Rohner, R. P.**
1976. Sex differences in aggression: Phylogenetic and enculturation perspectives. *Ethos,* 4 (1), 57–72.

**Rolfe, D. J.**
1977. Pre-marriage contracts: An aid to couples living with parents. *The Family Coordinator,* 26 (3), 281–285.

**Rose, J. D.**
1976. *Introduction to sociology* (3rd ed.). Chicago Rand McNally.

**Rosenfeld, J. P.**
1977. *Aging and wealth transmission: Inheritance and disinheritance.* Ph.D. dissertation, State University of New York at Stony Brook (forthcoming as *The legacy of aging: Inheritance and disinheritance in social perspective.* Boston: ABLEX Publishing).

**Ross, L.**
1978. Extra-marital relationships. Dubuque, Iowa: Kendall/Hunt.

**Rubenstein, J. S., Watson, F. G. & Rubenstein, H. S.**
1977. An analysis of sex education books for adolescents by means of adolescents' sexual interests. *Adolescence,* Fall, 293–311.

**Rubin, Z.**
1973. *Liking and Loving.* New York: Holt, Rinehart and Winston.

**Russell, B.**
1973. How do you share the responsibilities? *House and Garden,* July, pp. 49, 106–107.

**Ryan, M. L.**
1977. Effects of modeling, instructions, and personality on effective sensitivity behavior. *Dissertation Abstracts International,* 37 (12-B, Pt. 2), 6390–6391.

**Sanders, L. et al.**
1975. Child abuse: Detection and prevention. *Young Children,* 30 (5), 332–337.

**Satir, V.**
1967. *Conjoint family therapy.* Revised Ed. Palo Alto, California: Science & Behavior Books.

**Scales, P.**
1977. Males and morals: Teenage contraceptive behavior amid the double standard. *The Family Coordinator,* 26 (3), 211–222.

**Schachter, S.**
1959. *The psychology of affiliation.* Stanford, CA: Stanford University Press.

**Schachter, S. & Singer, J. E.**
1962. Cognitive, social and physiological determinants of emotional states. *Psychological Review,* 69, 379–399.

**Schaefer, C.**
1978. *How to influence children.* New York: Van Nostran Reinhold.

**Schlesinger, B.**
1970. Family life in the kibbutz of Israel: Utopia gained or paradise lost? *International Journal of Comparative Sociology,* 11, 251–271.

# References

**Schmidt, G.**
1975. Male-female differences in sexual arousal and behavior during and after exposure to sexually explicit stimuli. *Archives of Sexual Behavior,* 4 (4), 353–365.

**Schoen, R.**
1975. California divorce rates by age at first marriage and duration of first marriage. *Journal of Marriage and Family,* 37 (3), 548–555.

**Schoof-Tams, K. et al.**
1976. Differentiation of sexual morality between 11 and 16 years. *Archives of Sexual Behavior,* 5 (5), 353–370.

**Schulterbrandt, J. G. & Nichols, E. J.**
1972. Ethical and ideological problems for communal living: A caveat. *Family Coordinator,* 21 (4), 429–433.

**Schvaneveldt, J. D.**
1966. The interactional framework in the study of the family. In F. I. Nye & F. M. Berardo (Eds.), *Emerging conceptual frameworks in family analysis.* New York: Macmillan.

**Schwartzman, J.**
1974. The individual, incest, and exogamy. *Psychiatry,* 37, 171–179.

**Sebald, H.**
1968. *Adolescence: A sociological analysis.* New York: Appleton-Century-Crofts.

**Segal, J. & Yahraes, H.**
1978. A child's journey: Forces that shape the lives of our young. New York: McGraw Hill.

**Seth, M. & Khanna, M.**
1978. Child rearing attitudes of the mothers as a function of age. *Child Psychiatric Quarterly,* 11 (1), 6–9.

**Shorter, E.**
1975. *The making of the modern family.* New York: Basic Books.

**Shulman, A. K.**
1972. "The Schulmans have a 50-50 agreement that's down on paper." *Life Magazine,* April 28th, pp. 42–46.

**Sims, L. S. & Paolucci, B.**
1975. An empirical reexamination of the parent attitude research instrument (PARI). *Journal of Marriage and the Family,* 37, 724–732.

**Slater, P. E.**
1963. On social regression. *American Sociological Review,* 28 (3), 339–364.

**Smith, E. C.**
1964. *American surnames.* Philadelphia Chilton.

**Smith, E. M.**
1972. Counseling for women who seek abortion. *Social Work,* 17 (2), 62–68.

**Smrtic, J. D.**
1979. *Abnormal psychology: A perspectives approach.* Wayne, NJ: Avery.

**Sorenson, R. C.**
1973. Adolescent sexuality in contemporary America. New York: Harry N. Abrams.

**Speck, R. & Speck, J.**
1975. The urban commune—an alternative family style. *Family Therapy,* 2 (2), 181–186.

# References

**Spinetti, J. J. & Rigler, D.**
1972. The child abusing parent: A psychological review. *Psychological Bulletin*, 18–29.

**Spiro, M. E.**
1956. Is the family universal? *American Anthropologist*, 56, 839–846.

**Spiro, M. E.**
1958. Is the family universal?—The Israeli case. In N. W. Bell & E. F. Vogel (Eds.), *A modern introduction to the family* (revised ed.). New York: Free Press, 68–79.

**Spitz, R. A.**
1975. Hospitalism: The genesis of psychiatric conditions in early childhood. In W. C. Sze (Ed.) *Human life cycle*. New York: Jason Aronson.

**Spotnitz, H.**
1976. *Psychotherapy of preoedipal conditions*. New York: Jason Aronson.

**Srivastava, A. K.**
1977. Social-class interaction in the language effectiveness of bright secondary school students. *Psychologia: An International Journal of Psychology in the Orient*, 20 (4), 226–233.

**Steele, D. & Walker, E.**
1974. Male and female differences in reaction to erotic stimuli as related to sexual adjustment. *Archives of Sexual Behavior*, 3 (5), 459–470.

**Stein, H.**
1976. *Tiny Tim*. Chicago: Playboy Press.

**Stein, H. F.**
1978. The Slovak-American "swaddling ethos": Homeostasis for family dynamics and cultural continuity. *Family Process*, 17 (1), 31–45.

**Stein, P. J.**
1978. The lifestyles and life chances of the never-married. *Marriage & Family Review*, 1 (4), 10ff.

**Steinmetz, S. K.**
1978a. Violence between family members. *Marriage & Family Review*, 1 (3), 1–16.

**Steinmetz, S. K.**
1978b. *Battered parents. Society*, 15 (5), 54–55.

**Steinmetz, S. K. & Strauss, M. A. (Eds.)**
1974. *Violence in the family*. New York: Dodd, Mead.

**Stephan, C. & Tully, J. C.**
1977. The influence of physical attractiveness of a plaintiff on the decision of simulated jurors. *Journal of Social Research*, 101, 149–150.

**Stephens, W. N.**
1963. *The family in cross-cultural perspectives*. New York: Holt, Rinehart & Winston.

**Stetson, D. M. & Wright, G. C., Jr.**
1975. The effects of laws on divorce in American states. *Journal of Marriage and Family*, 37 (3), 537–547.

**Stewart, A. J., Winter, D. G. & Jones, A. D.**
1975. Coding categories for the study of child-rearing from historical sources. *Journal of Interdisciplinary History*, 4, 687–701.

**Stoller, R. J.**
1976. Sexual excitement. *Archives of General Psychiatry*, 33, 899–909.

**Strane, K. & Watts, C.**
1977. Females judged by attractiveness of partner. *Perceptual & Motor Skills*, 45 (1), 225–226.

# References

**Stuart, I. R. & Abt, L. E. (Eds.).**
1973. *Interracial marriage: Expectations and realities.* New York: Grossman.

**Stycos, J. M.**
1974. Some dimensions of population and family planning: goals and means. *Journal of Social Issues,* 30 (4), 1–22.

**Sussman, M. B. & Burchinal, L.**
1962. Kin family network: Unheralded structure on current conceptualizations of family functioning. *Marriage and Family Living,* 24 (2), 231–240.

**Sutton-Smith, B. & Rosenberg, B. G.**
1970. *The sibling.* New York: Holt, Rinehart & Winston.

**Tessman, L. H.**
1978. *Children of parting parents.* New York: Aronson.

**Thorson, J., Hancock, K. & Whatley, L.**
1974. Attitudes toward the aged as a function of age and education. *The Gerontologist,* 14, 316–318.

**Thorson, J.**
1975. Attitudes toward the aged as a function of race and social class. *The Gerontologist,* 15, 343–344.

**Townes, B. D. et al.**
1977. Birth planning values and decisions: the prediction of fertility. *Journal of Applied Social Psychology,* 7 (1), 73–88.

**Trainer, J. B.**
1975. Sexual incompatibilities. *Journal of Marriage and Family Counseling,* 1 (2), 123–134.

**Trost, J. A.**
1978. A renewed social institution: Non-marital cohabitation. *Acta Sociologica,* 21 (4), 303–315.

**Wagner, R. V.**
1975. Complementary needs, role expectations, interpersonal attraction and the stability of working relationships. *Journal of Personality and Social Psychology,* 32 (1), 116–124.

**Walshok, M. L.**
1971. The emergence of middle-class deviant subcultures: The case of swingers. Social Problems, 18, 488–495.

**Walster, E. & Berscheid, E.**
1971. Adrenaline makes the heart grow fonder. *Psychology Today,* 5 (1), 46–50.

**Wandersman, L. P.**
1973. A review and re-evaluation of the social class and socialization research. *Cornell Journal of Social Relations,* 8 (2), 197–218.

**Weathers, L. & Liberman, R. P.**
1975. The family contracting exercise. *Journal of Behavior Therapy and Experimental Psychiatry,* 6 (3), 208–214.

**Weber, M.**
1922. *The theory of social and economic organization.* New York: Free Press (1947).

**Weinstein, E. et al.**
1972. Empathy and communication efficiency. *Journal of Social Psychology,* 88, 247–254.

**Weisman, A. D.**
1973. Coping with untimely death. *Psychiatry,* 36, 366–378.

# References

**Weiss, R. S.**
1975. *Marital separation.* New York: Basic Books.

**Weitman, S. R.**
1970. Intimacies: Notes toward a theory of social inclusion and exclusion. *European Journal of Sociology,* Fall, 348–367.

**Weitzman, L. J.**
1975. To love, honor, and obey? Traditional legal marriage and alternative family forms. *The Family Coordinator,* 24, (4), 531–538.

**Wells, J. G.**
1976. A critical look at personal marriage contracts. *The Family Coordinator,* 25 (1), 33–37.

**Wenig, M. & Coffman, C.**
1978. Mothers and daughters break with tradition. *Journal of Cooperative Living,* 33 (July/August), 32–39.

**Westbrook, M. T.**
1978. The effect of the order of birth on women's experience of childbearing. *Journal of Marriage and Family,* 40 (1), 165–172.

**Westoff, C. F.**
1978. Some speculations on the future of marriage and fertility. *Family Planning Perspectives,* 10 (2), 79–83.

**Westoff, C. F. & Jones, E. F.**
1977. Contraception and sterilization in the United States, 1965-1975. *Family Planning Perspectives,* 9 (4), 153–157.

**Westhues, K.**
1972. Hippiedom 1970: Some tentative hypotheses. *Sociological Quarterly,* 13 (1), 81–89.

**Whelan, E. M.**
1978. *The pregnancy experience: The psychology of expectant parenthood.* New York: Norton.

**Whiting, B. B.**
1974. Folk wisdom and child rearing. *Merrill-Palmer Quarterly,* 20 (1), 9–19.

**Whiting, B. B. & Whiting, J. W.**
1974. *Children of six cultures: A psycho-cultural analysis.* Cambridge, MA: Harvard University Press.

**Widseth, J. C.**
1972. Reported dependent behaviors toward mothers and use of alcohol in delinquent girls. *Dissertation Abstracts International,* October 1972, 33 (4-B), No. 1833.

**Williamson, N. E.**
1976. *Sons or daughters: A cross-cultural survey of parental preferences.* Beverly Hills, CA: Sage.

**Williamson, S. Z.**
1970. The effects of maternal employment on the scholastic performance of children. *Journal of Home Economics,* 62 (8), 609–613.

**Winch, R. F.**
1958. *Mate-selection: A study of complementary needs.* New York: Harper.

**Winch, R. F.**
1967. Another look at the theory of complementary needs in mate-selection. *Journal of Marriage and the Family,* 29, 756–762.

**Winch, R. F.**
1974. Complementary needs and related notions about voluntary mate-selection. In R. F. Winch &

# References

G. Spanier (Eds.), *Selected studies in marriage and the family.* New York: Holt, Rinehart & Winston, pp. 399–410.

**Winch, R. F., Ktsanes, T. & Ktsanes, V.**
1954. The theory of complementary needs in mate-selection: an analytic and descriptive study. *American Sociological Review,* 19, 241–249.

**Wolfgang, M. E.**
1976. Family violence and criminal behavior. *Bulletin of American Academy of Psychiatry and Law,* 4 (4), 316–327.

**Wood, S. J., Bishop, R. S. & Cohen, D.**
1978. *Parenting.* New York: Hart.

**Woody, R. H.**
1978. *Getting custody: The last battle of the marital war.* New York: Macmillan.

**Yankelovitch, D.**
1969. *Generations apart.* New York: Columbia Broadcasting System.

**Yankelovitch, D.**
1974. *The new morality: A profile of American youth in the 70's.* New York: McGraw-Hill.

**Zajonc, R. B. & Marcus, G. B.**
1976. Birth order and intellectual development. *Psychological Review,* 82, 74–88.

**Zelditch, M. Jr.**
1955. Role differentiation in the nuclear family: A comparative study. In T. Parsons & R. F. Bales (Eds.), *Family socialization and interaction process.* New York: Macmillan, 307–352.

**Zelnik, M. & Kauter, J.**
1972. *Survey of female adolescent sexual behavior.* Conducted for Commission of Population, Washington, D. C.

# Glossary

**abnormal**

used within the context of the psychological perspective, refers to practices and behaviors that are considered by psychologists to be unhealthy.

**abortion**

the spontaneous or induced expulsion from the womb of the fertilized egg in a stage of development before it can survive on its own.

**abstinence**

refraining, in varying degrees, from sexual activity; as a method of birth control, the practice of not engaging in sexual relations at all.

**accelerated role transition**

when an individual is asked to take on a new role before he or she is capable of enacting it.

**acceptance**

the final stage in Kubler-Ross's theory of adjustment to dying; the final recognition of death and its acceptance by the dying person.

**afterbirth**

the material expelled from the uterus as the final stage of labor, including the placenta (the tissue through which the embryo transports its wastes and receives its nourishment in the uterus), along with all the accompanying material, including the roots of the umbilical cord.

**alcoholic**

a person with a physical and psychological addiction to alcohol.

**alternative**

used within the context of the sociopsychological perspective, refers to attitudes, practices, and behaviors that are not widely accepted by society, but are accepted by a certain segment.

**anger**

the second stage in Kubler-Ross's theory of adjustment to dying, characterized by the feeling of "Why is this happening to me?"

**anticipatory socialization**

process whereby a person learns about and rehearses the behaviors, values, and norms of a particular role or group as a preliminary to possible entry into that role or group.

**association**

the process of becoming more like another person through proximity and exposure (particularly in marriage).

**attachment**

a deep human feeling, originally experienced by the infant, characterized by lovingness for another person.

**authoritarian method of childrearing**

describes parents who are detached, controlling, restrictive, and overprotective; who discourage their children from asking questions, exploring, taking risks, and taking their own initiative.

**authoritative method of childrearing**
combines elements of authoritarian and permissive childrearing; a method where parents encourage exploratory, independent behavior, but also provide rules that, although enforced with mild punishment, are explained to the child and are subject to change depending on the child's reactions to them.

**avunculocal residence**
occurs when a married couple takes up residence with the maternal uncle of the groom.

**awareness**
accurately sensing and perceiving the people and things around you and understanding your relationship to them.

**awareness about one's partner**
knowing accurately what one's partner is experiencing in terms of his or her own self-awareness.

**awareness of the relationship**
understanding the interaction of the couple as a functioning unit rather than the behavior of each participant.

**bargaining**
the third stage in Kubler-Ross's theory of adjustment to dying, characterized by the dying person trying to work out a mythical "bargain" to assure his or her survival.

**battered-child syndrome**
a pattern of family disorganization characterized by child abuse, often repetitive from one generation to the next.

**behavioral contract**
a contract used in behavioral family therapy, which sets out acceptable and unacceptable behaviors and the consequences of such behaviors and to which the parties, in advance, agree to abide.

**bilateral descent**
lineage is traced equally through *both* the mother's and father's lines, in accordance with the laws of biology (as in the United States).

**bilocal residence**
rule permitting the couple to decide whether they will live with the bride's family or with the groom's family.

**birth control**
the intentional act of preventing live births, including contraception, abstinence, and infanticide.

**Caesarean section**
a surgical procedure in which the pregnant woman's abdomen is opened and the baby removed.

**calamitous death**
unpredicted, unexpected, and usually violent or degrading death (such as murder or suicide).

**chaperonage system**
a system whereby dating or courting couples are accompanied by another person (an adult); used in order to control the amount of symbolic and physical contact between potential marriage partners.

**child abuse**
violence against a child by or with the knowledge of the parent or caretaker; also has come to include extreme neglect of the child.

**child care**
a marital role associated with the spouse who provides the basic physical and psychological conditions to assure the normal development of a healthy child.

# Glossary

**child marriage**
the arrangements for marriage are made while the two potential partners are still children and romantic love is not present as a complicating factor.

**child socialization**
a marital role which includes the child care role (defined above), but also involves all other integrated efforts to produce a socialized, competent, educated individual.

**childbirth**
the termination of pregnancy with the delivery of a living neonate into the world.

**chronic phase**
the final phase in the development of alcoholism, in which the individual's life becomes dominated by drinking.

**coitus interruptus**
a method of contraception in which the man withdraws his penis from the vagina before ejaculation.

**commune**
a group of individuals living together, either in a single dwelling or within a prescribed area, sharing a common purpose and with assigned roles and responsibilities normally associated with the nuclear family.

**communication**
in marriage, when one partner can tell the other what is expected of him or her and the other partner can respond.

**communications theory**
in family counseling, the perspective which focuses on changing behavior through more effective communication.

**companionate relationships**
describes the type of marital relationship where the spouses are friends and companions to each other as well as marital partners.

**complex marriage**
a form of group marriage in the Oneida community established by John Humphrey Noyes in which there was a general attachment of all group members to each other.

**condom**
a thin sheath worn over the penis during intercourse in order to prevent the sperm from entering the vagina.

**congregate housing**
a dormitory-like arrangement for elderly people, where they share common facilities but have their own one-bedroom or efficiency apartments.

**conjugal courtship**
see marriage by consent.

**consensual relationship**
a relationship in which we enter and continue out of free choice.

**constitutional theory of homosexuality**
says that homosexuality is an inborn tendency, either neurological, glandular, or genetic.

**constructive emotional interchange**
providing another person with the kinds of selective but honest communications that are most helpful for them to understand and accept what you are saying in a way that will not hurt them.

**contraception**
the practice of preventing pregnancy.

**contraceptive**
a method of preventing fertilization from taking place during intercourse.

**contract**
something which establishes, either orally or in writing, the rules, regulations, guidelines, and goals of therapy.

**convergent feedback**
in communication, feedback which is consistent with our expectations (see also *feedback*).

**couple**
a socially recognized pair involved in a dating, courtship, or marital relationship.

**courtship love**
an intense emotional love that also parallels the rights and duties associated with the roles of husband and wife.

**crucial phase**
the third phase in the development of alcoholism, characterized by the individual's complete loss of control with regard to alcohol and including complete physical dependence on it.

**cue**
an internal or external stimulus that triggers a specific behavior or feeling (such as hunger or fatigue).

**dating**
a social process, comprising conventions that allow an individual to attract and interact with persons of the opposite sex.

**defense mechanisms**
psychological strategies for handling anxiety by distorting, blocking, or changing the reality of a situation.

**defensiveness**
the quality of distorting or blocking out parts of reality which are inconsistent with what one wants to see or believe.

**denial**
a general defense mechanism whereby we consciously refuse to accept, or even to see, something that is happening; in Kubler-Ross's theory of adjustment to dying, the first stage, characterized by the person's refusal to accept the fact that he or she is going to die.

**depression**
the fourth stage in Kubler-Ross's theory of adjustment to dying, characterized by the dying person becoming overpowered by depressing feelings.

**deviant**
an outsider who differs from the accepted social standards or norms; used within the context of the sociological perspective, refers to practices and beliefs that are not widely accepted by a particular society.

**diaphragm**
a supple cup with a springlike metal ring around its circumference inserted in the vagina over the cervix as a method of contraception (often used in conjunction with a spermicidal jelly or cream).

**dilate**
(in reproduction) the widening of the cervix which allows the baby to pass through the birth canal.

**divergent feedback**
in communication, feedback which is inconsistent with or contrary to our expectations (see also *feedback*).

**divorce**
a socially and legally prescribed method for ending a marriage.

**double descent**
a straight linear combination of patrilineal and

matrilineal rules of descent, which excludes females on the father's side and males on the mother's side.

**double standard**
refers to different attitudes and expectations regarding sex for boys and girls.

**douche**
the rinsing of the vagina by a jet of liquid, sometimes containing a spermicidal agent when used as a postcoital contraceptive technique.

**ego integrity vs. despair**
in Erikson's theory, the stage of development where one has to choose either to make some contribution to future generations or to despair of ever finding a purpose in life.

**ejaculation**
the process by which the male passes semen through the uretha and out of the penis.

**embryo**
the developing baby during the first three months of gestation (from conception to three months).

**empathy**
the ability to experience another's thoughts and emotions from the point of view of that other person.

**empty nest syndrome**
term used to characterize the typical difficulties parents experience when their grown children leave home.

**endogamy**
a regulatory principle of mate selection, requiring that one marry within a socially defined field of eligibles.

**endometrium**
the tissue lining of the uterus.

**episeotomy**
a small incision made during delivery in the childbearing woman's perineum in order to get the baby out more easily.

**equalitarian marriage**
in Blood and Wolfe's theory, both spouses have roughly equal resources and therefore the power is divided aproximately equally between them.

**equalitarian relationship**
a relationship in which there is a relatively equal distribution of authority in the family between husband and wife.

**equity**
the degree of equality with which two partners give to and receive from each other.

**Eros**
refers to passionate, romantic types of love.

**esteem building**
a type of communication from one partner to the other, with the intention of making the other feel important and worthwhile.

**estrogen**
an ovarian hormone, responsible for many of the woman's biological processes, including the regulation of menstruation and the preparation of the uterus for the implantation of a fertilized ovum.

**exchange theory**
in social psychology, the concept that each partner offers to the other an amount of emotional support roughly equal to what he or she gains from the relationship.

**exclusivity**
the practice of two people dating only each other.

**exogamy**
a regulatory principle of mate choice, requiring

marriage outside a socially specified group of people (contrasted with endogamy).

**expressive role**
the primary task of this marital role is to provide for the internal solidarity and harmony of the family.

**extended family**
a number of nuclear families, monogamous or polygamous, bound by the parent-child relationship and usually living together or in close proximity.

**external cue**
a stimulus outside a person that triggers a certain kind of feeling or behavior.

**family**
the conjugal (marriage) union and its kinship ties.

**family contracting exercise**
a five-step therapeutic learning experience in which family members learn to negotiate with each other with respect to needs, behaviors, attitudes, role expectations, etc.

**family counseling/therapy**
a range of related practices, including marriage counseling, sex therapy, child therapy, etc., designed to deal with more than one family member in a joint session in order to improve marital and family functioning and resolving family troubles.

**family planning**
a couple's decisionmaking regarding family size, spacing of children, methods of birth control, etc.

**family systems point of view**
the perspective that looks at the family as an organic, functioning unit.

**family violence**
the physical abuse of one family member by another.

**feedback**
a response to an individual's behavior that is reflected to the individual by specific others or by the environment.

**feedback loop**
a model of how feedback is used by individuals communicating with each other.

**fertilization**
the biochemical process in which the two reproductive cells of the male and female fuse and become one rapidly dividing and growing cell.

**fetishism**
the practice of attaching a sexual value to an inanimate object or to a part of the body (as opposed to the whole person).

**fetus**
the developing baby from three months until birth.

**field of eligibles**
the limited range of individuals who constitute the available population for socially approved mate selection.

**fraternal polyandry**
marriage between a woman and two or more men who are brothers (or otherwise related).

**gender-integrated gay community**
a community or subculture where male and female homosexuals interact with each other.

**gender role**
set of expected social behaviors specifically associated with one sex or the other.

**genealogy**
the tracing of one's family history.

**generation gap**
a presumed lack of communication between gen-

erations, involving differences of values, perceptions, and philosophies.

**generativity vs. stagnation**
in Erikson's theory, the conflict between the drive to prepare for future generations versus the tendency to become self-absorbed.

**gestation**
the period during which the fertilized cell, implanted in the uterus, grows into a fully developed newborn (in humans this lasts approximately nine months).

**gonads**
the sex glands: the woman's ovaries and the man's testicles.

**grief crisis**
a turbulent period of major psychosocial adjustment following the loss of a loved one.

**grief work**
the psychological process of readjustment to the environment and to living following a grief crisis, and involving emancipation from the psychological bondage to the deceased.

**grounds for divorce**
the specific legal criteria accepted for terminating a marriage by divorce.

**group marriage**
two or more men are collectively married to two or more women at the same time.

**HCG (Human Chorionic Gonadotropin)**
a hormone which is present in urine only during pregnancy, and thus is a reliable basis for pregnancy testing.

**heterogamy**
the marriage of people who are socially different.

**homogamy**
the marriage of people who are socially alike.

**homophobia (homoerotophobia)**
the irrational fear of associating with homosexuals or of homosexuality.

**homosexuality**
the preference for engaging in sexual activities with a person of the same sex.

**housekeeper**
a marital role associated with the spouse who cooks the food, cares for the clothing and furnishings and, in general, maintains a household.

**husband-dominated marriage**
in Blood and Wolfe's theory, where the husband has the greater amount of resources available and therefore holds the power in the relationship.

**hysterectomy**
the surgical removal of the uterus.

**hysterotomy**
an abortion technique involving the removal of the fetus and amniotic sac by surgically opening the abdomen and uterus.

**identity**
perception of oneself as developed through experience and the responses of others.

**identity development**
the formation of self-image and status identity as well as sex-role identity.

**incest**
socially prohibited sexual activity between two members of the same family.

**individuation**
within the context of the family system, the development of one's individual identity.

**induction**
in disciplining children, avoiding both physical and psychological punishment and explaining that certain behaviors, not the children themselves, are undesirable because of their adverse effects.

**instrumental role**
the primary task of this marital role is to provide the family with a means of subsistence and physical security specifically to deal with the environment.

**internal cue**
a stimulus inside a person which predisposes the person to a certain kind of behavior or feeling.

**intimacy vs. isolation**
in Erikson's theory, the period when a person has to decide whether to commit himself or herself to concrete affiliations and partnerships, even those calling for sacrifice or compromise, or to lapse into isolation or self-absorption.

**intraclass variation**
the variation within a socioeconomic class (with respect, for instance, to beliefs and life experiences).

**intrarelationship process of pairing**
the setting up of an implicit, unwritten, sometimes ambiguous, and often flexible, behavioral contract between the participants in a relationship.

**intrauterine device**
a soft plastic or metal device which is implanted in the uterus in order to prevent conception.

**IUD (IUCD)**
see intrauterine device (also called intrauterine contraceptive device).

**jealousy**
the belief that a person with whom we are in-

volved or in whom we are sexually or emotionally interested is involved with someone else.

**joint custody**
the practice of awarding custody of the children after divorce to both the mother and father.

**kibbutz**
a socioeconomic collective in Israel where many individual families work together to produce goods for the community.

**kinship**
a structured system of relationships, in which individuals are bound to one another by complex interlocking and ramifying ties.

**kinship role**
a marital role by which the spouse assumes the obligation to maintain contact and good relations with kin.

**labor**
the three-stage period before, during which, and immediately after the baby makes its trip from the uterus, down the birth canal, and out of the body.

**laparoscopy**
a surgical process of sterilization for women requiring two small incisions in the abdomen and a one- or two-day hospital stay.

**lesbian**
a female homosexual.

**level of content**
in communication, the superficial level of a message.

**level of intent**
in communication, the underlying feeling or intention behind a message.

# Glossary

**levels of disclosure and receptivity**
the ability and willingness of a partner to disclose feelings to a spouse and the ability and willingness of the spouse to be receptive to those feelings.

**levirate**
when a man inherits the wife and family of his deceased brother or other male kin.

**life change unit (LCU)**
a measurement (from 1 to 100) of the relative stress that events place upon people; the higher the number the greater the stress.

**liking**
an attitude a person holds toward another, contrasted with romantic love, and comprising affection and respect.

**love withdrawal**
in disciplining children, the use of psychological punishment such as ignoring or scorning children or telling them they will be unloved or unwanted as long as they misbehave.

**luteinizing hormone (LH)**
a hormone released by the pituitary gland, responsible for stimulating ovulation.

**marital form**
the socially specified arrangements between the adult members in marriage.

**marital role**
the set of attitudes and behaviors, reflecting cultural expectations and individual needs, a spouse is expected to demonstrate in the context of the marital relationship.

**marital rules**
explicit or implicit rules telling the marital partners who can do what, where, when, how, and under what circumstances.

**marriage by arrangement**
a frequent mode of acquiring a mate in which the choice is made by other than the two people to be married, often by the parents or male relatives.

**marriage by capture**
a rather rare mode of acquiring a mate, most often practiced in hunting societies having more men than women.

**marriage by consent**
an infrequent practice worldwide which relies on the voluntary consent of the marrying individuals (also called conjugal courtship).

**marriage by contract**
a marriage governed by a specific set of laws, either explicit or implicit.

**marriage by purchase**
a marriage whereby some form of economic exchange is made between the two individuals, their families, or their tribes.

**masturbation**
sexual self-stimulation.

**matriarchy**
a society where women are invested with power and authority over men.

**matrilineal descent**
genealogy is traced through the mother and all the women in the lineage.

**matrilocal residence**
the practice in which the newly married couple take up residence with the wife's family.

**matri-patrilocal residence**
the practice in which the newly married couple live initially with the wife's family for a specified period of time and then take up permanent residence with the groom's family.

# Glossary

**mature years**

the period of family life following the resolution of middlescence, from about 55 years of age onward.

**menarche**

a girl's first menstruation, usually signaling her entrance into puberty.

**menopause**

the period of a woman's life when menstruation ceases and she loses her procreative ability.

**metaneed**

in Maslow's theory, the higher needs of the individual, such as the needs for justice, goodness, beauty, unity, and order.

**metapelet**

on the kibbutz (see above), the person who functions as a caretaker, teacher, or substitute parent.

**middle years of family life**

the period of family life in which the children are in their adolescence and the parents generally in middle age.

**middlescence**

the period, from about 45 to 55 years, typically characterized by midlife change and sometimes crisis.

**midwife**

a person especially trained to assist during labor and delivery of the child.

**miscarriage**

an involuntary expulsion from the womb of a fertilized egg in any stage of development.

**modeled behavior**

behavior learned by observing other people and fashioning oneself after them.

**monogamy**

a marriage between only one man and one woman at a time.

**mothering one**

the individual assigned to and/or enacting the role of taking care of an infant, especially in providing physical attention and affection.

**myth of the cloaca**

the erroneous belief (usually by children) that there is only one opening through which urination, defecation, and the birth of the baby all take place.

**natural childbirth**

labor and delivery without medical control or intervention.

**neolocal residence**

the practice in which the newly married couple chooses its own residence and sets up a new household.

**neonate**

a newborn infant.

**nonfraternal polyandry**

a form of marriage between a woman and two or more men who are not otherwise related.

**nonmarital cohabitation**

where a couple lives together with the overt or covert idea of ultimately joining in marriage or forming a long-term relationship.

**nonmarital pregnancy**

pregnancy that occurs outside a socially recognized marriage relationship.

**nonmarital sexual preference**

a sexual preference outside a traditional marriage relationship and not involving one's spouse.

# Glossary

**nontraditional**
used within the context of the sociopsychological perspective; refers to attitudes, practices, and behaviors that are not widely accepted by society.

**nonunilineal descent**
form whereby descent is traced through more than one line, with each of the lines generally accorded equal kinship claims.

**normal**
used within the context of the psychological perspective, refers to practices and beliefs that are considered by psychologists to be healthy.

**normative**
used within the context of the sociological perspective, refers to practices and beliefs that are widely accepted by a society and expected of its members.

**normative sexual behavior**
refers to sexual behaviors widely practiced and accepted by a society and expected of its members.

**nuclear family**
family consisting typically of a married man and woman with their offspring.

**nuclear family of orientation**
the nuclear family as seen through the eyes of the children.

**nuclear family of procreation**
nuclear family as viewed from the parents' perspective.

**oral contraceptive**
(birth control pill) a method of contraception in which the woman takes a pill (regularly about 20 or 21 consecutive days a month) which introduces into her body a hormone or hormones which interfere with normal ovulation.

**ordinal position in family**
the birth order of a child with respect to his or her siblings.

**ovarectomy**
the surgical removal of the ovary.

**ovulation**
the reproductive process through which the ripened egg cell is sent from the ovary to the uterus through the fallopian tubes, during which time the sperm cell is given an opportunity to fertilize the egg cell.

**ovum**
(plural, ova) the female's mature egg cells which are involved in reproduction.

**paired relationship**
an ongoing relationship in which two individuals function together.

**pairing**
the process of forming a one-to-one attachment with another person.

**parapraxis**
also known as a Freudian slip; we say one thing when we intend to say something else.

**patriarchy**
society whereby the husband/father is invested with decisive authority and is accorded the best resources and privileges in the family.

**patrilineal descent**
descent is traced exclusively through the male line.

**patrilocal residence**
the practice in which the newly married couple lives in the same dwelling or a dwelling adjacent to that of the husband's family.

# Glossary

**permissive method of childrearing**
describes parents who have a *laissez-faire* attitude toward their children; who are noncontrolling, nondemanding, and nonpunitive toward their children, encouraging them to explore independently and try out new things.

**permissiveness**
refers to an open sexual standard.

**petting**
sexual activity that leads in the direction of and may or may not culminate in sexual intercourse.

**phalanx**
developed by Charles Fourier, a socially and economically cooperative community that would be related to other such communities around the world.

**Philia**
refers to love based on fondness, friendship, or respect.

**placenta**
the embryonic membrane through which the developing baby transports its wastes and receives its nourishment in the uterus.

**polyandry**
marriage of one woman to two or more men at the same time.

**polygamous family**
grouping of nuclear families bound by an extension of the husband-wife bond, that is, united through the presence of a common spouse.

**polygamy**
multiple spouses for either or both of the sexes.

**polygyny**
marriage of one man to two or more women at the same time.

**population control**
the deliberate manipulation of the size, composition, or rate of growth of a relatively large group of people (a community, ethnic group, nation, etc.).

**positive regard**
according to Carl Rogers, accepting another person as he or she is, and for what he or she is, without imposing judgments or stipulations.

**postdivorce reaction**
the attitude and behaviors often following divorce, characterized by mixed feelings of elation, depression, and confusion.

**power assertion**
in disciplining children, the use of punishment, including physical punishment, deprivation of privileges, and threats of punishment.

**prealcoholic phase**
the initial stage in the development of alcoholism, in which a person becomes a heavy social drinker and finds that drinking relieves tension and reduces levels of anxiety.

**pregnancy**
the condition of a woman carrying a developing offspring in her uterus.

**premature death**
refers to the death of a young person, especially a child.

**pre-ova**
immature egg cells which are inside the girl's ovaries when she is born and mature at puberty.

**press**
in Murray's theory, the realistic demands of the outside world (as contrasted with needs).

**problem drinking**
a step before total alcoholism; the problem drinker

is characterized by normal role behaviors most of the time but the need for alcohol as a regular part of the daily routine.

**prodromal phase**
the second stage in the development of alcoholism, in which the person begins to exhibit many of the behaviors we associate with true alcoholism, including sneaking a drink, denying the problem, and brief episodes of amnesia.

**profit**
in social exchange theory, the rewards each partner attempts to gain from a relationship minus the costs he or she must pay.

**progesterone**
an ovarian hormone, responsible in part for the reproductive cycle.

**projection**
the process of attributing to another person or to an object feelings that emanate from within oneself.

**promiscuity**
characterized by a completely open sexual lifestyle, with many partners and without commitment.

**propinquity**
the principle in mate selection that we tend to marry people who live near and are accessible to us.

**provider**
a marital role, associated with the spouse who assumes primary responsibility for the financial support of the family.

**psychoanalytic theory of homosexuality**
the theory that says homosexuality is a consequence of maternal deprivation or overprotection during the first five years of life.

**psychological menopause**
experienced by some middle-aged women who come to question some of their values that have remained unchanged since adolescence.

**psychopathological position**
(of child abuse) explains child abuse as symptomatic of a deep emotional sickness of the parents.

**puberty**
the beginning tf the adolescent period, marked by biological sexual development.

**rating and dating complex**
the model, proposed by Willard Waller, which suggests people make choices of whom to date based on external prestige factors, such as physical attractiveness, wealth, etc.

**rationalization**
a defense mechanism in which a person develops a false explanation for otherwise unacceptable actions, attitudes, or consequences.

**reaction formation**
a defense mechanism which involves acting in a way that is completely opposite to the way one really feels.

**reconstituted families**
hybrid families, in which there are one or more children from previous marriages living with a step-parent.

**recreational role**
a marital role associated with the partner who is responsible for organizing and carrying out family recreational activities.

**regression**
a defense mechanism where a person returns to a more childish type of behavior in order to deal with anxiety.

# Glossary

**relationship communication skills**
specific behaviors and skills that facilitate communication within a relationship.

**repetition compulsion**
the phenomenon in which we tend to repeat through life our earliest painful experiences.

**repression**
the most commonly used defense mechanism, which is similar to simple forgetting but designed to avoid remembering something painful.

**resource theory**
the theory which states that power in the family accrues to the partner who has the greatest resources at his or her disposal.

**rhythm method**
a method of contraception which works by avoiding intercourse at the time of month when the woman is most fertile.

**role**
set of behavioral expectations that accompany a status.

**role performance**
the actual enactment of role-relevant behavior of a status occupant.

**role prescription**
the behavior, values, and beliefs expected of the occupant of a particular status.

**role stage**
in Murstein's stimulus-value-role theory, the stage at which each partner tests the other's ability to function with a given role.

**romantic love**
an attitude, contrasted with liking, a person holds toward another which comprises attachment, caring, and intimacy.

**Romeo and Juliet Effect**
the phenomenon in which parental opposition increases a couple's affection for each other.

**secondary sex characteristics**
physical characteristics which differentiate boys from girls, men from women.

**self-actualization**
from Maslow's humanistic viewpoint, the process by which one fully uses one's talents and capacities in order to fulfill one's potential for creativity, dignity, and self-worth.

**self-awareness**
the ability to understand accurately one's emotions, sensations, and thoughts.

**semen**
the translucent liquid ejaculated by the male, which in a healthy person carries the sperm cells.

**serial monogamy**
having a number of spouses, one after another, though only one at a time.

**sex role**
see gender role.

**sexual attraction**
a bodily feeling of arousal that prompts fantasy.

**sexual potency**
for males, the presence of sperm in the semen, signalling the boy's entrance into puberty.

**sexual role**
a marital role which describes the spouse's functioning as a satisfying sexual partner within the context of a mutually enjoyable and usually exclusive sexual relationship.

**sexual stimulus value**
the sociopsychological quality of being able to arouse others sexually.

**significant others**
persons who have great influence on our behaviors as well as on our attitudes, values, and norms.

**singlehood**
used to describe a social status including an integrated social lifestyle based on the options an unmarried adult has.

**social class**
people sharing a similar life style and who occupy similar levels of recognized accomplishment and prestige with respect to economic, educational, or occupational achievements.

**social exchange theory**
the theory which states that people maintain social relationships when the rewards are greater than the costs involved.

**social learning theory of homosexuality**
a theory that says homosexual behaviors are learned through the behavioral processes of modeling or conditioning and that, under certain conditions, can be unlearned.

**social mobility**
the tendency of people to move from one social class to another.

**social position**
specific location within a network of social relationships.

**Social Readjustment Rating Scale**
a 43-item checklist of common situations that require a change in adjustment.

**social relationship**
an organized way of interacting between two participants, involving certain designated role behaviors.

**social reproduction**
see socialization.

**social symbol**
indicators (such as an engagement ring) that are recognized by others to have a specific meaning.

**socialization**
a lifelong process by means of which a human being becomes and continues to be a more or less adequately functioning and contributing member of a particular social group; a learning process.

**socioemotional intactness**
indicated by anything that preserves the unity of the family, either on a social or emotional level.

**sociological theory of homosexuality**
a theory that suggests homosexuality is an interaction of social, psychological, and economic conditions.

**sororal polygyny**
marriage between a man and two or more women who are sisters (or otherwise related).

**sororate**
the replacement of a deceased wife with her sister or female kin.

**spermatogenesis**
the process by which sperm cells are produced.

**spermatozoa**
(sperm cells) the male reproductive cells.

**spermicides**
chemical substances which destroy sperm cells.

**spouse abuse**
violence by one spouse against the other.

**status**

an individual's position in a network of social relationships.

**stimulus generalization**

extending the same response to phenomena generally considered to be similar (e.g., an extension of the incest taboo whereby those persons who are classified together in kinship terms with members of the nuclear family are called by the same term and are tendered similar obligations).

**stimulus value**

in Murstein's stimulus-value-role theory, the external, and rather superficial, value a potential mate holds for us at the beginning of the relationship.

**stimulus-value-role theory**

developed by Bernard I. Murstein, this perspective views mate selection as a fluid and dynamic process involving three sequential stages called stimulus, value, and role.

**surgical sterilization**

the process of preventing the reproductive functioning of a man or woman through surgical intervention (see also: tubal ligation; vasectomy; laparoscopy).

**swinging**

the pursuit of sexual activities outside the marital relationship by both spouses at the same time or in the same place.

**tender years doctrine**

a traditional (but changing) legal practice which says in effect that without compelling evidence to the contrary, children of divorce are better off in the custody of their mothers than of their fathers.

**testosterone**

a hormone manufactured in the scrotum (by the testes), which is responsible for the male's sec-

ondary sex characteristics, such as facial hair and deepening of the voice.

**theory of complementary needs**

developed by Robert F. Winch, this theory says that within our field of eligibles we seek out mates who offer the greatest promise of providing us with maximum need gratification by complementing our own personality needs.

**therapeutic role**

a marital role in which one partner assists the spouse in coping with problems of a psychological nature.

**topical awareness**

being aware of things outside the immediate personal or family situation.

**traditional**

used within the context of the sociopsychological perspective, refers to attitudes, practices, and behaviors that are widely accepted by society.

**transvestism**

the practice of dressing in the clothing of the opposite sex in order to attain sexual pleasure.

**tubal ligation**

a process of surgical sterilization in which the woman's fallopian tubes are tied.

**Type I complementarity**

in mate selection, where one person's need is complemented by a different need of another person in a way that brings about the gratification of the two different needs between them simultaneously.

**Type II complementarity**

in mate selection, where one person's need is gratifying to another person whose behavior satisfies the first person's need: in both cases the

need involved is the same though the level of
need differs.

**unconditional positive regard**
same as positive regard. According to Carl Rogers,
accepting another person as he or she is, and for
what he or she is, without imposing judgments or
stipulations.

**unexpected death**
death that occurs without preparation, such as a
death resulting from a sudden illness.

**unilineal descent**
lineage is traced through only one specific descent
line, the mother's or father's.

**unrequited love**
where one person loves another and the other
does not reciprocate that love.

**utility theory**
a general theory involving the costs and benefits
of an action; in family planning, a theory which
states that the more beneficial it would be for a
couple to have children, the more likely it is that
pregnancy will occur.

**value comparison**
in Murstein's stimulus-value-role theory, a stage in
which the couple begins to compare their respective values about religious orientation, political beliefs, attitudes toward parents, friends, interests in
sports, arts, hobbies, etc.

**vasectomy**
a surgical procedure for male sterilization in which
an incision is made in the scrotom and the sperm
ducts are tied.

**voyeurism**
the practice of becoming sexually aroused by
watching, either live or through some medium

(such as books, films, etc.), another person or persons in various states of undress or involved in
sexual activity.

**wheel theory of falling in love**
a developmental theory, proposed by Ira Reiss,
that conceptualizes falling in love and out of love
as a circular process comprising a number of connected stages.

**wife-dominated marriage**
in Blood and Wolfe's theory, the situation where
the wife has more resources at her disposal than
does the husband and therefore holds greater
power in the relationship.

**zygote**
a fertilized egg cell.

# Index